U.S. Chemical and Biological Defense Respirators: An Illustrated History

Christopher T. Carey

Schiffer Military/Aviation History
Atglen, PA

DEDICATION

This work is dedicated to Nazih G. Yousef, good friend and fellow expatriate alumni of the King Faisal Specialist Hospital & Research Center, Riyadh, Saudi Arabia, who as a young Captain in the Egyptian Army's Chemical Corps during the Yom Kippur War learned the importance of not unleashing the monster that is chemical and biological devastation. It is also dedicated to CSM George Murray of the U.S. Army Chemical Corps Museum at Fort McClellan, Alabama, for helping to preserve and maintain an important, if frequently overlooked and undervalued area of U.S. military history. Finally, it is further dedicated to the memory of Derek Griffiths, late of CBDE Porton and sorely missed by his friends and colleagues, for the many, many important contributions he made in the course of his life to the advancement and understanding of NBC protection science.

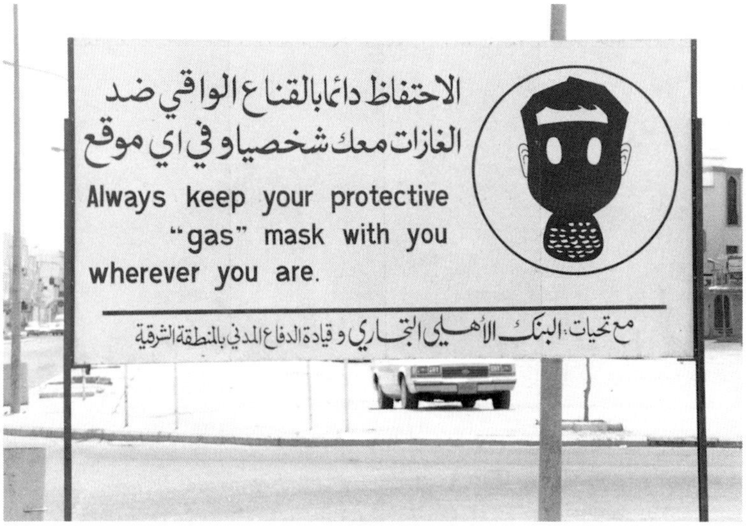

Public warning posted in Dhahran, Saudi Arabia, during 1991 Gulf War.

Book Design by Ian Robertson.

Library of Congress Catalog Number: 97-67596

Printed in China.
ISBN: 0-7643-0387-2

We are interested in hearing from authors with book ideas on related topics.

Published by Schiffer Publishing Ltd.
4880 Lower Valley Road
Atglen, PA 19310
Phone: (610) 593-1777
FAX: (610) 593-2002
E-mail: Schifferbk@aol.com
Please write for a free catalog.
This book may be purchased from the publisher.
Please include $3.95 postage.
Try your bookstore first.

CONTENTS

ACKNOWLEDGMENTS

Many thanks are owed to a number of individuals who have contributed insights, information and personal experi ence towards the writing of this book. One of those is James Sheldon, whose knowledge of and early interest in military respirators has proven a valuable resource. I wish that I could list a few of the others who have contributed, however, discretion requires respect for their anonymity. You who have so graciously provided anonymous encouragement and support for this book's preparation and production shall have to settle for a simple, if heartfelt, *thank you!*

Credit for any errors, mistaken assumptions, or incorrect representations of fact belong entirely to the author, and your critical communications are solicited to clarify any glaring errors present herein which might present themselves to individuals in the NBC world who are far more knowledgeable than myself. Despite one's best intentions and efforts, oversights will inevitably occur.

Thanks are owed indirectly to the Saudi Arabian National Guard, association with which as a 'hired hand' has provided lots of 'off time' from real-world occupational activities in which to revise and finalize this manuscript. Additionally, my wife (whose patience with and understanding of my many esoteric and doubtless at times exasperating interests has been substantial in the past several years) deserves praise for stoically putting up with the musty, *rubberish* aroma of hundreds of old respirator specimens, despite the allergic protests of her sensitive little Chinese nose, and for her unwavering encouragement throughout the duration of this project.

The excellent support provided by Schiffer Publications, most particularly through the skilled ministrations and encouragement of Military Editor Robert Biondi, cannot be commended too highly, since this book is largely a product of their expertise in fostering military history works for the benefit and enrichment of us all.

Finally, I suppose I also owe *some* measure of gratitude to my Siberian Husky bitch, *Laika*, whose great gusto in munching the original tasty manuscript of this book shortly after the first draft was completed further encouraged me to rewrite and revise it. At least she didn't choke on my words. It is my sincere hope that none of you do, either!

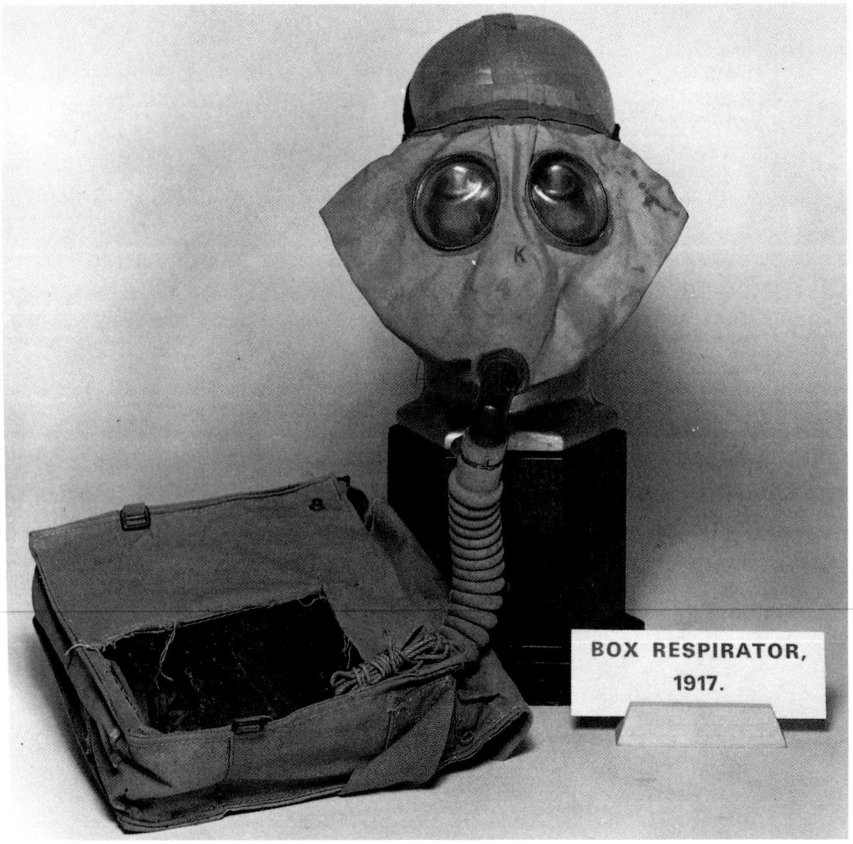

British Small Box Respirator (BSBR), displayed with carrying satchel and filter canister cut away so as to show filter contents. Courtesy of CBDE Porton Down, UK.

FOREWORD

The study of chemical warfare protective respirator technology is of necessity a very specialized area of defense science. Unfortunately, the average individual has about as much awareness of the nuances of the topic as he does knowledge of how to get along peacefully with his fellow man. This awareness invariably consists of one word: *"gasmask."*

For the informed specialist involved in current NBC protection technology work, the term *gasmask* effectively went out with the trench warfare days of the First World War and the appellation is furthermore usually a misnomer when applied to respirators used for protection against CBW agents, since most agents are not commonly found in legitimately gaseous form but rather as finely aerosolized particulates.

However, following the habitual practice prevalent in the medical world, wherein physicians use the terms "shot" instead of "injection" and "knife" instead of scalpel, the term *gasmask* is destined to remain a traditional verbal icon of the NBC protection technology world, as well as that of the layman.

My own initial associations with these respiratory protective devices began in an unusual manner, when as a child I discovered old derelict gasmasks strewn about and forgotten in musty bins at the local neighborhood army-navy surplus stores. At that tender moment in my life I regarded them merely as fascinating war toys, items with which to engage in playtime fantasies about all sorts of desperate adventures. By the time I had reached my freshman year of college, in 1964, such interesting, obsolescent *techno-artifacts* had been all but forgotten in the press of student concerns, such as maintaining a student deferment in the shadow of the escalating war in Southeast Asia.

My next encounter with a gasmask occurred shortly after I joined the U.S. Air Force, in the course of basic training. It was still, however, merely an incidental object with which I underwent the usual cursory NBC training and promptly forgot about soon after leaving basic training. Returning to Berkeley, California, in 1968, at the end of my service, the Free Speech Movement was in full swing, having evolved into the Vietnam War protest. Living in North Berkeley, I had to travel down the length of Telegraph Avenue to get to the Oakland hospital I was employed at and found the surplus Army M9A1 I had stashed under the seat of my VW *Käfer* useful on more than one occasion when tear gases were used to disperse the student protesters near Sather Gate.

Not until a considerable period of time after that did I return to a more prolonged and thoughtful contemplation of these interesting devices, subsequent to having been associated professionally with aeronautical & medical life support technology for a number of years. It was really the 1991 Gulf War in Southwest Asia which prompted me to swing somewhat away from conventional aerospace concerns to focus attention on the field of individual NBC protection technology. The necessity of having had to bring an American MSA manufactured M17A2 respirator to Riyadh with me (instead of the Avon S-10 which I would have preferred) stimulated a whole new—and this time very *personal*—awareness of the real life applications of protective respirator technology. The opportunities to participate peripherally in the NBC activities current at the time of the Gulf War further motivated my interests, and much of what has happened since then has encouraged me to produce this reference on American CBW respirator developments.

This book does not presume to attempt to constitute a comprehensive or fully authoritative history of the subject matter it addresses. The intent behind it is merely to provide a *general* and hopefully readable overview of the history of U.S. respirator developments in the *modern* chemical & biological warfare era. It awaits far more capable and scholarly experts in the field of NBC defense to develop this topic into a more complete exploration of the history of advances in U.S. respirator technology, since much of the subject's background is still classified or at the very least considered sensitive. A further basic intent behind this book was to provide a reference for a wide ranging audience, including recognized specialists in NBC defense, military historians and possibly even the average reader with somewhat eclectic interests. The photographic plates and supplemental illustrations selected to accompany the text should serve to provide a valuable visual identification key for recognition and categorizing needs relating to the many types of U.S. produced CBW respirators. This ought to be especially helpful in view of the fact that a comprehensive visual reference index of these masks spanning the past 90 years has never before been accomplished, to the best of my knowledge

In addition to this principal aim, it is hoped that some insight and appreciation of *gasmasks* as a general subject will have been gained from this effort and that it may inspire further, more detailed studies of the topic in future. It is also hoped that several impressions may become crystallized, subsequent to a read through of this book: 1) That individual protection against CBW agents is very much a currently vital and *continuing* concern—one which ought rightfully to be given proportionate priority in modern defense planning; 2) that advancement of the *state-of-the-art* in respirator research and development is a continuing process of shared evolution of concepts and methodologies which are firmly based upon, and interrelated with, *previous* respirator technology developments; and finally, 3) that human beings shall without question *continue* to resort to chemical and biological weapons of so-called "mass destruction" (I have always personally detested that overused and much abused *buzz phrase*, but it does seem to apply) so long as the means of producing NBC (*Nuclear*, *Biological* and *Chemical*) weapons remain easily accessed by any nation on Earth—no matter how impoverished or economically undistinguished. Interestingly, the terrorist use of Sarin nerve agent in the March 1995 attack on the Tokyo subway system amply underscores this point, at a time when general public attention is drifting away from NBC offensive weapons.

With a world wide chemical weapons moratorium now to be established by international consensus, the next major commitment remains stemming the growing threat of biological weapons in the present and subsequent decades. As an economical but terribly effective weapon of choice by terrorist groups, easily produced, stored and transported biological agents are just now being recognized for the potential they possess as a major menace to humanity.

Fortunately, the respirator filters in use today are generally effective against both chemical and biological agents. Filters and respirators, however, are only a part of the total protection envelope which modern defense technology must provide against these exotic weapons of war to completely insure the safety of military and civilian personnel who might be threatened by them. For this reason, and others equally as compelling, the search for effective respirator and filter design must continue despite the progress of international sanctions against use of such weapons.

This book documents the history of that process within the United States to date, to a modest degree.

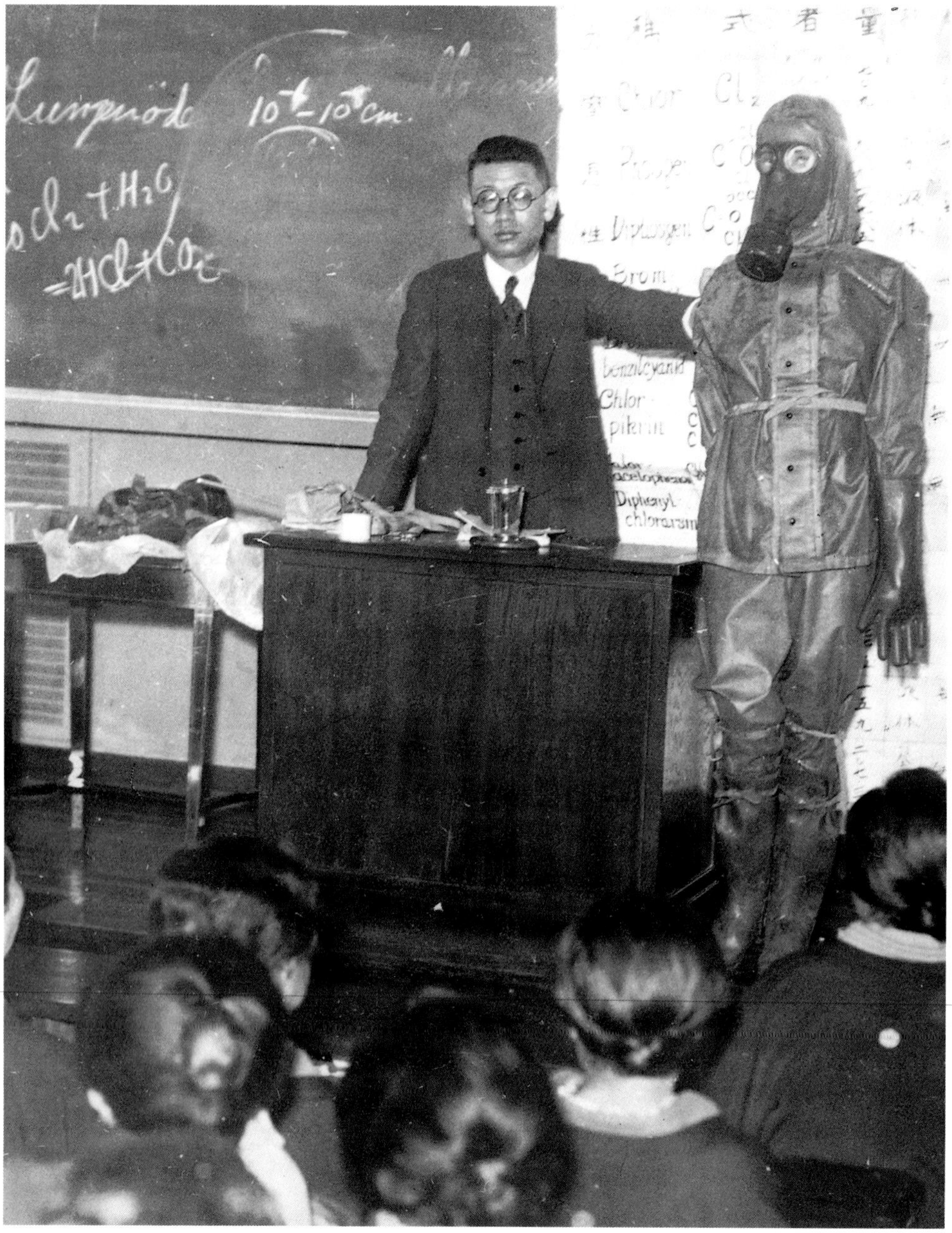

Japanese nurses being lectured on CBW protection at the Metropolitan Police Station in Tokyo, June 1939. Acme Photo, courtesy of Jim Sheldon.

CHAPTER ONE:
Some Historical Background on Chemical and Biological Warfare

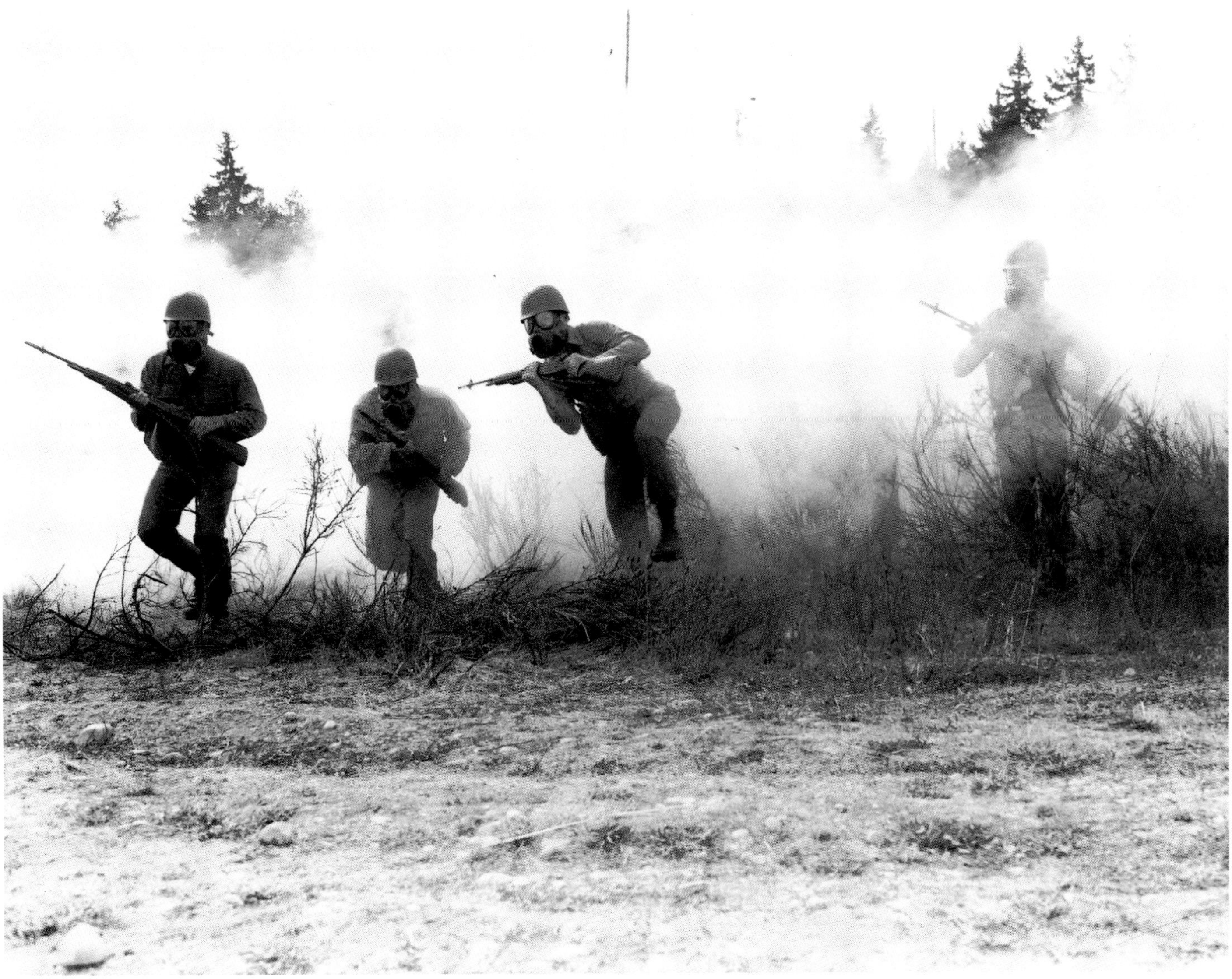

NBC training exercise at Fort Lewis, Washington. U.S. Army troops emerge from white phosphorus smoke screen wearing M17 Field Protective Masks. Note lack of protective hood, clothing and glove/shoe covers—in the 60s the threat was far more theoretical than it is now. U.S. Army photograph.

Chemical and biological weapons have been in use by humankind for centuries, contrary to common belief. Prior to the advent of man's ancestors, many forms of sea and land life evolved natural defense systems over thousands of years utilizing biological mechanisms which produced deadly chemical toxins, thereby effectively deterring would-be predators.

Man in ancient times could not help but take note of these apparently naturally occurring sources of severe injury inflicted by sea life and certain kinds of animals. The Greeks, in fact, referenced on several occasions in the course of discourses on philosophy, medicine and nature, instances in which fishermen were strangely injured—often with deadly results—by handling the fish they caught. So too, were references to injuries sustained by contact with spiders, snakes and lizards common in both Greek and Roman literature. The skunk's use of its natural body chemistry as a repellent agent was also well known and mentioned in the oldest surviving documents of early civilizations.

These numerous observations were not lost on ancient man as he developed his awareness that chemical and biological substances could be used offensively for his own purposes, after the example set by nature. Perhaps the very *first* instance of chemical weapons use is to be found in the prehistoric use of smoke to choke or burn out an enemy.

Among the earliest mentions of ancient chemical weapons used in organized warfare are Greek accounts which reference the soldiers of Sparta using a form of suffocating gas as early as 400 BC. The use of "Greek Fire" by the Athenians is also well documented in the same general period.[1] Later, in the early Middle Ages, historians note instances in which mention is made of decayed or diseased bodies being flung or catapulted over the walls of besieged fortifications, toward attacking forces; although it is possible the bodies were simply being catapulted away to *remove* a source of noxious odors and possible risk of communicable disease to the defenders, it is just as possible that the diseased bodies were themselves being hurled among the enemy forces as a rude but effective form of *biological* weapon to *spread* sickness.

Other documented accounts of early attempts to use primitive chemical or biological weapons in warfare include an instance in 1456 wherein the city of Belgrade apparently staved off advancing Turkish armies through the use of fumes given off by burning material which had been dipped in a chemical solution.

In the American west of the 1860s, several accounts exist of instances (some of which may be apocryphal), in which traders operating in cooperation with the U.S. Indian Agency spread smallpox among Native Americans by distributing blankets which were contaminated with the Smallpox virus.[2]

Later still, accounts tell us of a plan developed by the British during the siege of Sevastopol, in the Crimean War. A proposal to produce a toxic smoke by burning a mixture of sulfur and soft coal, which could be wafted into the city on a favorable wind, was finally rejected due to political disagreement on its ethics. A continent away, during the U.S. Civil War, a similar plan to attempt to asphyxiate the Confederate capitol, Richmond, using chlorine, was turned down by President Lincoln as being inhumane.

By the turn of the century (1900), lacrimating gases (tearing agents) were being used by Parisian police against anarchistic bohemian 'Apaches' to flush them out of their refuges in the Paris sewers and break up riots. Tear gas, well known by then to both the French and the Germans, was thus a likely substance for use by both sides in the earliest days of what would be first known—perhaps a bit ironically, viewed retroactively against the backdrop of today's mind-boggling arsenal of deadly weaponry—as 'The *Great* War.'

Tearing agents were employed to daze, confuse or disorient then as they are now. The escalation in the heat of 'modern' warfare, from use of simple, short-acting chemicals to incapacitate or reduce the ability among an enemy's forces to resist to the employment of more deadly agents specifically intended to kill, was inevitable, thus setting the stage for what we now regard as the era of *modern* chemical warfare.

The First World War was a time of experimentation and testing in this frightening new area of offensive and defensive warfare, as shall be seen in the next chapter. As the initial war experience with such weapons, much has been written about the use of chemical agents in this conflict, from descriptions of the terrible effects of chemicals upon unprepared armies to accounts of the scientific and technological advancements on both sides which brought chemical war agents into being. Of the over 3000 substances tested for possible war use during the war, only about 30 were used with appreciable success. Since the armistice of 1918 many thousands more have been investigated, but again with the discovery of relatively few which merit consideration as war agents with strategic potential.

However, the horror—both actual and psychological—which chemical warfare inspired in that first global conflict led to the first of repetitive efforts to outlaw their use. The Washington Disarmament Conference of 1921 was one such effort; the Geneva Conference of 1925 also addressed the use of chemical agents in war. Unfortunately, once introduced, this new form of warfare would not be easily dismissed, despite almost universal condemnation. Since the First World War several new types of deadly chemical agents have been developed; the most formidable of these are the nerve agents.

Whereas the older forms of chemical agents inflicted their damage by inhalation (choking gases, for example) or caused blistering injuries upon exposed skin (Sulfur Mustard), nerve agents acted upon the human central nervous system and caused immediate death by bringing about rapid respiratory or circulatory paralysis through disruption of nerve impulses. Furthermore, relatively small amounts of the deadly new agents could be fatal, either through inhalation or through skin absorption, and could be effectively dispersed as a war agent in a number of ways.

Tabun, the first nerve agent compound to be developed, was the discovery of I.G. Farben Industries scientist Dr. Gerhardt Schraeder, who in the course of research on organophosphorus preparations for use as contact insecticides in 1936, found one particular compound which seemed to be especially deadly. This fact was reported to the military authorities when it was determined that the compound was as effective on human beings as it was on insects. The German Wehrmacht immediately classified the entire research program as a national defense secret and initiated a study to uncover the compound's full potential as a possible weapon of war.

The result, in 1938, was the discovery of another even deadlier phosphorus based nerve agent, *Sarin*, and a still more deadly nerve agent in 1944 named *Soman*. Each of the new agents required smaller amounts to achieve logorithmically enhanced levels of effect. Full scale Tabun production was begun in 1942, with over 12,000 tons being produced in factories near the Polish border. Interestingly, Germany was alone in the world in possessing these deadly nerve agents through the end of the Second World War. In 1945 their existence became known outside Germany and today the agents are regarded as standard offensive weapons of effective mass destruction by all nations maintaining stocks of CBW agents.

Following the cessation of hostilities in 1918, the unsatisfactory resolution of national disputes in Europe created by the armistice set the stage for a slow drift back towards future armed conflict. Of all the new technological forms of warfare developed during the Great War, poison gas and the airplane were regarded as having the most potential for harm in renewed hostilities. Widespread anxiety was fostered and promoted among the citizens of Europe by pacifist prognosticators who foresaw massive fleets of aircraft, armed with chemical weapons, threatening the populated cities should a renewal of war come about. Disarmament efforts by these pacifist groups after 1918, unfortunately, were largely directed at nations with peaceful forms of democratic government and were not effective in discouraging the developing fascist nations from renewing research and development of chemical weapons.

As a result of the popular preoccupation with the horrors of the use of gas in a renewed war, much public awareness of the potential of chemical agents developed in the 20s and 30s. This resulted in a concern in Germany, England, France, Italy and other European nations with providing civilian defense capabilities against possible future use of chemical weapons. The United States, being far removed from the former European battlegrounds and safely isolated from similar anxieties by the expanse of the Atlantic Ocean, did not share the European fears to the same extent.

As events of the late 30s and early 40s turned out, the widespread fear of automatic and massive use of chemical weapons turned out to be groundless. Several instances in which chemical weapons were used outside of Europe prior to the outbreak of hostilities in 1939 proved to be localized, regional applications in which strategic or immediate tactical advantage was the motivating response factor—not humanitarian concerns or the pressure of world opinion.

Pre-war instances in which chemical weapons figured included several incidents involving planned use of "gas balloons" and chemical shells by the Red Army against White Russian forces in the Kakhovka region in 1920, and in the sailors' revolt at Kronstadt in 1921. In the late 1920s gas filled shells were apparently used against rebellious mountain villages in the Caucasus, and in the 1930s Soviet aircraft used aerially dispersed Sulfur Mustard sprays against the Basmatch tribes of central Asia.

The next significant use of chemical weapons took place in the mid 1930s when fascist dictator Benito Mussolini used aircraft to spray Mustard gas with devastating effect on the primitively equipped Ethiopian tribesmen who were harassing his expeditionary forces, under the command of General Badoglio. The largely naked Ethiopians lacked any form of protection against the harmful blistering effects of the Sulfur Mustard and the number of fatalities and disabling injuries were great. It is worthwhile to note that while the Italians had no compunctions whatsoever over using chemical agents against primitive, defenseless peoples, they later showed no inclination at all to use the same weapons against a formidably prepared and well-defended foe such as were the Western Allies.

In the far East, in its military incursions into Manchuria, Japan unhesitatingly used several areas in its captured *Manchuko* territories as field laboratories for active chemical and biological warfare research. Chemical agents were used in a number of actions, including the recapture of Ichang on the Yangtse River in 1937. Two excellent accounts of their research activities and use of biological agents are Williams' and Wallace's excellent documentary, *Unit 731: Japan's Secret Biological Warfare in World War Two,* and Sheldon Harris' *Factories of Death: Japanese Biological Warfare 1932-45 and the American Cover-up.* As in Ethiopia, the Chinese had little if any protection or defense against chemical and biological agents, and were regarded as something less than human, just as the Italians had regarded the Ethiopian tribesmen. There was muted world reaction to the known extent of these actions, but no serious protest was made by the rest of the world at the time. Having accomplished a great deal of research on the effects of chemical and biological agents on human beings, the Japanese wisely regarded American President Roosevelt's declaration that America would use chemical agents only if it were attacked with such agents by another power *first*, and downgraded their CBW research and development program thereafter to direct resources to other, more urgent priorities.

The only recorded incident involving chemical weapons use during the Second World War, among the Western powers, occurred in December of 1943 at Bari Harbor in Italy. A Luftwaffe air attack against Allied shipping, crowded into the harbor, blew up the American supply ship *SS John Harvy*, which was filled with more than 100 tons of Sulfur Mustard. The mustard agent had been sent in for contingency use, in the event the Germans used gas to slow up the Allied advance, and the explosion of the ship spread mustard liquid and vapor all over the harbor. Estimates of the casualties ranged from 83 dead and 534 severely wounded to over 1000 deaths. The symptoms of those afflicted presented a puzzle to the existing medical facilities present, owing to the strange symptoms present among the injured, and the incident remained classified by the U.S. Department of Defense until 1959.

Following V-J Day in 1945, dissemination of information on and the development of old and new forms of chemical war agents continued, bolstered as it was by the discovery of the new German organophosphate based nerve agents. The Soviet Union, long interested in the possibilities of chemical war agents, removed a whole Tabun production facility, along with its scientists and weapons stockpile and shipped it back to Russia. In both the West and in the Soviet Union research on chemical and biological weapons gained renewed strength as the new "Cold War" era began.

Since the 40s, reports of chemical weapon use have been few until recent years. Egypt reportedly used chemical agents against the leftist Yemeni forces in the mid 60s. During the Vietnam war, tear gases were used by the United States to flush Viet Cong from their tunnel complexes, as were herbicidal chemicals (2,4-D and 2,4,5-T—A*gent Orange*) for defoliation purposes.

In the late 50s and early 60s a new type of chemical agent captured the attention of the world. These were the psychochemicals, which act upon the brain to produce confusion, hallucinations, delusions, unreasonable fears and distortion of normal time-space relationships. Best known at the time was the Lysergic Acid group (LSD-25), the psillocybins and other hallucinogens. In subsequent years, information concerning secret military trials involving application of hallucinogens to unsuspecting test subjects has come out, revealing to some extent the extreme degree of interest which these psychochemicals produced among some researchers of the 60s and 70s. At that time it was strongly felt that the possible military application of psychochemicals to daze, disorient and confuse an enemy showed significant promise.

In the late 70s and early 80s, instances of the use of combinations of various toxins (described in the literature by the term *Yellow Rain*) against tribes in Southeast Asia were investigated; reports of chemical and biological agent use in Afghanistan also came to light in the same period. In perhaps the most flagrant use of chemical agents in recent years, Iraq employed chemical and biological agents against Kurdish civilians in communities on their northern borders, and later made widespread use of both Sulfur Mustard vessicants and nerve agents to inflict significant and wide-ranging injuries upon their Iranian enemies in the Iran-Iraq Conflict of the mid to late 80s.

Possibly the most comprehensive review of both the past and the present history of chemical warfare is expertly documented in distinguished historian Edward M. Spiers' several books on chemical warfare (*Chemical Warfare,* 1986, *Chemical Weaponry: A Continuing Challenge*, 1989, and *Chemical and Biological Weapons: A Study of Proliferation,* 1994).

Within the present decade, the 1991 Arabian Gulf War sparked the most recent renewed concern over the proliferation and use of chemical and biological weapons by belligerent nations; consequent to the Gulf War is the puzzle of the physical affliction known as *Gulf War Syndrome* which defies precise understanding but is *suspected* of being chemical or biological weapon related.

As the year 2000 draws nearer, incidents involving use of chemical and biological agents against civilians by radical groups, such as the Aum Shinrikyo Sect in Japan, have heightened awareness over the prospects of these weapons being used for terrorist purposes. Indeed, in view of their inherent simplicity to manufacture and store, biologicals appear to be the coming threat of most immediate significance in this regard.

Consequently, International efforts to bring about a Chemical Weapons Convention banning chemical agents appear finally to be nearing some sort of consensual closure. Unfortunately, a separate convention banning use of biological agents is nowhere near as ready to be put into effect, and it is the problem of cheap, simply made and easily stored biological agents that is most portentous. Although the major players in the chemical and biological warfare arena appear ready to consensually agree to eliminate CBW weapons, the question of how to keep these weapons out of the hands of terrorist groups remains unresolved.

As has been pointed out by researchers in chemical weapons development history such as Dr. Spiers, adequate answers *must* be forthcoming soon. Otherwise, the specter of CBW weapons use shall persist unchecked and the next major form of this potentially devastating threat shall continue to take shape covertly, elusively, somewhere in the shadowy corners of the world.

CHAPTER TWO: World War One: The Modern Beginnings

According to a mean spirited (possibly apocryphal) AEF joke, the first modern use of chemical war agents occurred in mid-1914 when unusually strong winds swept fetid air from the German trenches directly towards the French lines after the Kaiser's field kitchens had just finished serving a particularly spicy ration of *Bayerische Weisswurst mit Bohne*.

All humor aside, evidence suggests that the French may actually have used the first modern chemical munitions in the First World War.[1] Taking delivery of hand-grenade type weapons filled with ethyl bromoacetate (a non-disabling lacrimatory agent) in 1912, there are reports which suggest that these were used before (August 1914) the highly publicized Ypres Salient attack involving chlorine gas took place (in 1915). Due to rapid vapor dispersion of such harassing chemicals, the effect of their use was not recorded as being of particular significance at the time.

The Germans, for their part, used 105 mm howitzer shells filled with dianisidine chlorosulfonate in October of 1914, shortly after the French used their lachrymal filled grenades. Again, the results were ineffectual with regard to offensive consequence.

History records the date of 22 April 1915 as being the start of the so-called "modern" era of chemical warfare, for on that day a specially trained and deployed unit of Imperial German *Pionier* troops released a massive ground-projected cloud of compressed chlorine gas along a six to seven thousand meter segment of the French trenches at Ypres, between Langemarck and Bixschoote in Belgium. The French colonials and Canadian troops which took the brunt of this fearful and unsuspected new escalation in the horrors of modern war were faced with a dire predicament: either stand and be cut to pieces by the German machine guns, or remain in their shell holes and earthenworks and die of choking asphyxiation.

Colonel J.S.M. Auld of the British Army, who as a liaison witnessed the first two chlorine gas attacks, later gave an account of his observations to the American Academy of Sciences as follows. "Many men in the first attack, who had sufficient presence of mind, saved themselves by burying their faces in the earth, or by stuffing their mufflers in their mouths and wrapping them about their faces..." This instinctive reaction of desperate men saved a significant number of lives, for moist, porous materials tended to absorb some of the chlorine while admitting air for breathing. In fact, this primitive reflexive defense would later be referenced as an emergency measure, made even more effective if water, or even urine, were used to soak the material before use.

Dreadful surprise that it was, and responsible for the deaths of more than 5,000 unprepared men (more than 10,000 casualties total), this first large scale chemical attack in the annals of modern warfare was nevertheless an experiment.[2] Two previous and unsuccessful attempts had been made to use chemical agents on a large scale in Poland, during January of 1915, and had failed due to unfavorable (bitter and freezing) weather; the Ypres attack was in essence merely one final test of an unproven mode of warfare, regarded by the German High Command as of dubious and unpromising value. Consequently, unprepared for the monumental result of the experimental chlorine gas weapon, the Germans failed to exploit the resulting gaping hole in the Allied line. In so doing, they lost one of the few opportunities provided during the war for drastically changing the static nature of the conflict—an opportunity which might have even allowed the Kaiser's troops to drive completely through the Allies' defenses and reach the English Channel.

Therefore, the use of lachrymal agents by both sides ('teargases') had been intended to harass and disrupt only. The use of the new chemical agent marked a very new and different turn of events in that the chlorine attack was intended to produce fatalities by overt asphyxiation. Regardless of which side actually first used the more innocuous chemical agents (such as simple lachrymals), the Ypres incident shook the whole world as further irreparable damage was done to the "gentlemanly conventions of civilized war" to which both sides had previously given tacit recognition in the war's earliest phase.

Germany, mindful of the victorious brevity of the Franco-Prussian War, had prepared for a quick, decisive conflict. However, as the Schlieffen Plan for a rapid and successful capture of France became mired in the horrors of trench war, concern at the highest levels of the German High Command served to set the stage for the introduction of the new chemical weapon.

A letter, addressed to the High Command outlining "a new method of warfare" to resolve the costly stalemate, had been written by renown German chemist Fritz Haber. Haber had before the war successfully synthesized ammonia from nitrogen in air in practical quantities. In addition to resolving a chronic shortage of agricultural fertilizer, his breakthrough had also paved the way for expanded manufacturing of explosives at a time when Germany was experiencing a shortage of natural nitrate explosives materials.

Swept up in the turmoil of wartime mobilization, along with thousands of others, Haber formulated the concept of chlorine gas as a weapon out of his desire to remove himself from the unhappy and nameless fate of the ordinary trench soldier and play a part in the war more appropriate to his professional training and experience. Shortly after his letter was received by the High Command, he was invited to Berlin to develop his concepts of chemical agents in war (including asphyxiating gases), and was soon back at his former work with the Kaiser Wilhelm Institute (Berlin), where he began work with his colleagues on the development, production, handling and techniques for use of war gases.

Chlorine gas was selected initially by Haber's team due to the fact that it was already in substantial commercial production. The task turned to development of equipment to store and deploy the gas, and the details of training specialist soldiers (*pionier* troops) to use the new weapon. The first test of the Haber proposal was originally scheduled to take place against the Russian enemy, but poor weather prospects during the two Polish gas trials further accentuated the already objectionable nature of the gas weapon concept maintained by 'old school' traditionalists of the Imperial German Command. Finally, one additional test was permitted—this time against the Ypres Salient, a nominally quiet sector in the Belgian line. The result, as we all know, is history.

Germany was in a unique position to exploit Haber's historic proposals, for the German chemical industry at that time was monumental. Due to an immense and influential cartel of German chemical industry partners, Germany enjoyed an almost complete monopoly on chemical production in Europe. Shortsighted European preference for low-priced German chemicals by other neighboring nations strengthened the imbalance, with the result that German technology virtually controlled the pharmaceutical, commercial dye and industrial chemical business relied upon by thousands of manufacturing and scientific concerns.

As a result of the German monopoly, a sophisticated industrial manufacturing infrastructure was already in place in turn-of-the-century Germany for conversion of chemicals into a myriad of applications. Of particular importance was German mastery of the industrial dyes, which could be simply converted into a number of products—some benign and harmless coloring agents, and others possessing deadly toxicities. Thus, when this ideal combination of existing scientific resources, technical know-how and knowledge came together in the form of Fritz Haber's letter, the results were truly monumental both for the enemies of Imperial Germany and the history of modern warfare.

The devastating success of the German attack against the Ypres Salient prompted an immediate response by all participants in the 'Great European War,' and was responsible for the development of a new technical specialty in military organizations, the chemical warfare service. Individual defensive technology developed apace, starting with the first and natural act of the Ypres defenders of stuffing their mouths with cloth fabric, to improvised damp-soaked facepads tied to or wrapped around the face, manufactured and pre-soaked face masks (frequently with hoods & goggles), and finally to carefully conceived and produced full-face, impermeable facepieces with individual eye lenses and purifying canisters of filtering chemicals.

From the introduction of chemical agents as a significant weapon of war, the defensive aspect of chemical warfare services developed into a bilateral struggle to develop new chemical combinations which would render the enemy's existing offensive agent useless and simultaneously come up with corresponding advances that would successfully anticipate the enemy's next response. Much experimentation ensued, and the role of military intelligence in devising a suitable defense became significant. In fact, just before the infamous Ypres chlorine gas attack of April 1915, the Allies learned from a German deserter that the German forces planned to attack with a massive gas offensive; ironically, the vital warning had been disregarded by Allied officers well acquainted with so-called 'uncivilized' German conduct.

Meteorology was in its infancy, of course, and both sides were finding out about the vagaries of a capricious wind which might suddenly expose an offensive chemical agent to the deployer's own defending troops. It was also generally true that as soon as a new combination of chemicals was encountered by the enemy, he would be able to manufacture a similar substance and send it back shortly thereafter.

As the 'chemical front' developed and expanded, gas discipline became identified early on as a critical element in defensive strategy. Protective masks could be devised, but without stringent and continuing efforts to educate the individual soldier on the importance of maintaining and using protection, such technical defenses were rendered insignificant. More often than not, it was precisely this aspect of chemical defense concerns which would result in serious injury or fatality among personnel. In the front lines, where command and control frequently broke down or was poorly developed, this problem became second only to seeing to it that all individuals were provided with an effective defensive respiratory device which would protect against the latest enemy chemical combinations. Also critical, warning systems for alerting troops to use of gas were a tertiary concern of some significance.

German soldiers in the battle of Loos (September 1915), of the opinion that the British would be unable to counterattack with gas, evaded or disregarded Imperial High Command directives on gas defense training and precautions. Consequently, many more fatalities were sustained than could be accounted for through use of older style damp masks when the enemy troops did in fact respond in kind. The story remained the same through the entire duration of the war for both sides, through simple neglect or disinterest in accepting mandatory guidelines for gas defense.

One incident in particular exemplifies this situation through a humorous anecdote recorded in several war memoirs, involving a British General who was visiting the front trenches from his comfortable rear-echelon headquarters. As his party approached the gas discipline area of the front lines, he realized that he had neglected to bring his own gas mask along with him. Stopping one of the troops headed towards the rear, he asked the man for his gas mask kit to use temporarily on his tour. Concerned with gas precautions and how adequately his men were prepared for defense against enemy gas, the general stopped soldiers at random as he passed through the trenches to determine how well versed they were in the current gas discipline regulations. During one of these short inspections, he commanded several men to don their masks as if the alert had been sounded, while his adjutant timed their respirator donning procedure.

Both men fumbled through the unfamiliar mask donning process, provoking a snort of indignation from the General. "Here," he snapped, "I'll show you how to do it properly!" In response to his adjutant's hand signal the General then plunged his hand into his borrowed respirator satchel and withdrew a very dirty pair of socks![3]

The incident in reference, although amusing, highlights a very common situation encountered continuously throughout the war as soldiers disregarded gas defense regulations for various reasons. Of course, the use of the respirator satchel for carrying important but non-vital personal items (such as extra dry socks) was uniformly common, and resulted in uncounted incidence of gas injury.

Most of the offensive chemicals used by both sides were not 'gases' at all, but rather aerosolized liquids or finely powdered particulate matter. Accordingly, three primary methods were used to filter respired air containing war agents. The earliest of these was the chemically reactive method which involved exposing the war agent to a chemical element in the respirator filter to react with the chemical war agent so as to either neutralize it or render it harmless. This was the action of "hypo" on chlorine; it was also the function of urotropine against phosgene, and chemicals such as potassium permanganate and soda lime granules.

The second technique (used with chemically 'sluggish' chemicals such as chloropicrin) involved the use of charcoal granules to absorb, trap and retain poisonous particles as the inhaled air passed through them. Many hours of intensive effort were expended on the development of charcoal types which were more efficient, and this resulted in much debate and controversy centering on (among a considerable number of contentious items) the best ingredients for allied filter canisters for use with the latest full-face type respirators.

Towards the latter part of the war, when arsenic-based smokes (sternutatory harassing agents) were being brought into use in the form of Germany's "Blue Cross" gases, a mechanical element (such as a layer of felt) was added to filter canisters to trap and hold smoke particles against which charcoal and neutralizing chemicals were ineffectual. Germany had great hopes for the incapacitating potential of the Blue Cross shells, but their research had been hasty and premature for the explosive included as a component of the shells scattered the agent. This resulted in large particles, which were easily stopped by the Allied filters. Both sides used the Blue Cross type filtering materials from the onset of the arsenicals' use, which nullified its effectiveness.

As offensive chemical weapons research continued, the Allies found out (partly by accident) that slowed combustion of certain chemicals resulted in the production of smaller, finer particles which almost all filters were unable to stop. These 'smoke candles' were just about ready to be brought into action on a large scale when the war abruptly ended. While the Allied filters were also helpless against the new tactic, they had expected that the smoke candle weapon would bring about an abrupt German military capitulation before the secret of slow agent combustion could be discovered and countered.

Among the innovations of the so-called Great War were a number of interesting developments. One of these was labeled "skunk gas," and while it was essentially harmless, it forced the enemy soldier to keep his chemical protection mask on, thereby hindering and harassing him. The Germans also made great use of such types of harassing gases, and one of the reasons for their apparent successes of the 1918 German Offensive was the fact that the British respirator in wide-spread use at that time (the British Small Box Respirator, or BSBR) imposed a significant fatigue burden on the British troops. Aside from its increased respiratory resistance (hastening fatigue from the added work of breathing), the nose clip and mouthpiece elements were uncomfortable and irritating. Continued wear of the units resulted in prematurely tired troops, and harmless but foul-smelling "skunk gases" required prolonged use of the tiresome respirators which induced this condition.

By the time the First World War came to a close, over 3000 individual toxic chemical substances had been identified, developed and prepared for testing against the combatants of both sides. Most were subsequently found to be impractical or of marginal effectiveness as war agents; less than 30 or so were finally recognized as even being acceptable. Of all of them, several of the most persistent vessicant types (mustard & Lewisite) are still stockpiled and have been in use, off and on, since the early days of modern chemical conflict in Europe. The Iran-Iraq War spanning the mid to late 1980's saw much use of vessicant type blistering agents, and this chemical preparation remains a potentially formidable weapon against unprepared military formations. Of course since the beginning of the 'modern CBW period' in World War One, thousands of developments have taken place so that by today's standards, the state of the art as experienced then is now comparatively more than a bit primitive.

Since 1918, which was the 'end of the beginning' of classical chemical warfare as well as the start of the modern CBW era, chemical warfare has been placed together with biologicals and nuclear areas of weaponry to form today's 'NBC Warfare' branch of defense technology. In spite of the continuing concern over the use of such weapons and the numerous attempts to bring about worldwide political consensus on banning such weapons from war use (starting with the Washington Disarmament Conference of 1921 and the Geneva Conference of 1925), NBC weapons research, development and actual use of the weapons by nations around the world persists. Regardless of recent progress in establishing a Chemical Weapons Convention (CWC), which goes into effect in April of 1997, it is doubtful that a fully effective resolution of the problem of chemical weapons can ever be permanently guaranteed. This is especially the case as CBW agents find their way into the hands of terrorist or extremist groups.

It is against this interesting, if depressing, historical backdrop that *U.S. Chemical and Biological Defense Respirators: A Brief History* attempts to chronicle America's progress in the area of individual respiratory defense technology.

CHAPTER THREE: World War One: Early Respirator Development

Prior to the historically significant German chlorine gas attack against the Ypres Salient (April 1915), the occasional and largely ineffectual use of lachrymal harassing agents by both sides prompted no immediate recognition of the need for serious protection against chemical war agents. However, no one had predicted that these irritant agent incidents were an early portent of more ominous and deadly escalations in the battlefield application of chemicals which would soon follow. Perhaps the time-honored conventions of gentlemanly conduct under arms, lingering on despite the intrusive effects of science and technology, led leaders of both sides into the belief that such horrors would never be used in warfare.

In any event, German chemist Fritz Haber's inspiration forever dispelled such anachronistic notions, maintained by old school professional soldiers, with shocking suddenness. Literally overnight, nations on both sides of the "Great War" set about the task of providing protection for their armies against the new threat of gas.

Robt. H. Davis, in his fascinating and comprehensive work entitled *Breathing in Irrespirable Atmospheres* (St. Catherine Press, London, 1945), points out that prior to the advent of the First World War much significant work had been done in the field of respiratory protection—particularly for the purpose of providing protection systems for individuals engaged in mining work, underwater salvage work, and around industrial toxic substances. Most nations had done research of a similar nature for a considerable period of years prior to Ypres; therefore, there existed a fairly significant, if somewhat obscure and scattered, body of knowledge concerned with respiratory protection technology upon which to draw in addressing the new problem of battlefield toxic agents.

The major powers engaged in the conflict set forth on protective respirator programs, while simultaneously providing information to their troops about how best to deal with the new threat until adequate respirators could be devised and provided. Interestingly, each of these major powers would devise different approaches to the problem, as shall be seen.

The Earliest, Improvised Protection:

As mentioned earlier, some of the French & Canadian troops caught by surprise at Ypres in April of 1915 had reacted instinctively to the clouds of chlorine rolling towards them from the German line. Grabbing handkerchiefs, wool mufflers, and any fabric at hand, they had stuffed their mouths or alternately covered their eyes, mouths and noses with the material. A few, possessed of unusual knowledge of chemistry (perhaps college graduates who had taken such courses in school), had had the added presence of mind to briefly saturate the cloth with water first. This reaction saved many lives during the first German gas attack at Ypres.

After a bit of analysis of the situation, in the aftermath of the attack, suggestions were solicited and various stopgap measures were tested on an *ad hoc* basis by troops. These included filling handkerchiefs with moist earth to press over the mouth, keeping tins of soda solution around in which to soak handkerchiefs, and even filling a glass bottle (with the bottom broken out) with a mixture of straw and cloth which had been saturated with water or photographer's Hypo solution (an idea of noted Professor J.S. Haldane). Other improvised measures used lengths of hose as filtering columns, similarly stuffed.

All of these interim, makeshift measures were at best only partly effective. Some, like the bottle filter, were impractical and therefore, while theoretically sound, virtually useless. It was clear that some sort of formally conceived and produced respirator was the only realistic solution for effective, long-term protection.

Russian Protective Developments:

The earliest Russian attempts to provide individual respiratory protection mirrored those of the Western Allies. Gauze pads, wrapping, and similar barriers were tried with as little success as their counterparts' efforts.

Of note, among the protective respirator designs of the Great War, was the final Russian design, which was starting to be produced and used when the war ended. This design featured a thin, vulcanized, natural rubber hood fitting the whole head snugly. The (Selinski-Kummandt) mask, of which several variations have been noted, featured a canister of filtering charcoal only, which was connected directly to the lower front of the face-piece part of the hood and supported on the chest. A rubber 'flapper-type' exhaust valve appears on at least one version, while another appears to have no air-flow check valving, with both inhaled and exhaled air being directed through the filter can. This design, remarkable in that an only somewhat modified version is still in use in parts of the former

Soviet countries today (ShM series), provided a considerable level of protection, from available reports. The Russian "bathing cap" design saw considerable use during the WWII era, and was also adopted for use by Germany and other European nations at various times during the 30's and 40's (Finland, Sweden, and other Scandinavian countries). The German Volksmask 37 (VM.37) used this principle, and there were several experimental designs utilizing this concept which were discovered by an English intelligence team in the Drägerwerk facilities in Lübeck (at war's end in 1945). Despite the relatively high level of protection afforded by a whole-head rubber hood, this sort of mask is uncomfortable to wear for extended periods due to heat, humidity and pressure on the head.

Russian interest in and capabilities for protection against chemical warfare agents remained strong throughout the First World War, and endured long afterwards, under the Stalin regime.

French Protective Developments:

The French quickly developed their M-2 mask, which was made of face-fitting fabric. The M-2 had twin circular celluloid lenses, and consisted of multiple layers of muslin. Of the layers, 20 consisted of muslin (cheesecloth) impregnated with *Greasene* compound, and another 20 were impregnated with *Complexene* compound. There was no inlet or outlet valve, nor a filter canister. Air had to be drawn in and expelled through the layers of the mask itself. A weatherproof flap protected the mask from rain. Moderate protection was offered against the early war agents only, and for brief periods of time (Of interest is the fact that the M-2 French mask was issued to U.S. troops during the First World War for use as a "back-up," or secondary defense, while the British BSBR was relied upon as a first line of protection; this policy was later rescinded).

A significant French development, which figured later in U.S. developmental research, was the Tissot Mask. The Tissot mask first used what we call the "Tissot principle" of directed air control, employing twin ducts which ran from the inlet tube of the mask directly to just under the interior lower eyepiece rims for assistance in keeping the eye pieces demisted. The Tissot mask facepiece was made of relatively thin molded rubber, and featured a flapper-type rubber exhaust valve just above the inlet port on the snout of the facepiece. A flexible, fabric-covered rubber tube running over one shoulder ran back to a canister of highly hygroscopic chemicals which was worn via a harness on the back. The mask, while fitting the face very well, was of insufficient sturdiness to ensure continued reliability. American troops on liaison duty with French forces used the Tissot type mask, and reported favorably on it.

A later type of French mask, known as the ARS Mask (*Appareil Respiratoire Special*), was developed somewhat later (about 1919) and was not therefore used in the Great War. It drew somewhat upon the original German snout-type mask design in that it featured a face-fitting mask to which a replaceable filter canister of chemicals was fitted in a 'snout' configuration. Featuring an inlet (for the filter) valved with mica, and an outlet in the snout's metal filter attachment ring made from rubber, the mask used the Tissot principle for lens interior demisting. The facepiece itself was made from well-rubberized balloon material, with a liner of oiled or waxed linen. Circular twin eye lenses were made of thick cellophane, and fitted into metal lens rims. The ARS Mask remained essentially little changed (modification was made to the circular metal filter attachment component to allow a slightly downward angled inlet tube to be used) through the beginning of the Second World War, and examples dated 1939 were widely used by the French. Amazingly, news footage of the 1993 French farmers' strike shows several Frenchmen wearing the 1939 vintage ARS Mask as protection against the teargas used against them by the French Gendarmarie!

Italian Protective Developments:

The initial Italian protective mask was essentially similar to the French M-2 design, but a decision was later made to adopt the British Small Box Respirator (BSBR) when it finally came out. Prior to the first Italian (M-2 type) mask, the standard cotton pads soaked in water and or soda solution had been used—an experience apparently common throughout all military forces engaged in the conflict of the Great War. The Italians later developed their own CW masks of both the snout and canister/hose types.

German Protective Developments:

From a historical standpoint, in part due to the very early and important German participation in the development of chemical warfare technology, the evolution of German CBW respirators is extremely interesting. Several designs were developed and produced for use during the First World War. The earliest protection consisted of pads soaked in a solution of sodium thiosulfate & sodium carbonate. Following this was the issuance of masks made of absorbent cotton, shaped in the form of a snout that fitted the nose and mouth (also soaked in the same chemicals). Subsequently, two protective filtering systems were developed which are of great significance.

The first design consisted of a filter canister (the same as that used with the full face mask) connected to a rigid white mouthpiece by a flexible (corrugated) rubber tube of about 8 inches. The respirator was equipped with a metal nose-clip and was designed to be used with a separate set of goggles to protect the eyes. The mouthpiece was gripped tightly in the mouth and air was both inhaled and exhaled through the filter canister. Austria also developed a version of this type of respirator.

The second type, and perhaps the most interesting design, served not just as an archetype for generalized later respirator developments around the world, but remained essentially the same (albeit with updating and considerable refining of concept and components over the years) for decades. Known in the west simply as *The German Mask*, the facepiece was originally made of natural rubber. It was later made from proofed (oiled) leather, due to a shortage of rubber during the war.[1]

The twin circular eye pieces were made with two clear lens components—an outer one of a sturdy transparent celluloid-like substance, and an inner one of thin coated gelatin—which served to promote anti-dimming. There was no inlet or outlet valve, and air was respired both in and out through a squat, circular drum of chemicals which screwed into the metal snout-ring. The whole assembly of mask and filter drum fitted into a cylindrical metal carrying canister, and was worn suspended via a sling attached to it.

Several variant filtering chemical mixes were used in the German canister. The 1917 canister used three layers, consisting of one layer of Kieselguhr soaked in a solution of potassium carbonate and covered in a layer of powdered charcoal, one additional layer of charcoal, and a final layer of crushed pumice stone mixed with hexamethylenetetramine. The later (1918) type filter used a layer of charcoal and a chemical absorber only. With the advent of the arsenical smokes (sternatatory chemicals), a clip-on (or screw-on) filter extension was developed for the purpose of protecting against "Blue Cross" type shells.

It is interesting to note that from available evidence the Germans were the first to realize the effectiveness of breathing through a canister utilizing reactive and/or absorbing chemicals. Attaching the filter canister directly to the facepiece eliminated awkward hoses and separate canisters, but carried the disadvantage of limiting the size (and hence the durability) of the chemicals capable of being carried in the small snout-attached canister. It was after British forces captured the German Mask that a decision was made to develop a design incorporating the flow of respired air through a canister of filtering chemicals; this resulted in the subsequent British Large Box Respirator (also known as the *Harrison Tower Box*), about which more will be said later.

The basic design of the World War One German Mask set the style for decades of similar protective CBW masks of German design. Even as late as the mid-60s, German CBW respirators bore a startling resemblance to the original pioneering design of the Great War era (first used in 1915), and it was not until the advent of the German M-65 model that a truly different faceblank design was produced. The major improvements consisted of the addition of an exhalation valve, an inhalation one-way check valve, and evolved/improved materials for both facepiece and filtering canisters. As mentioned before, the WWI German Mask probably served to directly inspire the French ARS Mask development, previously referenced.

British Protective Developments:

The initial British response to the German gas initiative at Ypres was identical to that of the other Allied armies—makeshift fabric wadding saturated with water, urine or photographic "hypo."

Immediately thereafter, an interim protective device was devised which consisted of multilayered pads of cotton material which could be soaked in an aqueous solution of sodium carbonate and sodium thiosulfate and clapped across the mouth. Not long after these pads were made available, the women of Great Britain, in response to a call by Lord Kitchener, hand-prepared a similar form of protection to provide the troops. These cotton pads, wrapped in muslin gauze, were whimsically known as *mouth muffs* by the soldiers, and provided about the same degree of protection as the simple cotton pads originally used.

The first British respirator is generally recognized as being what is termed the *Black Veiling Respirator*. Produced in England by women's garment factories, this primitive 'mask' consisted of cotton waste enclosed in a length of black veiling material. After being sewn together, the Black Veil mask was soaked in a solution of sodium thiosulfate, washing soda, glycerine and water. The glycerine was added to keep the respirator moist, obviating the need to dip it into the chemicals immediately prior to use. Tied onto the face with the veiling fabric, it was adjusted over the mouth and nose. Although there was no provision for protection of the eyes, the cotton was able to be pulled up slightly towards them so that a small measure of protection in this manner ensued. The Black Veil Masks were used in the gas attacks of May 10 and May 12 of 1915, and achieved reasonable protection against the relatively low concentration of chlorine gas used in those instances.

The next British respirator was termed the *Hypo Helmet*, and is said to have been inspired by a Canadian sergeant who had seen a German pulling a bag over his head during an attack. This mask consisted of a hood, enclosing the entire head, made from the same muslin/flannel material used in the previous interim masks. The Hypo Helmet was initially fitted with a single pane of mica for vision, but this was later replaced by celluloid, and finally by glass eye-pieces set in metal rings. The lower skirt of the hood was tucked into the collar of the soldier's blouse, and air was inhaled and exhaled through the fabric of the hood. The Hypo Helmet mask was also presoaked in the same solution as the Black Veiling respirator, and reportedly achieved a fairly acceptable degree of protection against chlorine gas in actual trench use.

Next to be developed were what are referred to as the *Hypo P* and *Hypo PH Helmets*. With the first use of chlorine-phosgene mixtures in mid-1915, it became evident that the Hypo Helmet lacked adequate protection capability against phosgene. The Hypo P Helmet had, in the manner of the last Hypo Helmet versions, twin circular lenses, and also featured an early version of the rubber 'flapper' expiratory valve, which while serving to release expired air, also served to afford protection for the alkali of the solution against contact with carbon dioxide. Otherwise similar in appearance to the Hypo Helmet, the new Hypo P design was pre-soaked (immediately after manufacture) in a solution of alkaline sodium phenolate solution (carbolic acid). The chemicals served to neutralize the phosgene, and protected satisfactorily against concentrations of about 300 ppm. Two layers of flannelette were used in the Hypo P Helmet, as was the case with its successor.

Unfortunately, the Hypo P Helmet was not effective against high concentrations of phosgene gas, a failure quickly realized and exploited by the Germans. Therefore, a new version was produced which utilized a Russian discovery that the substance urotropine (hexamethylenetetramine) neutralized phosgene far more completely than the earlier solution of the Hypo P Helmet. Pre-soaked with a solution of urotropine, caustic soda, phenol and glycerine, a protection factor of 1000 ppm against phosgene for more than 24 hours was achieved. This modification of the Hypo P Helmet was thereafter known as the Hypo PH Helmet.

Masks of this type offered no protection against ordinary lacrimatory chemicals, however, and soon goggles were issued for use with them. Intended only for use inside the hoods during a lacrimatory attack, they were soon withdrawn from issue due to the fact that soldiers frequently wore them alone when regular gases were used. Hood type respirators used with such goggles have been referred to as *Hypo PHG Helmets*.

By this time (early 1916) it was apparent that protective hoods of this type had reached the extreme limit of their usefulness for a number of reasons. Among them were the discomfort experienced by users of the Hypo type helmets, lack of lacrimatory chemical protection, increasing concentrations of phosgene/chlorine gas combinations, and the introduction of artillery shell delivered gases such as Chloropicrin and superpalite.

Intelligence analysis of the various other respirators in use at that time, and especially a detailed examination of the standard German mask (described earlier, with its snout attached chemical filter canister), prompted the decision to develop a new type of mask, providing a higher level of protection. The result of this decision was a mask known as the *Large Box Respirator*. This mask is also known as the *Harrison Tower Box* (after Capt. Harrison of the English Anti-gas Lab).

It is amusing to note that several scholarly American chemical warfare references written in the mid-20's, by prominent U.S. experts in this field, contain a reference to what is termed the *British Tar-box Respirator*. This can only be explained by a misapprehension, more than likely based upon incorrect phonetic interpolation of the phrase "Tower Box," pronounced in an unfamiliar (English) accent![2]

As Robert H. Davis has shown in his book *Breathing in Irrespirable Atmospheres*, the preexisting body of English mine safety research was no doubt influential in developing the "box" style respirator for war use. The Large Box Respirator was a polyvalent mask of the hose & canister type, incorporating an oronasal mask made from multi-layered muslin. The facepiece was presoaked in a solution of sodium zincate and urotropine, and featured a rubber mouthpiece inside the oronasal mask which was gripped in the teeth. A set of rubber goggles were worn with the respirator for lacrimatory chemical protection, and a nose-clip secured the nose inside the muslin (a similar experimental type investigated prior to the Large Box Respirator's development appeared identical except that the muslin oronasal facepiece was omitted; nose clip and mouthpiece were uncovered and exposed). The filter box of the Large Box Respirator contained layers of charcoal, soda lime and potassium permanganate. Much of the work which Captain Harrison performed in the Large Box Respirator's design was done in France, although much of it also went on in the English Anti-gas Lab (later Porton). Captain Harrison was also responsible for the development of an absorbing chemical granule used in the filter which was built up of pumice, rolled in lime-permanganate (this followed the equally innovative work of one Major Lambert's discovery of making absorbent lime-permanganate granules).

Subsequently, a modification of the Large Box design resulted in what was termed the *British Small Box Respirator* (also known as simply the BSBR). The major difference between the BSBR and its predecessor was in the facepiece, which covered the whole face—eyes, nose and mouth. Made of fabric coated on the interior with gum rubber, the eyepieces were circular and identical to the last version used on the old Hypo PH Helmets. The rubber mouthpiece and nose clip of the Large Box Respirator were also retained, it being felt that in this manner a double element of protection was provided. In fact, due to the primitive fit of the facepiece, such a system was probably mandated.

Using a rectangular tin box of chemicals (layers of charcoal, soda lime and potassium permanganate), the BSBR filter was connected to the rubberized fabric facepiece via a fabric covered corrugated rubber tube. Lacking precise face fitting, and using flat sewn seams on either side of the face, the mask at first used celluloid lenses in circular metal frames. Later, splinterless glass was substituted for clarity of vision. Utilizing elasticized straps, a fairly good face-fit was achieved for protection against lacrimatory agents. A rubber 'flutter' expiratory valve was incorporated into the metal inlet duct in the snout of the facepiece (this type of expiratory valve is frequently referred to by a number of other terms, among them *Sadd valve*, *flutter valve*, and *spearhead valve*, all of which are used interchangeably), and at one point a protective metal frame was fixed to the flutter valve, although this was later removed due to complaints from the field of its being 'obstructive.'

In terms of construction, the BSBR featured a fabric facepiece (coated with rubber internally) characterized by two large folds (one at either corner, outboard of the eye lenses) to achieve a face-fitting shape. The spring nose-clip, secured to the inside of the facepiece used cotton gauze pads to pinch the nose closed. A head-harness of five straps was used: two on each side, above and below the ears, and one top strap coming back over the head from the center of the mask's frame. The squarish tin filter canister of lacquered natural metal color connected to the lower front of the facepiece via a stockinette-covered rubber hose (corrugated).

Of immense significance for a number of reasons (not the least of which being the fact that the BSBR was the first U.S. Army protective respirator adopted for general use in the First World War, as well as the design inspiration for all initial U.S. developments), the BSBR achieved a fairly high level of protection against the range of chemical war agents used in the 1914-18 period. Unfortunately, there were several aspects of the design which were considered liabilities by thoughtful chemical defense experts. Chief among these was the extreme discomfort of having to wear a BSBR for an extended period. The fatigue factor, imposed by the breathing resistance of the BSBR filter, augmented by the tiresome and difficult task of retaining the rubber mouthpiece for hours upon end (and having to endure having the nose clamped tightly for the same period), contributed to gas discipline laxities in the trenches when gases forced wear of the masks for lengthy periods.

(These problems were not overlooked by U.S. military officers whose troops used the BSBR in combat, and reports of discomfort and fatigue were passed up the chain of command to the U.S. chemical warfare officers responsible for research and development).

When the new mustard gases were first used in July of 1917 (36 times greater toxicity than chlorine), the BSBR provided fairly high effectiveness for their users, but again extended-wear discomfort factors contributed to casualties caused when masks were removed or the primitive face-seal was interrupted through motion artifact.

A square canvas sandy khaki carrier satchel was worn on the chest to hold the BSBR, which was divided into two compartments: one for the filter box, and the other for the mask facepiece assembly. Although well suited for the trench warfare fighting of the First World War, it was discovered to be awkwardly placed for prone fighting and firing postures, making mask donning in the horizontal (prone) plane difficult. This effect was particularly noted by soldiers who frequently had the impression that three inches of vertical exposure to accommodate the mask donning from such a posture was roughly the same as the vertical height of Mt. Everest—figured relative to the standpoint of making one's self a more conspicuous battlefield target.

Despite these problems, the place of the BSBR is assured in the annals of chemical defense technology, for while Germany continued its preference for a snout-type mask with directly attached filter (and influencing almost all of the other European nations' design preferences as well), the British school of design and development served as the foundation for U.S. Army styles of the succeeding decades. In 1926, a new design was adopted by the British which was called the Common Service Pattern. This was later standardized as the General Service Respirator, of which some 25 million units would be issued prior to and during the Second World War.

CHAPTER FOUR: Early U.S. Developments (WWI)

In spite of the obvious fact of eventual U.S. participation in the Great War, the actual opening of hostilities found America largely unprepared not only for war in general, but particularly for chemical warfare. Although gas had been in constant, growing use on the European battlefields for two years prior to U.S. entry in the war, the United States had no organization for either chemical defense or offense. As General Wm. L. Siebert (director of the Chemical Warfare Service) stated it in the annual War Department Report of 1919, *"The work of supply of the entire army with this equipment had to be developed from a starting point of nothing. There were no plants in existence when the U.S. entered the war, and we were utterly without experience."*

With no preexisting unified chemical command, the various services had initially attempted to handle the different aspects of chemical warfare in a piecemeal manner. In April of 1917, the U.S. Army Medical Service was charged with developing and producing gas protective devices (gasmasks, etc.). Earlier, in February of the same year, the U.S. Bureau of Mines had begun a study of air purification masks for industrial use. The experts involved with the latter work were immediately 'borrowed' for Army use.

By mid-1917, confusion reigned among many different army branches, which finally resulted in the establishment of the U.S. Army Chemical Service Section in October of the same year. Intended to coordinate activities only, it had no authority to control or apportion effort. This in turn led to the establishment of the U.S. Army Chemical Warfare Service, under terms of General Order No. 62 of the U.S. War Department on 28 June 1918. This was further underscored by President Wilson, under terms of the Overman Act of 1 July 1918. Through provisions of both, all activities associated with chemical warfare were united under the newly established branch of the U.S. Army.

At the onset of U.S. entry into the war, careful consideration was given to existing protective respirator designs. Three were generally available as of April of 1917. These were the French M-2, the British Hypo PH Helmet, and the BSBR. Of them, the decision was made that the BSBR provided the best overall protection. At the same time, a strong opinion was shared by U.S. gas protection experts that the BSBR had some very unfortunate characteristics, as well. Among these were the increased labor of respiration posed by the increased respiratory resistance of the BSBR canister (this resulted in precipitous and premature fatigue), the discomfort posed by the noseclip and mouthpieces, and the general discomfort of extended wear—now occasioned more frequently by use of the new mustard agents. The decision was made to concentrate on producing the BSBR for the time being, but to avoid the mouthpiece and noseclip design approach in future U.S. developments. Concurrently, a program was proposed for immediate initiation of efforts to produce a satisfactory U.S. chemical defense respirator.

By the end of the war, a total of over 5,692,499 protective gas masks had been manufactured in the United States (records show that of this total, over 4,210,586 of the U.S. masks were shipped to France).

The American Small Box Respirator (also known as The Training Gas Mask):

In May of 1917, the U.S. Army Chief of Staff requested the Surgeon General to supply 25,000 gas masks as soon as possible for provision to General Pershing's First Division, which was about to embark for Europe. According to General Amos A. Fries (later second Director of the U.S. Chemical Warfare Service, from 1920 through 1928), head of the AEF Gas Service, *"There were not half a dozen masks in the entire country. The prevailing idea at this time seemed to be that one could go out to the market and purchase them by the hundreds of thousands, like Halloween masks."* Disillusionment was quick to set in, as was soon seen subsequent to an order placed for 25,000 gas masks 'based upon' the British Small Box Respirator.

As the Surgeon General's medical organization had no facilities for the production of these masks, the matter was referred to the U.S. Bureau of Mines, which initiated the order and supervised the program. Despite the enormous effort and cooperative endeavors which resulted in the completion of the order in record time (less than a month), these 25,000 masks were produced without direct reference to the English models, and they were designed and manufactured without sufficient knowledge of British specifications and fabrication methods. Their inadequacy wasn't immediately apparent, however, and they were shipped to France along with Pershing's troops.

While still on the ships, en route and on the way to the front, it was discovered that the 25,000 hastily made American copies of the BSBR were seriously deficient. The mask fabric was found to be easily penetrated by lacrimatory gases, the nose clips discovered to be ineffective, the eye pieces found to be defective, and finally, the filter canisters were discovered to be unable to afford protection against chloropicrin! None of the 25,000 masks could be used.

Consequently, as an interim step, the AEF's First Division finally received the English BSBR for their use as some 100,000 of them were purchased by the U.S. in the summer of 1917. Meanwhile, back in the United States, thousands of masks similar to the initial order of faulty American copies of the BSBR were manufactured for use strictly limited to training purposes, pending further research into the precise specifications and parameters of the British mask. These masks were almost identical in appearance to the BSBR, upon casual inspection, and have been referred to both as the *American Small Box Respirator* (ASBR) and the *Training Gas Mask*. The ASBR (Training Gas Mask) used a black filter canister, the size of which was slightly larger than that used with the BSBR (the filter had been made to contain more charcoal due to the theory that American charcoal was not as effective as that used in the British filter—this was later shown to be untrue).

Early examples of the ASBR featured eye lens frames secured to the facepiece by twine, following the BSBR example, although some late models have been noted to feature green colored metal frames similar to those used on the subsequent C.E.M. respirator (ASBR eye lenses were made of celluloid reinforced glass).This is not unusual in view of the fact that refinements were frequently incorporated in WWI period masks midway during production, as continued developmental research suggested possible improvements in design. Occasional small variations will thus be noted in comparisons of similar models, such as the ASBR.

Generally, the ASBR facepiece appears very similar to the C.E.M. mask, which followed it, and also looks quite similar to the BSBR which inspired it.

The black filter canister, characteristic of ASBR models, had its top painted red to serve as a visible warning (viewable despite the fact that the canister was secured in the carrying satchel) that the ASBR was only to be used in training exercises. ABSR models also had "For Training Purposes Only" stamped on the inside of their carrying stachels.

The ABSR used an angle tube that was very similar in appearance to its counterpart on the BSBR (examples both with and without valve protectors have been noted); this was changed to a new design in the subsequent C.E.M. respirator. ABSR nose clips used rubber pads, also, instead of cotton gauze (as on the BSBR). ASBR carrying stachels were slightly taller than those issued with the C.E.M. and succeeding models, owing to the taller, black bodied ASBR filter canister.

In addition to the initial 25,000 faulty ASBRs initially produced, several thousand more of the same design were produced back in the U.S. strictly for training purposes and familiarization exercises, between July and October of 1917.

The Corrected English Mask:

In October of 1917, difficulties with obtaining exact design specifications for the BSBR were overcome and a respirator again patterned closely after the English BSBR was put into production. This respirator, of which more than 1,864,000 copies were produced before the Armistice, was known as the *Corrected English Mask* (C.E.M.). It incorporated an improvement in the facepiece which protected against chloropicrin and all other (then current) agents, the addition of a slightly changed flutter valve to the angle-tube component, use of coiled springs to retain eye pieces, a change in the angle-tube (which lowered breathing resistance), and substitution of activated coconut charcoal for the inactivated wood charcoal used in the BSBR. The noseclip and mouthpiece components were retained and were similar to those used in the BSBR except that rubber discs were used to pinch off the nose instead of cotton gauze pads. Early versions of the C.E.M. lacked a metal protective guard around the rubber exhalation valve; some later versions featured a narrow protector guard, while still later versions were provided with a somewhat more substantial (stronger and sturdier) guard. Both versions appear to have been numerous, based upon examination of surviving specimens. The C.E.M. mask was principally produced utilizing the yellow 'H' filter canister, although a few very late versions have been found to be fitted with the green bodied 'J filter.' Typical C.E.M. head harnesses were of the non-adjustable elasticized strap design, with one central strap affixed to the supra-forehead section and two lateral straps fitted to the face frame on each side of the head, all joining behind the head. A few versions appear to have been made using an elasticized five strap harness fitted with early metal slide-adjusters—modern but essentially similar versions of which are still in use on the latest U.S. masks today!

As noted before, in a previous chapter, the U.S. Army first provided a French M-2 type mask to First Division troops in the AEF as a 'spare mask' or emergency respirator for use in the event the primary BSBR or CEM type unit was lost or damaged (This policy was later rescinded when studies showed that soldiers had a tendency to change masks <u>during</u> chemical attacks. The urge to change masks was usually motivated by the discomfort experienced using the box type respirator's mouthpiece and noseclip for extended periods, which prompted a change to the far less effective but more comfortable French M-2 mask. A study of statistics after the change in policy, eliminating the issuance of the 'emergency' M-2 mask, demonstrated a significant drop in fatalities and serious gas-related injuries). Just about every respirator satchel also carried a spare pair of socks as a further emergency safeguard.

The C.E.M. carrying satchel was (as noted earlier) of a somewhat reduced size, and was provided with a small record card on which exposure to gas and consequent repairs could be documented. This card, which fitted into a slip-sleeve tied with a cord to the filter) also accommodated a small piece of repair 'plaster' for making repairs to the facepiece fabric. One of the primary reasons for provision of the service document with the mask was that at this time a satisfactory system for monitoring exposure to gas (especially for replacing exposed filters when needed) had not yet been devised.

C.E.M. masks have been noted with both celluloid and glass lenses.

The R.F.K. Mask:
In view of the still less-than-optimal characteristics of the Corrected English Mask, it was followed by an even further improved respirator that bore considerable resemblance to the CEM[1]. Significant changes incorporated in it included a slightly different shape to the facepiece and binder frame (to improve fit and comfort), reinforcing binder frame stitching and spun-in aluminum eye frames. A rubber backed fabric facepiece was used, similar in appearance to the C.E.M. mask, and internal nose-clip and rubber mouthpiece components were retained. This respirator was known as the *R.F.K. mask* (named after three personnel of the American Chemical Service named Richardson, Flory and Kops), and from February of 1918 until the armistice was signed, over 3,050,000 of these masks were produced. The RFK mask's khaki facepiece had a gum-rubber lining of approximately 1/64th inch thickness, and featured the same characteristic folds in the fabric on each side of the eye lenses as had the ASBR and C.E.M. masks. Stitching and interior joints were sealed by rubber cement, and the facepiece was made in 5 sizes, with sizes 2,3, & 4 being intermediate sizes. Originally, ordinary celluloid was used in lenses; this was replaced by various hygroscopic forms of celluloid known as 'non-dimming eyepieces,' and finally by various combinations of glass and celluloid known as 'non-breakable eyepieces'. It was recognized that despite the safety advantages presented by the last type of glass-celluloid-glass sandwich (called "Triplex" glass), the inner layer of celluloid would ultimately deteriorate with age; however, it was argued that the safety factor of Triplex glass balanced out the potential deterioration of the celluloid inner layer. Most R.F.K. masks were produced with the green 'J filter' canister attached, although variations have been noted in surviving examples (this fact may reflect field maintenance changes, or the fact that improvements were sometimes made to masks during production runs).

The R.F.K. mask featured an improved head harness of 6 elasticized straps to enhance fit—one on either side of the forehead, one above each ear, and one below each ear. The R.F.K. mask is immediately distinguished from the ASBR and C.E.M. masks by its two upper head harness straps, which are joined by an elasticized cross strap midway back to the juncture of all six straps in the occiput region. This head strap arrangement, with the addition of slip fit metal buckles, a headpad at the rear of the head, and some minor modification, would remain the basic model for *most* subsequent U.S. respirator harnesses, including the most recent ones.

The A.T. (Akron-Tissot) Mask:
The RFK mask was a moderate improvement of the basic BSBR design, but again, it retained the uncomfortable noseclip and rubber mouthpiece components which U.S. Chemical Service coordinators uniformly agreed were undesirable for sustained wear. Consequently, and in keeping with the American program of continuing to develop a suitable U.S. respirator while the BSBR based masks were in interim use, attention was being paid to the French innovations for possible inclusion. The French M-2 mask, while it was relatively simple and only moderately effective against increasing concentrations of war gas, pointed the way towards the desirable aspects of a simpler mask capable of being donned quickly. Awareness of this benefit was also reflected in the appreciation of some U.S. chemical warfare experts for the functional simplicity of the standard German Mask, with its integrated screw-on filter canister. The disadvantage of the German style mask, in the opinion of others, however, was that its size and weight limitations acted to prevent necessary changes in the type and quantity of necessary filtering components required to meet new chemical formulations (filter development was, of course, still in its infancy).

Most influential, however, was the French Tissot Mask, with its principle of channeled air deflection across the inner lens surfaces. Combined with the Tissot Mask's well fitting rubber facepiece, lack of need for a noseclip and mouthpiece, and the incorporation of an exhaust valve, the Tissot Mask presented an obvious inspiration for further efforts to improve the concept. Working with the Akron Rubber Company of Ohio, the U.S. Chemical Service designers came up with a new respirator design in 1917 which became known as the *A.T. Mask*. The A.T. mask featured a molded rubber facepiece (like the French Tissot Mask, but thicker and sturdier, and vulcanized to a cotton stockinet material on the outer surface) and used the Tissot type channeled air deflection principle for lens demisting, a flapper type rubber exhaust valve, and a stockinet covered corrugated rubber hose (like the BSBR) which connected a rectangular box of filtering chemicals. Due to the superior face-sealing capability of the A.T. mask, the troublesome mouthpiece and noseclip could finally be eliminated. A self-centering adjustable head harness (6 strap) was used. Between June 1917 and the Armistice in 1918 over 197,000 of these masks were manufactured, and the A.T. mask is today regarded (along with the subsequent K.T. mask) as the direct forebear study which eventually resulted in the final U.S. respirator design, the American Model 1919.

The K.T. (Kops-Tissot) Mask:
Working along similar lines of development, Kops produced another respirator design similar to the A.T. mask. Known as the *K.T. mask*, the respirator featured a semi-flexible facepiece binder frame, a butterfly shaped rubber interior air deflector (using the Tissot principle), and instead of the so-called "angle tube" (used in the BSBR and C.E.M. masks) it featured a separate inlet tube and exhaust valve outlet. In place of the rubber chin-rest used in the A.T. mask, it had an elastic chin-rest strap. The self-centering feature of the A.T. mask was incorporated into the K.T. mask, and a total of 337,000 of these masks were produced before the Armistice ended the war. The K.T. mask used the same yellow painted filter canister as the C.E.M., and featured a metal exhaust valve guard to protect the flapper type valve.

Additionally, the K.T. mask featured a more form-fitting, rubber-lined fabric facepiece (no folds in the fabric were needed), screw-frames for the eye lenses, and a 6-strap elastic harness of the type initially used on the A.T. mask (self-centering, adjustable).

While pointing the way to a final American design, the A.T. and K.T. models were difficult to manufacture (this was their most serious drawback), and a final U.S. respirator design incorporating elements of both respirators was finally produced, after a quick yet careful evaluation of all available respirator design experiences had been undertaken. Planned for issuance in time for the anticipated Allied Offensive of 1919, the new mask was designated The *U.S. Army 1919 Model.* This mask was also known as the *K.T.M. (Kops-Tissot-Monroe) Mask.*

The U.S. Army 1919 Model (K.T.M. Mask):
The original *U.S. Army 1919 Model (K.T.M. Mask)* entered production in October of 1919, and by the time the Armistice was signed only 2000 units had been produced. Production facilities had been developed so rapidly, however, that the necessary preparations were in place to produce over a million of the 1919 Models per month.

The facepiece of this first truly effective production respirator of the U.S. Army was manufactured from a special rubber compound, with cotton stockinet material vulcanized to the outer surface (as in the A.T. & K.T. masks). The facepiece material was cut from sheets of the stockinet covered rubber with a special die so that when folded and sewn along two short edges to form a chin seam, a properly fitting face-form was achieved. This method of fabrication greatly simplified mass production. Holes for the circular eyepieces were elliptical so that an uneven tension around the lenses caused the installed eyepieces to bulge forward, insuring an enhanced fit around the temples. The mask had an angle tube similar to that used on the A.T. mask, and an interior deflector similar to that used inside the K.T. mask, but had neither a chin-rest or chin strap, the mask being designed so that these were unnecessary. A head harness pad of canvas covered felt was used with six straps (three on each side of the head) and buckles to retain the mask on the user's face. The canister of the 1919 Model mask (designated the MI canister) was painted blue (the early, obsolesced ASBR canister was slightly larger and painted black; the canister of the R.F.K. type masks was slightly smaller again and painted green; the C.E.M. masks as well as the A.T. & K.T. masks used a yellow painted canister, for the most part, which was sized the same as the R.F.K.'s green filter). The 1919 Model mask used Triplex glass lenses which were press fitted (not held in by screw-threaded frames, as in the A.T. and K.T. masks) in circular metal frames with rubber gaskets. The length of the stockinet covered rubber hose connecting the mask's angle tube to the blue filter canister was approximately 24 inches, a lengthening required due to the placement of the U.S. Army 1919 Model's new side-secured canvas carrier.

The squarish, sandy-khaki colored canvas carrier, of the type used with the original BSBR, was adopted by the U.S. Army for use with all of its early respirators, up through the K.T. & A.T. models. Designated the MI carrier, it was not commonly used for the 1919 Model mask or subsequent developments. As mentioned earlier, the chest carried satchel had proven suitable for trench-style warfare, but had shown itself unsuitable for use in prone rifle-firing positions, making mask retrieval and donning difficult and potentially hazardous.

As a consequence, a new carrier was designed which would be placed on the soldier's left side, under the arm and just above the hip. Known as the MII carrier, this tan or OD (olive drab) canvas satchel was cut in an irregular conformation that has been described as a semi-kidney shape (despite its not resembling that organ by any stretch of the imagination). It was secured in place with two straps, the upper of which was looped across the opposite shoulder and the lower around the waist. The flap of the carrier, facing forward for easy access, was secured with what are best described as 'automobile curtain fasteners' ('snap' fasteners), and testing by all branches of the U.S. Army (cavalry, infantry, artillery and special gas troops) had indicated that it was acceptable for use without exception or objection. Most important, the carrier did not interfere with the standard U.S. Army field pack or gear harness in use at the time, and was relatively unobtrusive. Access to the mask was equally facilitated in any standard combat posture. Unlike the early MI carrier, which was divided into two compartments—one to hold the filter and an adjacent one to hold the facepiece—the MII style carrier was not compartmentalized, although the filter canister was secured with canvas straps inside the carrier which were easily released for access. The mask fitted into the carrier so that the hose was folded in a figure 'S', with the facepiece facing forwards. This would remain typical of all subsequent U.S. respirator carrying satchels and mask stowage configuration from the early 1919 Model until the advent of the new so-called "Lightweight" gas masks of the mid-WWII years (which used an entirely new carrier and stowing procedure).

Two years after its development (in 1921) the *U.S. Army 1919 Model* was standardized as the *U.S. Army Service Gas Mask MI.* The basic U.S. Army Service Gas Mask MI would see improvements over the next 15 years, in both faceblank and filter modifications, which would result in improved models designated MIA1 and MIA2. These developments will be covered in the next chapter (Chapter Five: The Progeny of Model 1919, and a New World War). Thus, the basic design of the Model 1919 would continued to serve U.S. armed forces through its refined MIA1 and MIA2 versions, for almost another 24 years (A detailed description of filter canister developments, from the early original models through the present, is to be found in Appendix III of this book).

CHAPTER FIVE:
The Progeny of Model 1919, and a New World War

As described in the previous chapter, the final result of the U.S. Chemical Warfare Service's protective respirator development program was the *U.S. Army 1919 Model Mask.* The 1919 Model was finally accepted as a standard issue item in 1921, and was designated *U.S. Army Service Gas Mask MI* with no significant change made in design or production.

As may be imagined (and especially in view of the then-prevailing opinion that "The Great War" was a war *to end all wars*), postwar demobilization and War Department budget reductions had a significant impact upon the protective respirator developments which ensued in the U.S. Fortunately, the lessons learned from America's complete lack of preparation for the First World War added to the War Department's recognition of the importance of chemical warfare in any potential future conflict, resulted in a moderate maintenance of the U.S. Army Chemical Warfare Service's operations. To a large degree this was due to the driving dedication and effort of USACWS directors, Maj. Gen. William L. Siebert and his successor, Brig. Gen. Amos A. Fries.[1] It was under their direction that the succeeding development of the new U.S. Army Service Gas Mask MI took place.

The Army Service Gas Mask MI (former Model 1919) underwent several developments over the period of time from 1921 through 1935. While the specifics of the variations will be discussed in detail shortly, it is helpful to consider the general events pertinent to the evolution of the Model 1919 in the 1920s and 1930s.

In about 1928, a modification of the faceblank of the basic mask resulted in the designation MIA1. Further modification resulted in a final MIA2 faceblank design which was almost identical to that of the MI and MIA1. Both of these models were accepted as standard in 1934 and 1935 respectively, and the United States ended the 1930s with these three basic service respirator faceblanks and two specialized variants. The specialized faceblanks were designated the Optical Mask and the Diaphragm Mask.

The Optical Mask design was developed (in the 30s) to accommodate the needs of soldiers using precision sighting devices, and had a distinctive appearance which resulted from the canister being mounted behind the head and connected to the faceblank by two tubes (one on either side of the head). The Diaphragm Mask (developed in the late 20s), so named for the large vibrating disc type voicemitter fitted to the front of the faceblank, was intended for use by officers and other personnel who needed to communicate clearly while protected by a respirator. Interestingly, the Army Optical and Diaphragm designs would be borrowed for use by the U.S. Navy, and more about that will follow in the chapter of the book dealing with U.S. Navy developments.

As the United States recognized in the late 1930s that it would ultimately be drawn into the new World War, the U.S. Army Chemical Warfare Service acknowledged that the older MI style respirators had major drawbacks which mandated priority for development of a new type of facepiece. Thus, a new generation of faceblank design began with what was designated the M2 style facepiece, the first fully molded U.S. designed rubber mask. Through the duration of the Second World War, major new respirator designs—all related to the new fully molded rubber M2 type facepiece—would be produced. Additionally, as may be imagined, advances in filter canister design would also take place concurrently. For a precise summarization of U.S. Army filter canister evolution, a full explanation of the major advancements is presented in Appendix III.

The U.S. Army Service Gas Mask MI:
As noted, the U.S. Army Service Gas Mask MI was virtually identical to the U.S. Army 1919 Model. The MI facepiece was cut from special sheet-rubber, vulcanized with a layer of stockinet material on the outer surface, in a manner that allowed the lower short edge of the pattern to be sewed, cemented and taped in a single seam under the chin. The eye holes were elliptically cut as described earlier (Model 1919) so that the eyepieces would bulge outward, enhancing the face-conformation of the mask. The lenses were of the Triplex safety type, and the circular eye frames were crimped around the lenses using a rubber gasket for gas tightness (not of the screw-thread type).

A cast aluminum angle tube inserted in the snout position of the facepiece housed the inlet and the exhaust outlet. Inside the facepiece, a 'butterfly' type Tissot style air deflector channeled air from the inlet across the interior lens surfaces for demisting. The expiratory rubber flapper type valve, designated type MI, was affixed to the angle tube's outlet duct and was protected by a stamped metal guard fastened to the outlet duct with screws. A 27 inch stockinet covered corrugated rubber hose connected the MI facepiece inlet to the filter canister, and a six-strap elasticized head harness (designated the Head Harness MI) was attached to adjustable buckles for fit. MII head harnesses were retrofitted to MI faceblanks in the event of repairs to that component, and the MI facepieces were stamped with the letters US and a number from 1 through 4 to designate the facepiece size. Size 1 was the smallest and fitted 5% of the population; Size 2 fitted 50%, size 3 fitted 35%, and size 4 10%.

When the Service Gas Mask MI was originally produced, it was fitted with the MI filter canister. This filter was painted blue for identification, and featured a pair of small button-valve inlets at the top of the container; this was protected by a metal rain-shield open at the sides ('slotted') which extended over the whole upper end of the canister (outlet end). The MI canister was an improvement over the last *principal* WWI type service filter (known as the *J filter*, which was slightly smaller in size and painted chromate green). It had a built in smoke filter pad (against "Blue Cross" type irritant smokes), but opinion held that the smoke element was still not fully effective, and subsequent filter types increased smoke protection.

Two carrier satchels were used with the Service Gas Mask MI. The most commonly used carrier was the carrier originally termed the '1920 Style Carrier,' which was standardized in 1921 as the Carrier MII. As previously described, the carrier was irregular in size and was worn on the left side. A 27 inch hose was used with the MII Carrier.

The other carrier used, less often, was the old type BSBR style MI Carrier. If the MI facepiece was used with one of the early WWI type J filters, it was used with a 12 inch hose and carried in the MI satchel. This carrier would accept any of the top inlet filters (such as the MI) or any of the bottom inlet carriers (WWI style). The early (green) J filters were subsequently designated for training use only with the advent of the MI filter, and were referred to commonly thereafter as "Training Filters." The basic design approach of the MI series masks was retained until the introduction of the new fully molded rubber M2 type facepiece, although stocks of the MI, MIA1 and MIA2 type masks were kept in war reserve stocks until released as surplus materiel in late 1944.

The U.S. Army Service Gas Mask MIA1:

The MI faceblank was slightly modified, with approval and adoption of the resulting MIA1 facepiece taking place in 1928. The major differences between the original MI facepiece and the new MIA1 version were found in the eye lens components and in the head harness. The MIA1 faceblank featured a new threaded circular guard ring to retain the Triplex safety glass lens. This enabled the lenses to be easily replaced in the field as occasioned, thereby reducing the likelihood that a soldier's mask would be rendered unusable through damage to the lenses. It also serves to immediately differentiate the MIA1 from the earlier MI mask. Further, a new head-harness assembly was adopted to replace the original MI design. Designated the MII head harness, the new harness was fully replaceable due to the fact that only the adjusting buckles were attached to the mask faceblank (the MI faceblank had a permanently attached harness). This facilitated replacement and maintenance requirements, and the combined modifications of the MIA1 resulted in lowered logistical and support costs—an important attraction during a time when the USCWS was having to conserve every penny of its allocated budget.

The new MIV filter canister was adopted at about the same time as the MIA1 faceblank, and it featured a number of improvements, the most significant of which was a lowering of the respiratory resistance of the unit. It also returned to the bottom inlet configuration similar to that used on the WWI filters, although internally the filtering elements were considerably rearranged and improved.

The carrier used with the new MIA1 mask assembly was designated the MIII. Similar to the MII, it featured an extra tuck in the material of the bottom of the carrier, secured by a rivet, which enabled freer access to the inlet port of the canister. It was in turn replaced by the MIIIA1 carrier, which had the hose-conforming curvilinear section of the satchel replaced by three linear sections which were easier to sew and manufacture. In 1935 the MIA1 was officially superseded by the MIA2 mask, but stocks were carried in war reserve status until released as surplus in late 1944. The faceblank of the MIA1 mask was produced in the same 4 sizes as was the original MI faceblank, further providing an immediately identifiable characteristic to set it off from the succeeding MIA2, which was produced in universal and small sizes only.

The U.S. Army Service Gas Mask MIA2:

In 1935 an administrative and manufacturing modification of the MI and MIA1 service masks took place. The previous system of 4 distinct facial sizes was eliminated. A necessity in the older two models due to use of relatively inelastic materials in the faceblank, the new MIA2 production standard incorporated thicker rubber and less restricting stockinet outer covering which allowed the faceblank to conform more readily to a greater number of facial configurations. The quality of available rubber had improved from 1920 to 1935, and partly due to increasing cost constraints brought on by the nation's economy, it was decided that a single uniform facepiece size would suffice to suit existing needs.

Unfortunately, this proved to be a hasty and erroneous assumption. Consequently a number of small facepieces were also produced, in addition to the so-called "universal" size. Facepieces of the MIA2 type mask were stamped with the characters US and either a U for universal, or an S for small. It was estimated that the universal size would fit approximately 95% of all faces, and the small size would cover the remaining 5%. Aside from this single change in production specifications, the MIA2 faceblank is essentially identical to that of the MIA1.

The filter canister MVIII was in service by this time, and it was shortly thereafter followed by the MIX filter for a brief period. The smooth-sided MIX filter featured a can that was a half inch shorter than the MVIII, and had an inlet on the bottom of the container that lacked a rubber disc valve. The MIXA1 filter soon followed (1939) and is the filter most commonly found in use on the first of the new M2 type "Heavyweight" gas masks of the early war years. The MIXA1 was 6 inches tall, had a rubber disc inlet valve on the bottom (in the conventional manner), and featured semi-corrugated ridges on the sides of the casing. Improvements in these canisters included advancements in particulate filtering fibers, and the use of chemical treatment of the charcoal to enhance effectiveness.

The MIIIA1 carrying satchel was issued originally concurrent with the MIA2 mask, but it was almost immediately replaced by the MIV model. In the MIV, the closure flap was reshaped to make it longer and narrower, and the lower closure snap was set into a fabric loop for easier access. The overall size of the MIV was slightly smaller than the preceding MIIIA1, as was the final MIVA1 version which was identical to the MIV save for the addition of 4 inches of length to the waist strap. (It was the MIVA1 carrier which was most frequently used with the later fully molded M2 "Heavyweight" type masks that replaced the MI series masks, although a final MIVA2 carrier was also issued with the latter).

The U.S. Army Diaphragm Gas Mask (MI through M3A1): The so-called Army diaphragm type gas mask originated at about the same time as the original Army Service Gas Mask MI. There were 4 subsequent developments of the diaphragm mask up through 1945. The earliest of these was the U.S. Army Diaphragm Gas Mask MI. It corresponds to the Service Gas Mask MI (standardized Model 1919), and was used concurrent with that model by those with communications requirements. With the Service Gas Mask MIA1, a counterpart Diaphragm Gas Mask MIA1 was produced, reflecting similar improvements but remaining very similar in external appearance to the Diaphragm Mask MI. When the 1935 production changes took place resulting in the Service Gas Mask MIA2, a corresponding communications mask was produced designated Diaphragm Mask MII. With the advent of the new fully molded rubber M2 type facepiece in 1940, a communications mask counterpart designated Diaphragm Mask M3 was produced (corresponding to the new M2A1 service mask) that used a circular metal voicemitter situated over a rear-facing protected (MVI type) flapper valve, located under the bifurcated inlet tube. A further communications counterpart to the service gas mask was produced in 1942, with the addition of an entirely new speech diaphragm/exhalation valve to the molded rubber faceblank, resulting in the Diaphragm Mask M3A1 design. This final design used a molded plastic voicemitter housing with a caged plastic mushroom exhalation valve situated directly below, and retained the bifurcated plastic inlet tube attaching the filter hose used in the M3 Diaphram mask.

For visual identification and conceptualization of the physical changes which set the diaphragm models off from the conventional 'service' masks, see the photo plates (The 'standard service mask vs. diaphragm mask' approach to gas mask design ended with the production of the new M17 series masks in the late 1950s, wherein for the first time it was recognized that a communications capability was an important, mandatory component of all respirators. As a consequence of that change in design concept all contemporary protective chemical & biological respirators from that time forward feature a communicator of either the horn or the vibrating disc type. This component is commonly called a "voicemitter").

The early Diaphragm Masks (MI and MIA1) featured a slightly different type of inlet and exhalation valve block on the facepiece. Unlike the Service Gas Mask counterparts (MI and MIA1), the MII rubber flapper type valve was used on the outlet, protected in the conventional manner with a standard stamped metal valve protector. In congruence with the standard Tissot air demisting principle, incoming filtered air was directed to the interior of the eye lenses, although the imposition of the speech diaphragm required a slightly different physical ducting configuration. On the Diaphragm Masks MI and MIA1, the Tissot deflector ducts are internalized, whereas on the Diaphragm Mask MII, the duct is conspicuously placed externally in the form of a metallic 'Y' tube, coming off the inlet angle tube and skirting the diaphragm and exhaust valve (protected by the metal Y shape). The Diaphragm Mask MII also used the MVI (spearhead) type flapper valve instead of the MII type. The Diaphragm Mask M3 (corresponding to the new M2A1 fully molded type faceblank) used a different style metal voicemitter housing, separate from the Tissot air channels, and the even later Diaphragm Mask M3A1 facepiece (corresponding to the Lightweight Service Gas Mask M4) used a fully molded plastic voicemitter housing. The exhaust valves on the Diaphragm Masks MI, MIA1, and MII, as mentioned, were of the (MII) rubber flapper type. The exhaust valve of the M3 diaphragm mask consisted of an MVI rubber flapper (spearhead) situated below the circular metal speech diaphragm housing, which was protected by being located between the bifurcated inlet assembly. The Model M3 and M3A1 Diaphragm Masks used fully molded rubber faceblanks made of gray-green color, and the M3A1 mask featured a plastic caged (M8) exhalation valve as part of its speech diaphragm assembly, that eliminated the need for the flapper (or MVI spearhead) valve between the complex bifurcated inlet duct on the facepiece.

All diaphragm gas masks were issued in carrying satchels similar to the standard service gas mask carriers, but were imprinted with the legend "Diaphragm Gas Mask" in almost all cases. As with standard specifications of the period, the carriers were constructed of tan or OD colored canvas duck, and except for the identifying legend are identical to the service respirator satchels.

The U.S. Army Optical Gas Mask M1: With increasing use of optically sighted weapons and surveillance systems in the military forces, it was recognized that the standard eye lenses used with the Service Gas Masks were unsuited for this application. Consequently, a special mask was designed which we know as the U.S. Army Optical Gas Mask. This mask had a very distinctive appearance from both the conventional service models and the diaphragm masks, although it incorporated a speech diaphragm in its basic faceblank design. First produced in the very late 1930s (contemporary with the first fully molded M2 type faceblanks), this molded rubber mask featured twin, small, circular lenses of high-grade, ordinary optical glass. Twin 11 inch corrugated rubber hoses attached to both ends of a cylindrical filter canister, worn behind the head, joined the facepiece on either side of the small eye lenses to deliver filtered air incorporating the Tissot principle. A speech transmitting vibrating disc unit is located in the lower front of the mask (which is molded of gray-green rubber), below which is a metal frame protected MVI (spearhead) type rubber exhaust valve. An adjusting screw between the lenses enables the intraocular distance to be custom tailored for use with binoculars and other visual sighting instruments.

The U.S. Army Optical Gas Mask of 1940-41 is virtually identical to the corresponding U.S. Navy model identified as the USN Model NDO Mk. I, except that the latter is fabricated from black rubber instead of gray-green rubber. Both used the M3 (coiled spring straps) head harness assembly.

The U.S. Army Optical Gas Mask M2:
A somewhat later development of the optical mask was designated Army Optical Gas Mask M2. This mask, molded originally of gray-green rubber, featured a fully molded faceblank in which the Tissot style air channels were integrally combined. The result was a very different appearance from the distinctive profile of the earlier Optical Mask M1, with its prominent bilateral rubber hoses and filter situated behind the user's head.

The Optical Mask M2 featured a combined diaphragm voicemitter & exhalation valve (C15 type) assembly known as the "Diaphragm Angletube Assembly C11." This mask used a single rubber corrugated hose running from the mask's chin inlet to the M10A type cylindrical filter canister (identical to that used with the "Lightweight Gas Mask" designs of the mid-40s), and featured head-harness assembly M7 for retention. The M2-10A1-6 Optical Gas Mask, later molded in black rubber, was manufactured and used up through the 50s. Examples are now occasionally found available, still sealed in their original tin storage cases.

The New M2 Fully Molded Gas Mask Design:
With the realization that U.S. involvement in the 'new' war was very likely inevitable (late 1930s), the USCWS pressed for development of a newer respirator design which would more fully reflect advances in methods and materials. Improvements in rubber compounds and identification of the need for better visual field of vision, among other criteria, permitted the design of a mask which would feature for the first time a fully molded, one piece faceblank. Among the distinct disadvantages of the original MI series was the fact that the central seam under the chin presented a potentially weak and vulnerable area for penetration of chemical agents. Additionally, use of stockinet type coverings on faceblanks and hoses presented serious decontamination challenges. The exposed and vulnerable MI type flutter exhalation valve, in use since the earliest WWI respirators had been designed, also presented a potential for failure due to possible physical damage to or malfunction of the rather fragile component.

By the time the 1930s were ending, considerable progress had been made in the molding of rubber products by several companies, including B.F. Goodrich, Goodyear, and the Acushnet Company (which was fulfilling U.S. Army Air Corps contracts for rubber oxygen masks and components at the time). A design project was set in motion by the U.S. Army Chemical Corps (formerly the U.S. Army Chemical Warfare Service) to produce a new generation of faceblank and hose assembly. This reached fruition in 1938 with the introduction of a new facepiece known as the M2 series. Featuring a one-piece, seamless and fully molded faceblank of gray-green natural rubber, the new design marked a significant advance in protective mask state of the art.

The U.S. Army Training Mask MI/M2:
The new fully molded rubber facepiece design was first used in production of a new training gas mask.[2] Due to the fact that the U.S. Army nomenclature underwent a change with the development of the new style masks (September of 1940), the original designation of the Training Gas Mask was *Training Gas Mask MI*. In September of 1940 in compliance with the new system and to eliminate confusion, the designation was changed to *Training Gas Mask M2* (prior to that date Roman numerals were used for model designation identification; after that date, Arabic numerals were substituted for the earlier Roman numerals). The earlier MI, MIA1 and MIA2 type masks retained their original Roman Numeral designators, but all new types, including the Training Gas Mask MI, were designated under the new system. Hence, the possibility of some understandable confusion over the "MI/M2" identifier under discussion here.

The Training Gas Mask MI/M2 used a faceblank that was identical to the subsequent Service Gas Mask M2 in every respect. The characteristic differences of the MI/M2 training mask facepieces from the later M2A1 type Training Gas Masks are twofold; 1) the shape and inclination of the eye lenses vary somewhat, and 2) the type of exhalation valve utilized is different. Aside from this, the MIA1/M2A1 Training Gas Mask used the same smaller, cylindrical MI Training Filter as the earlier MI/M2 mask. As was typical of the period, the MI/M2 Training Mask underwent the same sort of upgrading of its exhaust valve as the service mask counterparts, and the change was reflected in the mask designation in a similar fashion as the latter. Hence, the MI/M2 Training Gas Mask used the older MIV Acushnet valve, and the M2A1 Training Gas Mask employed the Connell type MV exhaust valve. The correct designation of the Training Gas Mask, using the standard Army Nomenclature system (outlined fully in Appendix II), was the Training Gas Mask MIA1/M2A1-I-I.

The training gas mask was used extensively by troops who were in basic military training, prior to seeing action, and it was intended to be used only for that purpose. However, allowance was made for its use in the event of an emergency as primary protection against chemical attack, and later in the war there were instances of the training masks being carried by troops in the South Pacific in preference to the bulky service respirators. The training gas masks were also issued on an emergency basis to civilians for chemical warfare protection in the Hawaiian Islands, during the war, after the canisters had been replaced with new units and the masks had been checked and refurbished for serviceability.

The Training Gas Mask MI/M2 and MIA1/M2A1 were issued and carried in a snout-type tan canvas duck gas mask satchel MI, which resembled the frustum of a cone, and was similar to the carrying satchel issued civilians with their Noncombatant Gas Mask MIA1 and MIA2 respirators.

It is interesting to see what U.S. Army Field Manual 21-40 had to say about the use of the Training Gas Mask just before the start of the Second World War, keeping in mind that this mask would serve as the design inspiration for a newer, lighter generation of designs:

"Limitations and use: The Training Gas Mask is intended for training purposes only. However, the canister will protect against all standard chemical agents; but it should be noted that the amount of protection furnished against the standard casualty type agents is equal to many of the canisters used in the WWI period (1917-1918), and in the case of irritant smokes, superior. The life of the training canister (MI) is slightly less than that of the latest standard (military) canister, but less than WWI types. In case of emergency, it may be used for protection against a chemical attack."

The U.S. Army Service Gas Mask M2:

Although intended at the onset as a supplementary training mask, the excellent features of the fully molded rubber M2 faceblank quickly became apparent, and a service mask version was devised in which the standard MIVA1 filters were mated to the new facepiece. The new mask featured twin, curved, semi-triangular eye lenses made of transparent plastic material which increased the field of vision, minimized reflected light and allowed the lenses to be positioned closer to the eyes. The left and right lenses were identical and interchangeable, while the faceblank eye holes were cut smaller than the lens frames so as to assure a gas tight fit when the metal eye frames were crimped over the lens units from the outside.

The new rubber facepiece design decreased internal dead air space, and a pair of molded in air channels—running from the integral rubber inlet at the chin of the mask to just beneath the interior of each lens—provided demisting in the accepted manner (Tissot). The chin inlet was joined to a pure, rubber hose of 27 inches which connected to the MIVA1 type filter. Initially, the type MIV exhalation valve was used on the Service Mask M2; this was also known as the "Acushnet" valve, and featured a flat circular mushroom valve, unprotected on the front side, and set into an annular mount of plastic or metal. The MIV valve seat assembly was inserted into the front lower part of the faceblank, in the orifice provided, and secured using wire and tape.

A group of 6 buckle sets were secured to the edges of the faceblank component, to which an M4 type head-harness was attached. Using a system of rivets and rubber retainers, the buckles were secured by short woven canvas straps (two of the rivets penetrated the faceblank, constituting a theoretical potential for leakage although this was apparently never formally recognized or corrected, and the same system continued to be used through the 1950s for mask retention).

An important but easy to overlook detail of the M2 type molded masks was the inclusion of small rubber extrusions just below and in front of the lower harness retention points on the faceblank. These were "rifle skids" and helped prevent a rifleman's shoulder stock buttplate from catching on the harness mount while firing a rifle in the prone position. Obviously, such a mishap occurring during use of the mask under attack from gas would result in the compromise of the gastight face-seal.

The original M2 and subsequent M2A1 masks were used with the MIVA1 carrier (as previously described), and used the MIVA1 filter. The M2 type facepieces used with the MIVA1 carriers and MIVA1 filters were together known as the "Heavyweight Gas Mask," an allusion to the substantial weight of the complete new service mask and filter design (over 5 pounds for the entire assembly, with carrier).

The U.S. Army Service Gas Mask M2A1:

The differences between the M2 service mask and the subsequent M2A1 mask design were slight; they consisted of the use of a different type of exhaust valve in the facepiece, very slight conformation variance in the molded form of the rubber facepiece in the lower frontal region, a different exhalation valve, and subtle revision of the inclination angle plane of the eyepieces. Whereas the M2 facepiece had used the Acushnet type, unprotected MIV exhaust valve, the M2A1 facepiece employed the so-called "Connell" type valve (MV type). The Connell valve was a modification of the original MI flapper valve and consisted of a flat flapper valve, seated in a vertical plastic protective mount (metal was also used for the mount) and secured in the exhaust orifice of the faceblank with wire and tape, the valve was still largely unprotected on its outer surface. Although slight, a comparison of the MI/M2 and M2A1 facepieces, side by side, highlights the subtle but distinct differences in appearance. As mentioned earlier, these distinctions apply equally to both the early and late training masks and the early and late M2 type service masks.

The U.S. Army Service Gas Mask M2A2:

In 1942, the substitution of a still more recent exhalation valve in the basic M2 faceblank resulted in the new designation of U.S. Army Service Gas Mask M2A2. The new exhaust valve was known as the Outlet Valve Assembly M8, and consisted of a mushroom type circular check valve which was seated in an annular plastic housing with a plastic slotted grill cover (featuring plastic spokes radiating to the periphery of the guard, from the center). This new type of exhaust valve is described in U.S. Army TM 3-205 Changes, dated 30 March 1943, and remained in use on the subsequent M3, M4 and civilian MIA2 type masks which were developed later in the war. Aside from this single change in faceblank components and a more smoothly molded lower frontal area, the M2A2 facepiece was virtually identical to the M2A1 variant.

U.S. Army Service Gas Mask M2A3:

The M2A3 faceblank was largely similar to that of the preceding M2, M2A1 and M2A2 masks except for the use of a new expiratory valve, designated the Outlet Valve C15. This valve used a metal seat with a rubber 'mushroom disc,' the entire assembly of which was covered by a rubber air deflection cover which directed exhaled air out in a downward vector. The new valve (C15 type) would be used on most of the later type masks issued during the war, and was also used on the later M9 series masks of the early 50s.

(One of the most confusing aspects of the introduction and evolution of the fully-molded rubber [M2 type] facepieces is the fact that owing to unanticipated design and production contingencies encountered during the mid-war years, a huge number of the very early M2 type facepieces ended up being incorporated into and reused on later, 'newer' models due to complications relating to rubber supplies and formulation of compounds in actual production [such as the M3 and M4 Lightweight Gas Masks].

Perhaps the most serious of these complications was the "cold set" tendency of synthetic (Neoprene) rubber used in the M3 and M5 series masks to seriously deform under the severe cold conditions characteristic of European winters. Lacking both adequate supplies of natural rubber and the ability to quickly manufacture new replacements for the unsatisfactory synthetic mask facepieces, a massive effort to salvage, refurbish and recondition the older, natural rubber M2 type faceblanks was carried out from early 1943 onwards. For this reason, among others, the dates of manufacture found molded into WWII gas mask facepieces are frequently unreliable for purposes of determining the precise age of the respirator model they are found to be used on. Expediency and wartime exegeses were the overall motivations which dictated these actions. Just as the press of WWI wartime developments in gas mask design had been reflected in changes made among similar models in production together, so too had these factors influenced manufacture and production practices in near-similar ways in the Second World War.)

CHAPTER SIX: World War II: Evolution in the 1940s

With the introduction of the new generation of U.S. respi rator (M2 Series), fully molded from rubber, a whole series of developments began which would ultimately result in the emergence of the first true 'ABC' military respirator (the M9 Series) in 1947. The Second World War was a period of innovative evolution, driven by trial and error, and spurred on by actual experience in all areas of chemical warfare defensive concern (i.e., requirement, design, production and field use of CBW protective equipment). Although the individual protective mask was never tested in actual attack by chemical agents during the new war, there had been no assurance that chemical agents would not be used by the Axis powers and consequently the assumption had to be made that continued progress on the "chemical front" must be made. This was, of course, especially true of protective equipment such as respirators, and the filter canisters which were the essential component of defensive masks.[1]

By the time the U.S. formally entered the conflict in December of 1941, the U.S. Army Chemical Corps had once more been enervated by the recurrent prospect of chemical warfare in Europe (and the South Pacific). Correspondingly, and in coordination with the overall marshaling of U.S. military and industrial strength, research and development once more flourished at the U.S. centers for such work (Aberdeen, Edgewood Arsenal, and others) after more than a decade of marginal activity.

At the time of its declaration of war against the Axis, Great Britain had sought assurances from the belligerents that they would observe the 1925 Geneva Protocol, which prohibited the use of chemical and biological agents in warfare. Germany, Italy, Bulgaria, Rumania, Finland and Japan all responded in the affirmative. In the Japanese surprise attack against Pearl Harbor in 1941 gas was therefore not used. On 5 June 1941 President Roosevelt warned Japan that the use of chemical war agents by U.S. forces was reserved, *but would only be considered for active use in the event that Japan used this form of warfare against China.* Of course, the Japanese had already used chemical war agents against the Chinese in Manchuko (Manchuria) in the late 1930s, but evidence of this was difficult to prove sufficiently to warrant action, and in any event had taken place prior to the President's statement of policy in this regard. Great Britain's gas policy mirrored that of the U.S.: offensive use of chemical agents would be considered an option only as a retaliatory act, and would not be prompted by 'normal' escalation of hostilities.

The overall result of this was an accentuation of U.S. effort towards defense, rather than offensive chemical warfare development, and for this reason the U.S. was (as was determined after the war, during post-war intelligence assessment) better prepared to defend against chemical agents use than any of the other major nations involved in the Second World War.

The new M2 series faceblank was a major advance in individual protective equipment for U.S. soldiers. It eliminated the vulnerable chin-seam, fragile air deflectors, angle tube and multiple metal parts found in the earlier MI series masks, and it brought the lenses closer to the eyes of the wearer for enhanced vision and consequent reduction of mechanical dead-space, a further benefit that drastically lowered production costs and greatly simplified mass production (eliminating the tedious handwork required by the MI series). While the new molded rubber faceblank was heavy, especially in combination with the standard Army metal canister, it provided excellent protection against toxic vapors.

Because the demand for the new faceblanks was so urgent, the CWS provided only three sizes of mold for the contracting manufacturers (which included the Industrial, Dryden, Continental, Sun, Acushnet Process, Firestone, Goodyear, General Tire, and U.S. Rubber Companies). These face molds were based upon fitting tests on a limited number of workers at the Edgewood Arsenal. Variations in the manufacturers' molds made it possible to fit 90% of the troops with the so-called "Universal" size, with special large and small sizes to fit the remaining 10%. Wear and serviceability of the new M2 facepieces was tested on over 1000 soldiers; difficulties encountered in tooling for facepiece production precluded further changes in design for the time being.

Although the technical staff of the CWS regarded the M2 mask as an excellent protective respirator, evidence from actual field use suggested that the respirator, weighing over 5 pounds complete with MIVA1 carrier and MIXA1 filter canister, was bulky, heavy, and ill suited to the highly mobile combat requirements of the new war. Known as the "Heavyweight Gas Mask", in training trials conducted during the early 40s troops wore the mask unwillingly and resistance to it was noted. The reaction of troops required to wear it for extended periods while on combat maneuvers was so strong that the decision was made to further develop respirator design, and in January of 1942 a new requirement was issued.

The new requirement resulted in a smaller, lighter and less cumbersome respirator which became known as the "Lightweight Gas Mask." With a smaller cylindrical canister, shorter hose, and a simpler carrier, the new respirator weighed less than 3.5 pounds. [The same degree of protection was obtained from the new mask, although filter protection was not as prolonged as that provided by the older canister. A noted shortcoming was slightly increased respiratory resistance of the new filter canister; however, uniform tests of the new mask resulted in acceptance by all units involved in field use, and the mask was produced in several variations (covered in the following text)].

Despite the apparent success of the new lightweight system, further experience with field operations—notably those involving amphibious or jungle warfare—resulted in requests from South Pacific Commands for an even lighter, smaller and more compact chemical respirator. The requirement suggested a mask design similar to that of the German military forces, with a compact, snout-attached filter, which would eliminate the bulky hose, match the protection already offered by the older system, be easy to protect against moisture, but not interfere with a soldier's need to fire in the prone position.

The USCWS turned the problem over to the CWS's MIT Development Lab for analysis and recommendations, but meanwhile reports noted that some fighting elements were carrying the Training Mask MI/M2 type respirator in jungle fighting situations. After a series of experimental models of mask were tested by the MIT unit at Camp Edwards, evidence suggested that a cheek-mounted filter would best meet the new criteria for an ultra compact assault respirator. This was further reinforced by word that the English had just introduced a new "Lightweight Type Respirator" among English military units, which consisted of a reworked General Service Respirator faceblank configured to mount a screw-on aluminum canister on its cheek. Finally, a prototype U.S. mask design was produced after a similar manner, and a new lightweight aluminum canister (designated the M11 filter) was developed for use with the new faceblank. The M11 filter concept was borrowed from the German FE 42 type canister, and featured a water-repellent smoke filter and a wide, deep bed of activated charcoal. The new respirator used a new style carrier, fabricated of butyl proofed canvas and incorporating a folding closure flap which made the carrier watertight. The improved lightweight respirator (Assault Gas Mask M5), however conceptually excellent and the direct forebear of the final M9 design of the late 40's, suffered severely from problems related to a shortage of rubber and the use of synthetics which rendered it unusable during extreme cold (more about this in the subsequent text).[2]

In addition to the "optical gas mask" and "diaphragm gas mask" series (described earlier), a design for headwounds was also developed (M7 Headwound Gas Mask) which consisted of a plastic hood with single flexible visor and used with the M11 filter .

Additionally, an M6 gas mask for dogs was developed, and protective gas masks for horses and mules were also produced earlier in the war years.

The last World War Two design was known as the Service Gas Mask, Snout-type, M8. This mask used previously issued faceblanks in combination with an adapter assembly which enabled the new M11 filter to be fitted directly to the snout of the mask. The M8 design was not produced until 1945, and consequently never saw actual field issue.

The final U.S. Army gas mask produced in the 1940s (1947), and the ultimate product of a continuing refinement process throughout the war years, was the M9 mask. The M9 mask, bearing a striking resemblance to the earlier and unsuccessful M5 assault mask, was the first genuine 'ABC' (Atomic, Biological, Chemical—now referred to as NBC) respirator produced in the United States. Although it was first introduced in 1947, well after the end of the war but still during the 40s (and therefore directly linked to wartime research and development), the M9 will be discussed in the next chapter.

U.S. Army Service Gas Mask M2, M2A1, M2A2, M2A3 (Heavyweight Gas Mask):
(For a description of these respirators, please see the previous chapter).

U.S. Army Service Gas Mask M3 (Lightweight Gas Mask):
The new "Lightweight Gas Mask" design requirement referenced in the text above resulted in the M3-10-6 service respirator (initial standard designation), which entered production in 1943 after being standardized in September of 1942. This first of the new lightweight designs consisted of a molded rubber faceblank virtually identical to the earlier M2 faceblank except that it incorporated an internal oronasal cup—the first time such an addition had been used in a U.S. mask for more precise air flow (& anti-misting) control purposes. The 18 inch long M3 rubber hose (corrugated, as all U.S. gas mask hoses were) was used with the facepiece, as was the M7 head-harness assembly. The facepiece was produced in the previous three sizes (Universal, Small and Large). There were no 'rifle skids' molded into the faceblank of the M3 mask. Inside the facepiece, the oronasal cup was either vulcanized or cemented into place, for further security.

The new style lightweight cylindrical filter canister first used with the M3 masks was designated M10. A subsequent change in interior filtering components resulted in a new designation of M10A1. The weight of the whole M3-10-6 gas mask was under 3 pounds, and a new style M6 carrier of tan/OD canvas duck was used, which was smaller than the earlier MIVA2 ('kidney') satchel, yet was carried in the same manner as before (under the left arm and secured by a shoulder strap and a waist strap). The closure flap of the M6 carrier was secured by three pull snaps fitted to fabric loops (for ease of use). The standard expiratory valve used on the M3-10A1-6 was the plastic caged M8 'mushroom' type valve.

Due to rubber shortages, most surviving M3 type (Lightweight) gas mask specimens found today feature synthetic (neoprene) rubber facepieces. Some are found with all neoprene components while others were apparently manufactured with neoprene facepieces and natural rubber hoses.

The U.S. Service Gas Mask M3A1 (Lightweight):
The M3A1-10-6 respirator's faceblank was identical to that of the M3 except for use of the rubber shrouded C15 expiratory valve, secured as all others were with wire and tape in the standard lower frontal mask orifice. It should be noted that field repairs frequently resulted in newer components (particularly expiratory valves) being retrofitted to older or existing respirators. The new M10A1 filter was later used with the earlier M3 masks, resulting in M3-10A1-6 and M3A1-10A1-6 designators.

By the middle of the war (1943) several problems were encountered which had pronounced effects on gas mask development and production. One of these had to do with a lack of a single standard face mold for the production of all faceblanks by contractors, due to their being several manufacturers producing masks from similar but not identical master molds. Steps were taken to rectify this difficulty, which ultimately resulted in a specification for the facemold which all gas mask fabrication contractors would conform to in their production of faceblanks. For this reason and several others, serious delays were encountered in producing the new M3 series masks. Further complicating the matter was a shortage natural rubber with which to make the faceblanks. The rubber supply reserves deficit resulted in faceblanks being fabricated from the newly developed synthetic rubber, neoprene. Neoprene rubber was thought to be an acceptable substitute for natural rubber at the time, but as was later shown during use of this mask (and the M5 Assault Gas Mask, made from the same synthetic material) in the winter severe cold of the European Theater of operations, selection of neoprene was a serious mistake.

While production delays of the new M3 lightweight masks were being resolved (in 1943), an interim version of the lightweight mask was produced which was known as the M4 series. Intended as an emergency measure, the M4 mask was later produced alongside the M3 series, sharing many similarities. It should be noted in passing that the oronasal cup feature (used by the M3 and M4 series, thereafter to be a standard mask component) was a technical breakthrough of great significance in gas mask development (Although the M4 series masks were originally intended as an interim contingency until the M3 production problems were resolved, they continued to me made concurrent with the M3 until war's end).

The U.S. Army Service Gas Mask M4 (Lightweight):
Initially produced as a stopgap measure, pending resolution of the M3 production problems, the new M4-10A1-6 lightweight mask was put together piecemeal style, using older, reconditioned and refurbished M2 style rubber faceblanks (of natural rubber, not neoprene) fitted with a cemented-in oronasal cup and attached via an M3 type rubber hose to the new small-sized cylindrical M10A1 (improved M10) filter canister. A vulcanization process was later used for installation of the oronasal "nose cup" component (Note: Some examples of the early M4 masks have no internal oronasal cup fitted).

Due to the vagaries of rubber supplies, the temporary use of neoprene rubber in faceblanks, and complex distribution logistics, a number of 'mix and match' combinations will be noted on older examples of the M3 and M4 masks which survive today. Such curiosities as a natural rubber M4 (M2 type) faceblank fitted with a neoprene oronasal nosecup and hose are not uncommon, as are occasional examples of the rubber shroud on the C15 expiratory valve being made of the same (neoprene) material.

The M4 mask shared the M7 head-harness with the M3 series masks, and except for the complications which delayed M3 mask production (and the use of natural and synthetic rubber compounds for fabrication of components), the two respirator series are essentially near-identical in overall configuration. The M4-10-6 and M4-10A1-6 masks were produced in a single Universal size only.

The U.S. Army Service Gas Mask M4A1-10A1-6 (Lightweight):
The M4A1-10A1-6 faceblank was identical to the M4 except for use of the newer C15 expiratory valve in place of the earlier M8 type valve. *Most* M4A1-10A1-6 mask faceblanks were produced entirely from natural rubber and included natural rubber hose, facepiece and rubber component parts. The C15 exhalation valve was used on this mask, as was the M7 harness. As with all of the earlier series following the MIA2 masks (except for the M4 mask), the M4A1 masks were produced in Small, Universal and Large sizes.

Approximately 13 million of the new lightweight style service gasmasks (field repaired, modified M3, improved M3A1, refurbished M4 & production M4A1) were produced from 1943 through 1945; both types remained in continuous service until the war ended, due to problems with the new style, innovative but inherently unserviceable M5 Assault Gas Mask, which suffered from the severe and unforeseen "cold set" deformation characteristics of neoprene rubber (Note: in the 1950s, the standards for the M3 and M4 masks still in use were changed, allowing for the inner oronasal cup to be considered an 'optional' component; removal of the cup was considered to be in full compliance with this change in functional use criteria and therefore masks kept in reserve capacities or non-strategic use frequently had their nose cups removed for comfort).

The "Assault Gas Mask" M5 (later standardized as Combat Service Gas Mask M5):
As mentioned above, a further need for an even lighter, more compact and more easily water-protected gas mask led to the production of a mask initially known as the "Assault Gas Mask." Inspired by the need for a less cumbersome gas protective design and intended principally for amphibious assault troops to use in the upcoming invasion of Europe, the new mask was to retain the same general rubber-molded facepiece characteristics of the M2, M3 and M4 precursors; it was, however, to be molded of neoprene synthetic rubber with a cheek-site fitted female screw thread orifice of approximately 58 mm width, to which the new aluminum M11 lightweight 'drum' canister could be attached (the former chin-sited orifice was sealed closed during the molding stage).[3] The canister screw fitting featured a one-way rubber disc check valve on the inner side for one-way air flow control. The new facepiece used the new C4 head harness, and was originally produced with the M8 plastic caged expiratory valve. Versions were apparently also fitted with the newer C15 expiration valve, although field retrofitting may also have taken place. Inside the M5 faceblank an oronasal cup was fitted in the conventional manner of the earlier M3 and M4 masks; this cup was

either vulcanized, cemented or riveted in place (also initially fabricated from neoprene)

A new style carrier was developed for the M5 mask consisting of a butyl-proofed canvas duck material; the closure flap enabled it to be closed in a water-tight manner and then used as an emergency flotation device. Reports were received after the Normandy invasion that the mask satchel had actually saved a number of soldiers' lives in this manner, as they waded ashore heavily overburdened with equipment from the landing craft.

As a bellwether concept, pointing the way to future developments, the M5-11-7 Assault Gas Mask was a *theoretical* success, but proved to be a functional failure. The cheek-sited filter (influenced, it is felt, by the British "Lightweight Type" gas mask design roughly contemporaneous with it) would remain an advanced feature for decades, and is in fact still generally employed by almost all of the most recent chemical respirator designs. As a practical, successful field service respirator, however, the M5 (neoprene) mask was a dismal failure. The main problem centered not on the design of the mask, but rather on the material used in its manufacture. A shortage of natural rubber at the time it was due to begin production runs (late 1943, with first issue to troops in December) resulted in the new synthetic rubber, neoprene, being used for faceblank manufacture.[4]

Neoprene appeared a reasonable substitute for natural rubber initially, but serious problems resulted from its use. Among them were difficulties in molding uniform thicknesses of neoprene rubber for faceblanks. Added to this were problems with impurities and other irregularities. The final, and most serious problem centered on neoprene's unanticipated physical response to low temperatures, or what is known as the material's "cold-set" tendencies (deformation due to unusual cold).

M5 assault gas masks were produced using neoprene faceblanks in which neoprene oronasal cups were secured. The unsuitability of neoprene as a gas mask material was not discovered until the invasion troops issued them found out that in the unusually cold weather of Europe the masks developed a cold-setting tendency to deform (and thus not seal effectively). So serious was this problem that the masks were regarded as completely unusable, hence many were discarded outright after the invasion forces forged inland without convincing evidence that gas would be used by the retreating Axis forces (a very famous Bill Mauldin cartoon of the period referenced this unhappy matter).

Thus, the Army was forced to entirely abandon the new M5 design (as well as those early M3 lightweight masks which used neoprene faceblanks or oronasal cups), and the continued need for interim M4 type respirators became more critical. The Assault Gas Mask was finally standardized on 7 July 1944 as the Combat Service Gas Mask M5-11-7, just in time for further production to be canceled. Apparently, a few of the M5 neoprene masks were sent to the South Pacific for evaluation in that milder climate (cold-setting was not a problem in the tropics, of course), but the war ended before a proper evaluation of their use in that theater could be carried out. A total of 520,000 of the M5 neoprene masks were delivered prior to cancellation. [It is interesting to note that it has been theorized that the frantic replacement of the faulty M5 masks with hastily produced M4 masks came to the attention of the German intelligence around the time of the Ardennes Offensive, late in the war. This coincided with a general re-equipping of the Allied forces with chemical warfare protection equipment, owing to the fact that higher headquarters was concerned about the rate at which invasion forces had been discarding their masks and CBW gear after a feared German chemical threat failed to materialize. Apparently, the Germans, lacking knowledge of specifically *why* the new masks were being distributed (their own Model GM-38 had, after all, been fabricated from synthetic rubber), and aware of the CBW protection build-up interpreted this as evidence that the Allies were greatly stepping up chemical warfare protection capabilities for possible offensive purposes. The educated *surmise* is that this interpretation by the OKW (*OberKommando Wehrmacht*) served to further inhibit any inclination which may have existed on the part of the German High Command to deploy their own substantial stores of chemical weapons, and strengthened their belief that the Allies were exceedingly well prepared for a chemical conflict, should one be initiated by Germany.]

Despite the failure of the neoprene rubber M5 Assault Gas Mask (due to the unsuitable nature of that synthetic rubber for facepiece use), the M5 design had great promise. It would eventually inspire one of the most successful gas masks ever produced, the U.S. Army M9 respirator.

The U.S. Army Service Gas Mask, Snout-type, M8:

The final wartime attempt to produce a more convenient, lightweight gas mask resulted in a model identified as the Snout-type Gas Mask M8-11-10. The M8 used a rubber faceblank of M2, M3 or M4 fabrication together with a special M11 drum filter canister adapter connector that enabled the new aluminum housed filter to be attached directly to the lower chin inlet orifice. The combination appeared not dissimilar to the early Training Gas Mask MI/M2, except that the MI filter canister used on the MI/M2 training mask was visibly different in shape (the MI training filter and the M10/M10A1 lightweight service mask filters had quite a similar appearance). There were two main types of M8 faceblank, the difference being slight and related to the details of the lower head-harness attachments on the faceblank; this may be attributed to use of older, refurbished facepieces to produce some of the M8 assembly units.

The M8 type gas mask used the late model C15, rubber shrouded expiratory valve and the C4 head harness, and the carrier satchel, made in the snout-style shape of a cone-shaped frustum from khaki canvas duck, was designated *Carrier M10*.

All of the standard Army service type respirators made from the M2 through the M8 were fabricated of gray-green natural rubber, except for the M3 and M5 facepieces, hoses and oronasal cups which used black neoprene rubber (an older black-colored U.S. mask's faceblank or component—hose, exhaust shroud, etc.—is almost immediately identifiable as either an M3 or M5 production item). Once again, the M8 Snout-type mask was not intended as an advancement in respirator design but rather as an emergency, interim contingency. It remains a very seldom encountered U.S. respirator today and examples when located are usually in very poor condition.

CHAPTER SEVEN: U.S. Navy Developments: 1915-1921

United States Naval operations had highlighted divergent requirements for maritime chemical warfare protection, in contrast to those of the land forces.[1] In the latter years of the First World War, cooperative chemical warfare defense research, which included Naval personnel, dedicated much attention to an analysis of the available protective respirators for use against chemical agents. Opinions were divided, based upon examination and limited testing of requisitioned protective mask designs from both sides, as to which chemical defense mask offered the most expeditious protection from the extant chemical agents in use (1915-1918).

Respirators evaluated included the French M2 design, the BSBR from England, the French Tissot type, and the German 'snout-type' mask. While U.S. Army chemical personnel ultimately decided that the BSBR mask, with its face-piece, hose and filter canister, was the most effective and substantial expression of the state-of-the-art for emulation, the U.S. Navy maintained the opinion that the German design, featuring a compact filter fitted to the snout of a facemask, was more suited to the needs of the sea-going forces than was the bulky canister on a hose configuration..

Discrete design concepts, borrowed from both the British and German masks, were finally combined by Naval chemical research personnel to construct a mask which would be identified as the first official U.S. Navy chemical respirator. This mask, which used the British SBR type facepiece (retaining nose clip and rubber mouthpiece inside a rubber coated fabric full-facemask) with a modified German-style filter canister attached in the German manner to the snout of the mask, was refined and finally designated the U.S. Navy Gas Mask Mark I (Mouth Canister Type).

Concurrently, recognizing the especial need for unconstrained range of motion by seamen in performance of their duties aboard ship, experimentation continued with a very different type of protective respirator which featured a cylindrical filter canister worn behind the head. Termed at first simply as the "Navy Head Mask and Canister," this mask appears to have used a modified Akron-Tissot (AT) Mask facepiece to which a non-corrugated rubber hose (joined to the mask between the eye lenses) led over the ears and around to the back of the head, where it connected with a cylindrical filter canister worn immediately behind the occipital region of the head. The AT type facepiece was worn in conjunction with a type of skull-cap which served as a suspension harness and support for the metal filter canister. The major components of the mask's facepiece appear to be of the conventional AT Mask type (eye lens, flapper-type rubber expiratory valve protected by a metal guard located where the angle-tube of an AT Mask was normally sited), although the normal AT type head-harness had been modified in that it was sewn to the fabric skull-cap along its upper-front and secured by a strap to the lower rear part of the cap.

General Amos Fries' book *Chemical Warfare* (co-authored with Major Clarence J. West, and published in 1921) makes the briefest mention of this design on page 48 and illustrates it in a side-view on page 194.

Further documentation of the early Navy gas mask development is found in a small (53 pages) booklet published by the U.S. Navy Bureau of Construction & Repair (in collaboration with the U.S. Navy Bureau of Medicine and Surgery). In this book, which was printed in 1920, excellent information is presented on not just the U.S. Navy Gas Mask, Mark I, but on an apparent development of the "U.S. Navy Head Mask and Canister" design known as the U.S. Navy Gas Mask Mark II (Head Canister type).

The head canister type mask, derived from and differing from the original behind-the-head filter mounting concept, is described in the following section.

U.S. Navy Gas Mask, Mark I (Mouth Canister Type):
This design was the result of the original U.S. Navy efforts to develop a suitable chemical protective mask, and was produced in late 1917 or early 1918. The mask is a combination of discrete design elements borrowed from both the British Small Box Respirator and the WWI German Mask—both of which were recognized as the preeminent chemical defense masks to emerge from that war period (while the French Tissot Mask was also very significant, it was not widely used as were the German and English masks).

Superficially, the U.S. Navy Mark I Mouth Canister Mask bore close external resemblance to the standard German/Austrian snout-canister mask of the period. The facepiece of this original U.S. Navy Mark I mask was quite similar to the standard BSBR counterpart, and to certain Austrian versions of the German mask, in that it used a gum-rubberized thin fabric facepiece which contained circular metal rims holding glass objectives; internally, and unlike the German/Austrian masks, it employed the British style rubber mouthpiece connected directly to the snout-mounted filter, in conjunction with the use of a noseclip. Inside the fabric facepiece of the Navy mask, two lateral fabric ligatures extend from the upper part of the mask's facepiece—outboard of the eye lenses—to help support the weight of the filter canister (a photograph in Fries' and West's *Chemical Warfare* on page 231 exists which shows these two lateral supporting fabric ligatures on the *outside* of the facepiece). The circular metal lens frames were secured to the mask with strong cord, a common feature of early masks with circular lenses and a design feature of the BSBR, early ASBR and German masks.

The overall facepiece was secured to the head by 6 black fabric straps—two on each side of the temple and two joined into a single head strap coming from the upper front edge of the mask. The snout of the mask, unlike the BSBR with its angle tube, was fitted with a wide (8 cm) circular connection disc, perforated in its center by a female screw-threaded orifice 3 cm in diameter, which was secured to the mask by cord and tape.

The slightly tapered metal filter (drum style) canister, used by screwing its male screw-threaded connector to the connection disc of the mask, was visually very similar to the metal German filter canister of the same period. It measured about 7 cm in diameter at the bottom, and was 4 cm tall. The filter material used in the drum consisted of two layers of absorbents (one of soda lime and another of charcoal, separated by a cotton wadding pad), of 6-20 mesh size (instead of 8-14 mesh). According to available references, the filter drum used with the Navy Mark I mask was charged for a capacity of about 2 to 3 hours of total exposure to the chemicals and concentrations typical of the First World War period.

Unlike the German mask, which lacked an expiratory valve (air was breathed both in and out through the filter), the Navy Mark I mask used a rubber flapper-type expiratory valve attached directly to the filter drum's outlet connector (affixed at a right angle to the connector tube, and situated therefore between the mask connector plate and the body of the filter drum—a location which provided some protection for the valve's delicate rubber tube). The exhaust valve worked in conjunction with a one-way check valve built into the canister, which prevented exhaled air from reentering it. This served to prevent degradation of the filter chemicals by carbon dioxide, and also served to prevent accumulation of harmful moisture within the filtering elements. It also eliminated the 'bellows' effect demonstrated by the leather fabricated German Mask, which swelled and collapsed with each breath (no expiratory valve or check valve for one-way air flow control), and served to prevent humidity from the breath from accumulating on the inner lens surfaces. A last benefit was to prevent lacrimatory gases, potentially unabsorbed by the filter, from being allowed to concentrate within the mask.

An earlier version of the Mark I mask apparently used a filter drum that was of a slightly larger diameter on its bottom surface (9 cm). The inlet end of both filters was perforated with small holes (much like the 1930s style German filter canisters). One additional aspect of the original Navy Mark I gas mask was a metal figure-eight wire frame which could be used inside the mask to help keep the lenses in a favorable viewing position; the accessory was inserted before use and removed before the mask was returned to its stowage container. Provision for wear of corrective lenses was apparently not yet configured into the early protective mask designs.

U.S. Navy Gas Mask, Mark II (Head Canister Type): The second type of U.S. Navy gas mask of this period appears to be an advanced version of the "Navy Head Mask and Canister" design described earlier. This mask was designated the U.S. Navy Gas Mask, Mark II (Head Canister Type), and is described in the Navy brochure referenced above (dated 1920). [2]

Perhaps the single most unusual design of the era, the U.S. Navy Mark II type respirator presents a somewhat strange sight in that the mask consisted of a rubberized facepiece to which a lightweight (aluminum) headpiece was fitted. The metal headpiece gives the appearance of an inverted colander, and held a tin ducting gas filter canister directly on top. The facepiece, of rubber proofed fabric, was attached at its upper margin to a fabric skull-cap, which was also secured to the metal headpiece bearing the filter box. Elasticized straps attached to the facepiece, and also secured to the metal headpiece, joined at the rear of the head. The metal filter canister was connected to the rubber facepiece via twin rubber tubes that exited separately from just behind and above each eye lens before joining together and entering as a single tube to the metal filter box on the metal headpiece. The main canister drew air from a set of flat, distinctive, rectangular smoke filter elements worn one on each side of the headpiece, via connecting inlet tubes exiting the metal filter can via a screw-port at its rear and attaching to the bilateral smoke filter pads at their rear margins.

Two standard filter cans were interchangeably used with the Mark II mask; one was gray in color and was used for standard war gases (of the WWI period), while the other can was black painted and was used for carbon monoxide protection. The gray war agent filter provided about 6 hours of aggregate protection against lethal gases (example: 50 ppm of chloropicrin, etc.), and the black canister provided protection against CO in concentrations of 5000 ppm or less, with relative humidity of 80% at 60°F. The smoke filtering elements consisted of a sandwich construction of rectangular shaped felt pads separated by a wire mesh, and were replaceable, as would be expected.

The rubber facepiece, with twin circular Triplex type safety glass lenses, featured a rubber flapper-type expiratory valve situated on the upper forehead atop a rubber tube extended upwards from the facepiece's front section. Limited protection was afforded to it through placing it close to the forward part of the head assembly, where it did not protrude greatly.

With the rubber facepiece folded into the dome of the metal headpiece, the respirator was stowed in a (box-like) carry case which contained spare smoke filter elements, and presented a relatively compact aspect despite the singularity of its design and fabrication.

The U.S. Navy Gas Mask, Mark II (Head Canister Type) had just started production shortly before the First World War ended, and an insufficient quantity of the smoke elements had been fabricated by the time the Armistice was signed. Reference was made in the Bureau of Construction and Repair booklet that while the land-based gas defense protective masks could be rather easily modified and updated to maintain pace with improvements in offensive chemical munitions, the Navy (Mark II) mask could not be updated with as much ease. Further statements were made asserting the Mark I and Mark II types interfered as little as possible with shipboard activities, but that the head canister type mask "was superior" in this context as well as in that of chemical defense & protection between the two types. Visual aspects of the Mark II were commended (glass enabled clarity of vision), but communication needs and concerns were not addressed (the Mark II provided little if any facility for communication—important on a wartime seagoing vessel). The U.S. Navy (old) Mark I and (old) Mark II protective masks are to be carefully differentiated from the later U.S. Navy "ND" Mk I, Mk II, Mk III and Mk IV (Navy Diaphragm) and the "NDO" Mk I (Navy Diaphragm Optical) masks, which came into being in the 30s and 40s.

U.S. Navy Ammonia Gas Mask:

This was the standard Navy Mark I (mouth canister type) fitted with a special filter drum for use against ammonia gas fumes. Before use against ammonia, the bottom cap of the ammonia filter drum was removed and the sponge and 25 component layers of cotton padding were removed from the filter and soaked in a saturated solution of tartaric acid. Excess solution was squeezed out from the material, the cotton elements were replaced in the canister and the perforated end plate resecured.

CHAPTER EIGHT: Later U.S. Navy Developments: 1930s and World War II

Prior to the end of the First World War, the U.S. Navy had early on identified special needs which chemical defense res pirators designed for use by sea forces ought to properly address. These included enhanced communications and vision features which would permit Navy gas masks to be used while operating visual sighting systems, range-finding equipment, and speaking sets.

The First War had ended with the development and initial adoption of the old style Mark I (mouth canister type) and Mark II (head canister type) masks.[1] Neither permitted ease in using communications gear, although they did achieve the goals of accommodating physical range of motion activities engaged in by seamen carrying out shipboard duties while underway.

The first two Navy masks (original Mark I and Mark II) were developed prior to the appointment of two special boards appointed by the Secretary of the Navy (first in 1918 and second in 1921). Among the results of the recommendations arising from the two special investigative boards was the appointment of the Navy's Bureau of Ships as the responsible agency for chemical warfare protection in all its phases.

Both during and increasingly after the First War, the U.S. Navy had established significant ties with the U.S. Army's Chemical Warfare Service facility at the Edgewood Arsenal in Maryland for purposes of sharing information, assistance and support. Consequently, in February of 1922, it was decided to establish a full time Naval office of chemical warfare research at the Edgewood facility, which has remained in place since that date. The establishment of this close interaction between the U.S. Army's Chemical Warfare Service and the Naval Office of Chemical Warfare Research at Edgewood enabled the subsequent design and production of the optical and diaphragm masks to be used by both services, and also supported the U.S. Navy Mark III and Mark IV respirator development programs of the early to mid-40s.

During the ensuing years following the Armistice, renewed attention was given by both services to mask designs which enhanced speaking and more readily permitted visually coordinated tasks. The U.S. Army Chemical Warfare Service had already developed their 1919 Model design into what became the first standard Army gas mask after the war—the U.S. Army Service Mask MI. Through cooperative planning and interservice liaison, the Navy's need was identified as being complementary with a similar Army need for better communications capability. This resulted in the development of the first so-called 'diaphragm mask,' standardized by the Army as the Diaphragm Gas Mask MI in the early 1920s. The MI version of this diaphragm mask was adopted by the U.S. Navy as its ND Gas Mask Mark I.

The changes between the Army version and the navy version were few, and consisted for the most part of the use of a gray stockinet material vulcanized to the rubber facepiece instead of khaki, and substitution of a U.S. Navy filter canister, similar in shape and function to the Army counterpart. A similar type of carrying satchel as the MIII Army sack was used with the U.S. Navy mask.

When the Army produced a new version of the Diaphragm Gas Mask, designated the MII (a diaphragm equipped version of their MIA2 Service Gas Mask), the Navy adopted the new (Army) MII model to replace the earlier (Army) MI diaphragm mask, although both masks continued to be used concurrently for a considerable period of time. This redesigned communications type mask was designated the Gas Mask, ND Mk.II. Again, it used an elasticized M3 type cable head-harness and a U.S. Navy filter canister, but was otherwise almost identical to the Army counterpart. The metal bifurcated Tissot tube assembly on the front of the MII mask distinctively sets it apart from the circular annulus type diaphragm assembly on the MI model.

Meanwhile, attention was still being focused on the need for an enhanced optical mask which would facilitate wear while operating shipboard sighting, ranging and surveillance duties. Consequent with Army identification of a similar need for use with specialized units of its land-based forces (artillery and communications battalions), a new type of mask was developed in the late 30s which featured small circular, optically correct glass eyepieces. This mask was developmentally related to the original WWI Navy "Head Mask and Canister type" gas mask in that it used a refined version of that design featuring twin rubber tubes joined at one end to a canister positioned behind the head and at the other to inlets below each eye piece.

The new mask was produced for both the US Navy and the US Army (the former in black rubber, the latter in gray-green rubber), and came into use in the very last year prior to US entry into the new war. The Navy version of the mask was designated Optical

Gas Mask, NDO (Navy Diaphragm Optical) Mk. I, while the Army version was designated the Army Optical Mask MI.

It was obvious to U.S. Navy personnel involved with gas mask development that the new optical style mask featured some important advantages, and the behind-the-head canister location appeared to be far better suited to shipboard use than the somewhat cumbersome hose and canister mask which restricted range of motion. The result was a decision to remain with the behind-the-head canister type of mask and expand upon the concept for improved general use. This resulted in the next generation general purpose Navy gas mask, which was very similar to the optical mask except for placement of the filtered air inlet ducts and size of the eye lenses. The new mask, designated by the Navy Department as the Gas Mask, ND (Navy Diaphragm) Mk III, had redesigned safety lenses shaped somewhat like aviators' goggles, and fresh air inlet ducts positioned under the eye pieces rather than to the rear of the lens on each side (in the manner of the optical mask). The U.S. Navy ND Mk III came into use in the first year of the war.

A still later refinement of the new Mk III mask resulted in the Gas Mask, ND Mk IV, which was identical to the Mk III except that it featured the same style, larger semi-triangular lenses (with enhanced field of vision) that all Army masks from the M2 series onwards had featured. This final upgrading of the WWII Mark Series came into use in late 1942 and remained in use without any further revisions or modifications until the late 50s. Both the Mark III and Mark IV navy masks, as well as the Optical Mask Mark I, were carried in a carrier of gray canvas duck, featuring a single adjustable shoulder strap for transport. The satchels are clearly stamped in black ink with the designated mask intended for carry (i.e. "ND Mark IV" or "NDO Mark I") therein. During the middle years of the Second World War (1942-43), the ND Mark III, Mark IV and NDO Mark I masks were issued to ships equivalent to 105% of the ship's complement, and of that total number approximately 15% were of the NDO Mark I type.

With the end of the Second World War in 1945, U.S. Navy participation in protective chemical defense research declined to a significant degree for the usual reasons association with post-war demobilization, although the Naval liaison office at Edgewood Arsenal was maintained. With the final adoption of the ND Mark IV and the NDO Mark I, the Navy had come close to accomplishing its agenda of perfecting the gas defense respirator for sea duty (insofar as they had met the needs extant in the war years of the 1940s).

The next major development in U.S. Navy chemical defense respirator development would not occur until the late 1950s, when the Navy introduced its Chemical/Biological Mask, ND Mark V. The Chemical/Biological Mask, ND Mark V, was a considerable departure from the older style Mark III and Mark IV masks in that it used twin, cheek mounted filter discs and a large single visor made of flexible transparent plastic. There was no small interior mouth cup, in congruence with the earlier Mark masks, but the mask featured a sophisticated face-seal about which more will be discussed later, and had a simplified, efficient voicemitter. It was made from black rubber, and used flat rubber straps as a harness instead of the spring-filled elasticized cable harness of all the earlier Mark series masks (including the World War One Mk. I and Mk II masks). A molded-in Tissot type air deflection system was used to aid lens demisting, and the mask featured an Army C15 type exhalation valve below the voicemitter. The Mark V NBC mask (U.S. Navy Mask, Chemical, Biological, Mk V) remained in service until the late 80s, at which time it was replaced by the controversial "new" MCU 2/P design.

The current U.S. Navy NBC defense mask, designated the MCU-2A/P, came into service in the late 80s, replacing the old and new Mark series masks. It will be discussed in a separate chapter, in view of the fact that its design and development is part of a larger story concerning the current generation U.S. Military respirators.

The Navy also produced, during the Second World War, a civilian chemical defense respirator which was intended for wear by those individuals who were performing non-combatant duties. This mask bears a curious resemblance to the Mark V mask of the 60s in that it featured a single large transparent plastic lens and used twin disc-like filtering elements in a similar manner to the later Mark V. The mask was known as the Civilian Gas Mask, NC (Navy Civilian). This mask is also known as the NC-1; both designations were used to refer to this mask, which was intended for use by civilian personnel working for the Navy Department on shore installations.

The U.S. Navy Gas Mask, ND Mark I:

This first Navy mask adopted after the First World War was virtually identical to the Army Diaphragm Gas Mask MI. It featured a gray stockinet vulcanized rubber facepiece made from a molded rubber sheet. The circular eye lenses of the ND Mark I were made from Triplex type safety glass (celluloid inserted between two sheets of glass) around which metal lens frames were crimped to form a gas-tight seal. The faceblank of the ND Mark I was manufactured in 4 sizes (small, medium, large, and very large). It was estimated that the number 2 size would fit approximately 50% of all naval personnel.

The voicemitter, housed in a perforated circular metal housing on the lower front of the mask partly hid the (MIII) flapper style rubber expiratory valve, which was situated behind and slightly to the right of the diaphragm type speech transmitter, pointing downward. A 27 inch stockinet covered corrugated rubber hose was joined to the mask via the combined diaphragm, inlet, and expiratory component fitting, attaching a filter canister very similar (minor changes to the container and U.S. Navy data label) to the corresponding U.S. Army type in use with the Service Mask, MIA1. The Mark I was carried in a carrying satchel identical in shape and function to that used with the U.S. Army mask, using the same shoulder and waist strap arrangement for wear under the left arm at the side. The head harness is slightly different from the Army service mask head harness component, and is the Army M3 elasticized cable arrangement. A similar harness was used on almost all the later navy masks.

The U.S. Navy Gas Mask, ND Mark II:

The ND Mark II naval gas mask was virtually identical to the U.S. Army Diaphragm Gas Mask MII and used gray stockinet vulcanized to the rubber facepiece. As with the Army mask, a singularly unique appearing metal 'Y' tube assembly branches around the recessed diaphragm to enter the faceblank centrally, just below each eye lens. The bottom of the 'Y' tube connects the stockinet covered corrugated rubber hose (27 inches) to the standard box-shaped style filter canister used by the Army MIA2 Service Masks.

The ND Mark II faceblank was of the universal size type, and the circular metal eye frames containing the Triplex type safety glass were screwed into place, thereby permitting replacement of broken lenses in the field without difficulty. The flapper type rubber (MII) expiratory valve was situated in front of the speech perforated diaphragm housing where it was well protected by the twin branches of the inlet's 'Y' tube assembly. The head-harness is the same elasticized cable assembly as that used in the ND MkI, and most other aspects of the mask, hose and canister are, as has been pointed out, of virtually identical size and shape to the Army counterpart (filter canister is readily identified by U.S. Navy data label). The carrying satchel is also identical in this context.

The U.S. Navy Gas Mask, ND Mark III:
A completely new design, inspired by the Army Optical Mask MI/ US Navy NDO Mark I, the Mark III faceblank was molded entirely from black rubber and featured a cylindrical filter canister situated behind the neck, to which were joined twin corrugated black rubber tubes (one from each end of the filter) that passed around the side of the head to enter the facepiece just below each plastic eye piece (one on each side).

The facepiece eye lenses were made from transparent synthetic plastic, and were secured with crimped-on metal frames. The Mark III head-harness used the identical fabric covered spring cable network joined to short canvas straps (on the mask) which is used on the Navy optical mask for retention, and the gray metal, cylindrical canister was fixed to a retaining steel clip at the rear of the harness, widthwise, for support behind the neck. The lenses might be replaced if damaged, and a rearward facing, downward positioned flapper-type expiratory valve (MVI spearhead) was located in the front of the mask below a prominent, circular, perforated speech diaphragm disc (of a new and different design from previously featured speech diaphragms). There was no inner oronasal cup, but the Tissot principle of anti-misting air direction was employed through molded in air ducts opening up inside the mask under each lens and a small mouth cup enhanced utterances into the voicemitter. A gray carrying satchel of canvas duck material was used to carry the mask, via single adjustable shoulder strap that featured a snap-closure flap opening upwards and outwards. The carry sack was stamped "Gas Mask, ND Mark III," and inside the canvas carrying satchel a small cylindrical anti-misting impregnated cloth container was provided, secured by a loop of fabric.

The Mark III mask was provided with either a metal or pressed fiberboard face form used inside the facepiece to maintain its shape when the mask was stowed. When stowed, the filter can fitted inside the faceform and the hoses were secured under the head-harness straps. In the event the mask was prepared for use, the faceform was taken out to permit rapid donning and stored in the mask carrying satchel.

The U.S. Navy Gas Mask, ND Mark IV:
Aside from very slight changes, limited to enlarging the eye lenses, the Mark IV mask was virtually identical to the earlier Mark III model. Both used identical filter and hose components, as well as identical MIII cable-type head-harnesses which joined to short gray canvas straps secured to the faceblank via rivets and rubber retaining loops. The chemical filter contents of the canisters were identical, admitting unfiltered gas through a series of holes placed lengthwise along the lower seam of the cylinder. These holes were covered by a length of adhesive tape until the mask was ready for use, and were subsequently uncovered when the tape was removed. This filter featured a lowered resistance to breathing than that imposed by the army style MVIII and MIX type filters and was more suited to the naval exertional applications required of it.

As with the Mark III mask, the carrying satchel was virtually identical and made of gray canvas duck material that featured a snap-closed upwards opening flap, with an adjustable single shoulder strap. A fiberboard faceform, as described above, was provided with the mask and was used in a similar manner, through use of a length of white cord attached to it.

U.S. Navy Optical Gas Mask, NDO Mark I:
Like the Mark III and Mark IV masks, the NDO Mark I faceblank was made from fully molded black rubber, and was very similar in overall configuration to them. Owing its origin somewhat to early WWI "Head Mask and Canister" designs, it had a slightly different arrangement of the corrugated rubber hose inlet sites (behind, rather than under the eye lenses) and was distinctive in its use of small circular, optical grade glass lenses with an adjustment screw for setting intraocular distance. The NDO Mark I faceblank was of the universal size type, and was otherwise identical in every major respect to the Mark III and Mark IV masks, including the style and type of carrying satchel provided. [At least one limited standard NDO Mark I variant carrying satchel has been found, fabricated exactly as the standard navy mask carry bags are, but in a khaki canvas material instead of navy gray; the imprint on the bag features the U.S. Army Chemical Corps crossed retort insignia with "U.S. Navy NDO Mk I" lettering in black ink instead of white].

The U.S. Navy Civilian Gas Mask, NC-1:
As mentioned earlier, the Navy NC-1 mask for civilians is constructed of brownish-gray stockinet covered rubber sheeting, with a single seam under the chin which was sewn, glued and taped. Twin type metal filter element containment discs were located on each cheek which could be unscrewed for replacement of the circular filter cartridges carried therein. The single large and flexible plastic lens was cemented and heat-sealed to the faceblank after being stitched in place. There was no inner oronasal cup, although the Tissot principle was employed for demisting. An elasticized head strap harness, similar to that used by Army masks, was used for retention.

The NC/NC-1 facepiece was issued in two sizes, a universal size and a small size, with a flapper type rubber expiratory valve situated at the chin, pointing downward, and somewhat exposed to physical damage.

The U.S. Navy Gas Mask, Mark V:

The ND Mark IV and NDO Mark I masks remained in use through the years immediately following the Second World War. With the development of atomic weapons, and awareness of a new need for complete ABC (Atomic Biological and Chemical) protection, the Navy recognized that a new ABC type respirator capable of affording better protection from radioactive particulates was needed. By the time of the mid-50s, it was also apparent that the old stocks of WWII type gas masks were physically deteriorating, due to various deleterious environmental and storage factors.

Thus, in the late 1950s, the old Mark IV masks were finally replaced by the introduction of a new ABC defense respirator. Designated the ND Mark V, the new mask was molded from black rubber and featured a large, single, flexible and clear visor thermochemically joined to the facepiece. A newer speech diaphragm component disc was situated at the lower front of the mask, over the mouth, and below the speech diaphragm an Army type C15 style expiratory valve was located, with its rubber shroud facing rearward, under the chin.

In addition to a rapidly adjusted rubber strap head-harness, twin metal C-1 filter containment discs were affixed, one on each cheek, to hold the replaceable filters used with the mask. The initial impression conveyed by the mask brought to mind the earlier WWII civilian NC mask, but the resemblance was purely superficial, for the major innovation of the new Mark V mask was found inside the facepiece, in the area of its face seal.

The Mark V face blank was molded with a pneumatic face seal design, not dissimilar to the British S-6 respirator. This enabled the mask to conform to a wide range of facial configurations, and although it worked quite well when the mask was new and the rubber well conditioned, the potential effects of aging on the integrity of the semi-pneumatic air sack which constituted the face seal were something to consider carefully. Once punctured or worn through, the primary face-seal mechanism which the air-filled bladder constituted lost much of its effectiveness.

It is of interesting relevance to cite an informative and astute analysis of face seal mechanics as they pertain to CBW masks—given the similarity of the Mark V's face seal to that of the British S-6 mask—which was thoughtfully provided by an internationally respected scientist and expert in respirator design and development from the UK:

> "The most important thing about a face seal is that it is a waterseal. Sweat rapidly accumulates around the contact area between the rubber surface and the skin, and this makes the seal. With the British S-10 respirator, tests were never conducted on a man until the mask had been worn for 10 minutes. This was to allow the sweatseal to develop completely. When this is done, then dynamic protection factors of about 20,000 are quite possible.
>
> The water seal, from personal experience, must be at least 1 cm in width. In the old molded rubber respirators (e.g. Canadian C-3 and British Light Type), the rubber forms the seal as it is pulled reasonably tight, and you get a good effect because of sweat build-up; as you move the mask, however, leakage can occur. The first major advance after this was the British S-6 "airbag" which had a slight positive pressure inside to force the thin rubber of the airbag wall against the face and help to give improved performance for people with an uneven facial profile (a whole book could be written about this subject, alone). When the S-6 mask was moved, the seal was rocked on the airbag, and was much more difficult to completely dislodge. Hence, the S-6 was a very good mask! The snag with the "airbag" was that it was difficult and expensive to make, a valve was required to equalize the pressure at altitude, and the naturally thin rubber airbag wall perished in 5 to 7 years time (due to natural environmental effects).
>
> In the British S-10, the object was to create a 'Ford,' and not a 'Cadillac;' additionally, an airbag in halogenated butyl could not be made affordably. The next best thing was a reversed peripheral seal which sat down upon the skin to give an adequate width of sweat seal, and was of predetermined cross-sectional wall thickness variation for the rubber to hold the surface close to the skin in the expected dynamic motion. The chosen wall thickness variation worked very well indeed, and is one of the main secrets of success for the British S-10 respirator.
>
> *Finally, it is vital for a reverse peripheral seal to lie snugly on the cheek, forehead and chin skin in operation, for a good waterseal to form. A reverse seal which digs into the skin, as is the case with some designs examined over the years, is quite useless."*

Re-examined in the light of these interesting remarks, the face seal of the ND Mark V mask takes on a significance that would otherwise be overlooked or ignored. Of especial interest is the fact that the Mark V mask was replaced later by a mask (MCU-2A/P) which features a reverse peripheral seal, much like the British S-10, but being made from silicone rubber instead of halogenated butyl compound (as in the S-10), lacks the penetration protection necessary for protection against vessicant agents. This will be discussed in a subsequent chapter, dealing with the latest generation masks.

The last of the U.S. Navy *Mark* series (Mark V) was introduced into service at the beginning of the 1960s, and it is interesting to think about how long the WWII masks remained in service. The Mark V mask was issued in a differently shaped gray canvas carrying satchel, internally reinforced on its outer side with an angulated plate to help protect the mask. A top opening flap, secured by snaps, allowed access to the mask while carried via the single adjustable shoulder strap fixed to the satchel. As before, the type of mask contained within was stamped in black ink on the outer surface of the carrier, Gas Mask, ND Mark V (this was changed to read *Mask, Chemical Biological, ND Mark V* on the last Mark V carry-satchel issues).

[Note: It should be mentioned that one of the primary antagonists of proper filter canister function is ambient water vapor (overt moisture, or extreme humidity). For obvious reasons this difficulty is more pronounced at sea. Storage of both protective equipment (such as respirators themselves) and their filtering components must therefore be far more stringently secured against environmental contamination by these elements (as well as the abnormal salinity of the ocean air). Thus, CBW protective equipment intended for sea use requires very careful storage and handling. On ships this is frequently accomplished by securing the CBW equipment in sealed compartments until needed. This contrasts with the land based requirement of the individual having to carry his equipment with him constantly. In both situations there are different forces acting in which personal CBW equipment may suffer performance degradation, and loss of or lessened protective capability. Factors of variation in temperature, ambient humidity and condensation remain critical elements to consider with regard to storage of protective masks and filters, whether on shore or at sea.]

CHAPTER NINE:
U.S. Civilian Defense Developments: 1937 to the Present

During the Second World War period, several variant types of U.S. civilian defense (noncombatant) protective respirators were developed and put into production. Awareness of the need for civilian protective masks was spurred by knowledge of the extensive preparations which had been made in both Germany and England in the 1930s to provide chemical protective equipment for their non-military populations.

The Germans in particular had set an example of note in the mid-1930s by coordinating a comprehensive program of civil air defense under the administration of the Ministry of Air and the Air Defense League. Volunteer members of the latter civilian organization (*Luftschutze*) were encouraged to privately purchase their own gas respirators. Additionally, under supervision of the Air Ministry, a uniform civilian respirator design was produced in sizes for men, women and children, which was designated the *Volksmask 37* (or VM. 37). The German civilian protection programs continued to provide combined gas and air raid protection throughout the war of an exceptional level.

Along similar lines, the British Ministry of Home Security (Air Raid Precautions Department) had undertaken the development and distribution of civilian gas protection respirators of several types as part of a larger program of British chemical defense preparation in the 30s. Committed to a program of providing comprehensive protection for its civilians against chemical agents and air attack, the British government distributed some 38,000,000 gas respirators during the "Munich Crisis" alone.[1] An anti-gas helmet for babies was approved in 1937, and distribution of a final version was initiated in 1940. In additional to the principal Civilian Duty Respirator, a General Civilian Respirator was developed which could be made cheaply in large quantities.

Following suit, the French encouraged the purchase of gas respirators as the threat of war approached during the late 30s, although their respirator policy relied upon private purchase of respirators which were fairly expensive. The Italians followed a similar policy, but did distribute them *gratis* to state, civil and Air Raid Protection personnel.

Japan, a nation which had developed significant offensive chemical weapons capabilities (as well as adequate military protection equipment), did provide civilians with respirators, but by the end of the war had distributed merely 9 million of them to civilians in the principal Japanese cities. This strangely contrasts with their awareness of chemical weapons effectiveness, fostered by actual limited use of agents in the conquered *Manchuko* (Manchuria) province of mainland China against unprotected Chinese civilians and soldiers (mid-30s).

It is not difficult to imagine the motivations behind such acute awareness of the threat of "gas warfare," in view of the part played by chemical war agents in another European war which took place just two decades earlier. The memory of the horrible effects of war gas was still strong in Europe, and in Germany the new chancellor himself had a very personal recollection of his own encounter with mustard agent in the German trenches of 1918 (Hitler's gas injury was relatively minor, but the experience left him with a soldier's deep-seated abhorrence of chemical warfare weapons).

With the studied and well-conceived models of the British and German civilian gas protection programs to take note of, and mindful of the 'gas hysteria' which was sweeping Europe as a new war threatened to develop, the U.S. Army Chemical Warfare Service identified the need for similar protection for U.S. civilians, despite the fact that the U.S. was geographically somewhat isolated from the next apparent theaters of war (Europe and the South Pacific). The need for civilian gas respirators was first formally recognized in 1937, with exploratory development initiated of a suitably efficient, low-cost and easily manufactured protective mask design.

This early design was designated the Noncombatant Gas Mask MI, which used a faceblank constructed from a *Zapon* coated fabric material. For technical reasons, the mask was considered not fully suitable, and an improved model was developed which became standardized as the Noncombatant Gas Mask MI-I-I (using the MI gas mask filter which would shortly be used with the new fully molded rubber M2 face blank to produce the Army Training Gas Mask MI/M2) in 1940. This second mask was enhanced with adhesive-treated, laminated fabric, and had twin circular transparent eye pieces which were sewn and cemented to the facepiece. It used an elasticized head harness and had an early type expiration valve and used a 'minimum' amount of rubber in its construction.

A still further modified version was developed designated the MIA1 facepiece, which used sheet rubber and provided a chin seam for greater comfort. Finally, further work resulted in a third version standardized as the MIA2-I-I, which used an improved laminated fabric facepiece and conformed to the same general design configuration of the earlier models. This last mask was produced in substantial quantity (about 8 million), and stocks were maintained against the possibility of use of gas agents against the general population; the MIA2-I-I mask is still found today as new and unissued surplus materiel, in that substantial quantities were never distributed.

A final, further advanced version of this basic mask was developed which used plastic-impregnated felt, found to be superior to the previous masks in both fit and comfort, while delivering an equivalent level of protection. Designated the MIA3-I-I, this mask was never standardized and produced. When the war ended, remaining substantial stocks of the MIA2 masks were retained by the Office of Civil Defense, although in the late 1940s defense memorandums noted that the WWII vintage civilian protective masks were unsuitable for protection against 'ABC agent threats.'

The MI civil defense masks were surprisingly simple and fairly well-designed for protection against war agents common in that period. The facepiece of the widely produced MIA2-I-I was gray in color, rubber coated and of a moderately stiff, though flexible, construction. The gray metal MI cylindrical filter canister was secured to the facepiece through the use of a large circular clamping ring around the proximal part of the filter body. The MIA2 facepiece used the plastic caged M8 type expiration valve, affixed to the left lower, forward side of the facepiece, and the twin circular transparent lenses were made of vinyl plastic, which were cemented into place. The built-in filter canister rubber check valve at the MI filter's distal end served as the sole inlet check valve for air flow control. A gray elasticized head-harness was stitched directly to the facepiece, using the conventional strap-style arrangement of the military masks (but non-replaceable, with no buckles such as those featured by the latter).

The MIA2 respirator was packed with a brief 16 page pamphlet entitled *Your Gas Mask*, and came packaged in a cardboard carton. A snout-type sandy-olive colored canvas carrying satchel was also provided with the MIA2 mask, very similar in appearance and function to the carrier provided with the U.S. Army Training Gas Mask MI/M2. A single shoulder strap could be adjusted to suit the wearers' needs and enabled the mask to be slung at the side. The MIA2 Noncombatant Gasmask was produced in three adult sizes (Small, Medium and Large) and in one slightly smaller size for older children.

Several other civilian type respirators and/or protective respiration devices were also designed and developed by the Army CWS during the Second World War period. Included among these was a small rubberized fabric respirator designed for use by very small children. Known only as the Gas Mask, Small Child MI, the gray laminated facepiece featured a single, large transparent vinyl eye lens, oblong in shape, and used a gray elasticized, 6-strap harness which could be removed (using buckles). A small gray metal filter canister, labeled M2, was fitted to the chin portion of the facepiece; about two-thirds the length of the MI canister, it functioned and was attached in a similar manner. A rubber disc check valve was located in the distal end of the filter can. The mask used the plastic-caged M8 type expiration valve situated directly over the nose portion of the facepiece, and immediately above the filter inlet connector.

One of the chief concerns among the CWS design personnel, regarding the development of chemical respirators for use by children, was the matter of claustrophobic-type adverse reaction of children to the prospect of having their faces covered by a mask. Not uncommon among adults as well, the claustrophobia-producing nature of a face mask might provoke children to attempt to remove a mask inappropriately. It was decided that providing as large a visual area as possible would eliminate most of this anxiety among children, therefore a large transparent panel was used in the MI Small Child Gasmask, instead of twin circular eyepieces as incorporated in the adult MIA2 mask.

A similar concern had prompted the Army CWS to enter into consultation with the Walt Disney Studios concerning the design and possible production of a children's protective respirator which featured a facepiece molded in the shape of Walt Disney's well-known and much loved cartoon character, Mickey Mouse. The mask would use a filter similar to the existing MI unit (or the M2 filter used on the above children's mask), and consist of the molded cartoon character's face fitted to conventional elasticized head straps.[2]

No word is available concerning the fate of this project, but it is assumed that the design was never procured or put into production. The small child respirator described above appears to have settled the need for such as mask, although the Disney design is unquestionably one of the most interesting and curious gas mask designs ever to be conceived.

Another design for very young children (babies) too small to be fitted with a face-mask type respirator was known as the Infant Protector MI. This device consisted of a large proofed fabric bag, about three feet long, featuring a large transparent vinyl viewing panel in the upper surface. A standard gray metal Training Filter MI was used to filter air entering the bag through an attached hose which was connected to a hand bellows mechanism. The infant was placed within the bag, after which it was closed and sealed through the use of a folding flap and drawstrings; filtered air was then admitted through use of the bellows and filter component assembly by the child's parent or custodian. A similar design used material described as "pliofilm." This type of infant bag respirator was produced and distributed in limited numbers in the early 1940s. Much of the manufactured stock was held in reserve until the war's end and was not circulated due to the unlikely prospect of the civilian population of the continental U.S. being subjected to actual gas attack.

As the war neared its conclusion, it became increasingly apparent that the anxiety over chemical war agent use, with which the U.S. had entered the war, had been greater than circumstances had demonstrated was necessary. While it was recognized that a strong defensive capability had a significant deterrent effect, the end of the Second World War resulted in a lessening of concern with preparedness planning for civilian defense against gas attack in the subsequent post-war years.

However, a new threat had surfaced with the development and initial use of nuclear weapons in the final days of the war with Japan. In the late 1940s the beginnings of the new 'cold war' with the Soviet Union, combined with attendant concerns over protection from the new ABC weapons (atomic, biological and chemical), resulted in renewed emphasis on civilian defense. With the introduction of the Army's new M9 series military respirator in 1947, attention was given to the development of a new civilian defense respirator for both noncombatants and the population at large.

Initial specification discussions were initiated in 1948 by a directive which reviewed the previous (WWII) developments in civilian respirator design. The new design, officially designated as the Mask, Protective, Noncombatant, E51R15-11-22R, was later to be standardized as the Mask, Protective, Noncombatant, M16-11-14, and had been prompted for the most part by recognition on the part of the Army of the need for a protective respirator for use by military noncombatant personnel working at U.S. installations and bases. U.S. Army Chemical Corps Technical Committee communications on Project Number 4-80-0212 (dated 7 Sept 1948) outlined this requirement, and initial specifications were reviewed and discussed.

The goals and objectives of the new noncombatant mask included low-cost, ease of manufacture and procurement, and protective efficiency adequate to meet ABC threats. The mask would be designed to utilize the new standard aluminum cased M11 filter (as used on the military M9 series mask) or the lightweight E3R3 filter canister in a snout attachment configuration. At a projected procurement cost (per mask, in quantity) of about $9.50, the mask was to be considered (initially) expendable, although this attitude later changed.

Produced in 6 sizes when introduced (2 were for children), the mask was later produced in only 4 (1 child size and 3 adult sizes). It was gradually recognized that the mask would be suitable for widespread use by the general population, rather than just by non-fighting military personnel, and eventually a total of about 60,500 of the masks were manufactured. Principal using agency ultimately became the U.S. Civil Defense Agency (FCDA, formerly Office of Civil Defense or OCD), although a vastly smaller quantity was also procured for the FBI (about 300). With adoption for civil defense preparedness, the mask had finally become standardized as Mask, Noncombatant, Protective, M16-11-14 for Army use and designated CD Mask V-800 by the Federal Civil Defense Agency.

The M16/V-800 respirator used a facepiece of moderately stiff, yet flexible fabric, coated on both sides with black "G-8" rubber. It featured a single large transparent vinyl plastic eye piece (similar to the WWII U.S. Navy NC-1 civilian respirator, and the Small Child Mask of the same period) vulcanized in place, with the standard military type M11 (rubber shrouded) expiratory valve (E17R1, in experimental designation) situated on the left lower side of the front of the mask. A black 6 strap elasticized head-harness, adjustable through use of buckles and replaceable, completed the assembly. In the lower frontal area of the mask, below the transparent visor panel, a metal screw-type connector assembly was secured for attaching the M11 type aluminum-bodied filter.

The M16/CD V-800 civilian mask was issued with an olive drab colored carrying satchel (designated E22R1 experimentally and standardized as Carrier, M14) which featured a single shoulder strap and a two-position snap-closure flap; it was similar to, but not exactly like, previous "snout-type" mask carrier satchels. The M11 filter canister was packed in a sealed metal can, and in many cases these M11 filters (which were produced in late 1945 for use with the ill-fated M5 assault mask) were retained in storage, and issued at this later date with the M16 respirator.

The CD V-860 civilian mask, a variant of the CD V-800, was identical to the CD V-800 in appearance except that a rubber hose, connecting an M10A1 type filter, attached to the front of the facepiece; additionally, the exhalation valve was sited at the front of the nosepiece, instead of on the left cheek (as on the CD V-800 mask)

Although organized U.S. civilian defense remained active throughout the later post-war period, and extending through the cold-war era of the 50s and 60s, it languished considerably through subtle neglect. Although effort was maintained to designate and stock collective CD shelter protection throughout the U.S., individual protection equipment was given a far lessened priority (presumably due to budgetary constraints, in view of the massive cold war budget appropriations needed for offensive weapons development and maintenance). Consequently, only a small number of higher-placed civil defense functionaries and immediate "reaction teams" were provided with CBW protection equipment and garments. Stocks of the M16 type respirator were maintained at central distribution points in the U.S., but due to the prevailing view that chemical warfare was unlikely, much of this stock was never distributed beyond regional storage areas for CD materiel.

The new threat of the 50s, 60s and 70s was nuclear war. The possibility of sustaining a general chemical attack against the general population of the U.S. was thought to be extremely remote, again due to the physical isolation of the American continent. However, respiratory protection against nuclear contaminants remained a recognizable requirement, and therefore a further civilian protective mask development took place in the late 60s.

In 1975, the M16 /CD V-800 respirator was officially reclassified as being technologically obsolescent, and steps were taken to discontinue maintenance of existing stocks of the mask through cooperative agreement with DoD (Department of Defense) and DCPA (Defense Civil Preparedness Agency, which is what the original OCD and former FCDA had become). In the meanwhile, a new civil defense protective mask design had come into use. This mask, standardized as the U.S. Army Civilian Protective Mask M22 (developmentally known as the E52R27 mask), had been developed between 1957 and 1959 (Project 4-80-02-031-02, resulting in Mil Spec M-50023, dated 23 June 1959). The mask was designated by the DCPA as the CD V-805 respirator.

The new adult M22/CD V-805 mask was unique in several ways. It was the first 'canisterless' protective mask produced by the U.S., and featured filter elements which were integrated into the basic assembly of the facepiece itself. The faceblank was constructed of grayish vinyl plastic material, incorporating twin "pie-slice" shaped eye lenses made of transparent plastic. The mask, viewed in either frontal or lateral aspect, bears a striking resemblance to the U.S. Army's all silicone riot agent protective mask, the M28 (formerly XM-28), prompting the remark that it had a 'grasshopper' look, or animal's muzzle appearance.

The filtering elements incorporated in the M22/CD V-805 mask used C17 Type II filter material consisting of a core of pulverized ASC charcoal, with fiberglass and plastics laminated and fused between external layers, heat-sealed on both sides, with fiberglass screening. The filters were reputed to be capable of multiple use, and an interior fiberboard air deflector aided lens antimisting while serving as a mask structural former. The M22/CD V-805 mask was produced in 6 sizes designed to fit all faces in the U.S. civilian and military population except those of some children of less than 4 years of age, and bearded personnel. The mask used the 'civilian protective facepiece assembly' C18 (MIL-F-50022 in 6 sizes), the C19 (E19) expiratory valve, and C22 multistrap head-harness.

Estimated cost of the mask on a complete per unit /volume basis (as of 1960) was estimated to be approximately $6.50, thereby making it suitable for disposable or expendable use status. The U.S. Chemical Corps' initial plan was for a primary production run of about 25,000 units, with the civilian (private) industries taking over production thereafter and making the masks available to the public on a "for-profit" basis.

One other type of CBW defense respirator produced roughly concurrent with the M22/CD V-805 mask was designated the Infant Protector CD V-815. Little information is available about the production or possible procurement of this protective item, except that it was apparently intended to function in a manner similar to the WWII type Infant Protector MI, using more modern materials and fabrication techniques.

As of 22 Sept 1987, the M22/CD V-805 civilian protective mask was reclassified by the U.S. Army and the OCDM (Office of Civil Defense Management) as obsolescent, and no longer suited to the existing requirement (NBC protection for noncombatants). Remaining stocks of the mask were disposed of as surplus materiel. The opinion extant at this time (1987) was that it was extremely unlikely that the U.S. general civilian population would sustain a broad-based chemical attack and civilian defense research and development had assumed a very low priority. Certain projects were continuing with the development of several new designs, however, including one which would be suitable for use by personnel with beards (a particular concern, as the popularity and acceptance of facial hair gained public acceptance in the 70s and 80s). Research at Edgewood would also continue in several related areas, although the concept was more to provide a new form of protection for non-fighting military personnel such as those handling special fuels, or engaging in work around non-war agent toxic substances.

At present, several recently developed civilian NBC respirator proposals have been evaluated and tested, in work being accomplished by the U.S. Army Chemical Systems Laboratory facilities at Edgewood, in cooperation with commercial contractors such as the ILC Corporation. Among the new NBC capable respirator proposals are several which provide whole-head cover, specifically intended for adults with beards, and possible modification for use by children. A few of these are the ILC DERP (Disposable Eye Respiratory Protection) Mask, and the new U.S. Army NBC Mask for Dependents (modified from an off-the-shelf commercial product). The International Latex Corporation, with its extensive defense and space-related research and development in life support systems, has figured prominently in this area, as work of this sort continues.

One of the results of the chemical threat encountered during the recent (1991) Gulf War was focused awareness on the key importance of user-training and familiarity with civilian protection equipment to assure effective defense against CBW agents. Both Israel and the Arab nations experienced numerous problems associated with these topics (user training and familiarization, user anxiety and equipment distribution), and all nations have hopefully benefited from this modern example of the importance of maintaining a formidable CBW defensive posture—for civilians as well as for military personnel.[3]

The favorably isolated geographic situation of the United States remains, however, considerably different from that of nations in Europe and elsewhere, in that we do not share our borders with traditional enemies or known belligerent nations. Therefore present strategic defense planning does not place a high priority on development of civilian defense equipment for mass protection of the public against internal (domestic) chemical, biological or nuclear threats; nor is it likely that this attitude will change to an *appreciable* extent in the future.

CHAPTER TEN:
Nerve Gas and Nuclear War: The Late 1940s and 1950s

One of the great, unanswered questions of the Second World War is "Why didn't the Third Reich use chemical weap ons?" This question, the cause of never-ending speculation and conjecture among students of military history, will probably never be answered fully or completely.

While the standing policy of the United States and Great Britain toward the use of chemical weapons was one of *retaliation only*, Germany certainly did not have any such inhibiting policy of similar substance. There was certainly Hitler's personal antipathy towards chemical warfare and there appeared to be an apparent unofficial consensus against Germany's initiating chemical war; this was based, to all reasonable assessment, upon several complex and interactive factors.

Fear of retaliation from an enemy who *appeared* to be extremely well prepared to defend against or wage chemical war seems to have been a particularly strong element in German policy on use of chemical weapons.[1] In addition to a feeling that Allied chemical defensive equipment was superior to that Germany possessed, an important assumptive error was made in German intelligence assessment of the Allies' *offensive* chemical weaponry capability. Germany had succeeded in developing new and deadly nerve gases (Tabun/GA and Soman/GD), a consequence of research in organophosphates conducted by the I.G. Farben Company in an earlier search for effective insecticides. Germany estimated a *similar capability* on the part of the Allies, although the Allies did not in fact have these agents either in development or production throughout the war.

A curious sequence of events may have prompted this erroneous assumption, in that reports of organophosphate insecticide research had been briefly circulated in U.S. chemical journals shortly before the war began; but when U.S. scientists had decided that there was no promise in their development, research in this area promptly ended. One opinion is that German intelligence noted the rather sudden cessation of any further reports of work with organophosphates and interpreted this as evidence that the formidable war applications of these compounds had been discovered, resulting in complete censorship of any further information in the chemical or scientific journals being imposed.

Further, due to early, overwhelming successes in battle which continued until 1942-43, there was no logical, rational advantage to be gained through the use of such weapons. Later, when the tide of the conflict was clearly turning against Germany, the ominous threat of 1918—at which time the Allies were finally prepared to use massive quantities of war gasses against the German Army—was recalled; this again reinforced German fear that the Allies were not only extremely well prepared for chemical warfare, but that they possessed the deadly organophosphate nerve agents, as well.

Hitler's personal experience as a German soldier in the First World War had left him with an intimate and deeply seated aversion to the use of chemical agents. As a result, the overall responsibility for research, development, strategic planning and procurement of chemical agents by the German Chemical Warfare Service was left, for all practical purposes, in the hands of the OKW (German High Command), professional soldiers with a traditional distaste for such unconventional weapons. As the war continued, and as acute shortages of strategic materials began to be more profoundly felt, production and quality standards for chemical warfare protection equipment languished, leaving Germany less well prepared for defense against such weapons. Items such as protective masks for horses were discontinued in 1941, and individual protective clothing distribution ended in 1942. By the time the Allied invasions began in 1944, Germany's defensive capabilities for defense against CBW weapons were severely diminished.

When Hitler, late in the war and in the throes of his insane determination to bring Germany down with him, finally issued authorization for the use of chemical weapons, the OKW undoubtedly disregarded the order or otherwise ignored it, properly recognizing it as the desperate act of a mad man.

Another curious twist in the matter occurred during the German Ardennes Offensive (Battle of the Bulge). In the midst of the cold winter following the Allied invasion of Europe, American soldiers discovered the so-called 'cold-set' tendency of their new (M5) Assault Gas Masks (made from synthetic neoprene rubber). Consequently, many of the useless masks were discarded; this was augmented by a generalized attitude in the field that Germany would not initiate chemical warfare. Alarmed by this trend, a directive from American Headquarters prompted a surge in issuance of new chemical defense masks to the troops and a renewed effort to re-equip units with chemical defense gear to replace lost or unusable items. Speculation has it that German intelligence, which had to have known of this, interpreted the issuance of new gas masks and equipment as evidence that the Allies were expecting use of gas and were taking extraordinary precautions to defend against any possible German gas initiative as they continued to advance.

Whatever the real reason or combination of reasons why Germany did not use the formidable new nerve agents it possessed—which the Allies were *completely* unprepared for—the known fact that Hitler did in fact finally sign a directive authorizing its use late in the war remains. We can only presume that the directive was deliberately or inadvertently mislaid, miscommunicated or otherwise not transmitted down the chain of command for reasons we may only guess at. The critical elements of devastating surprise and the results of horrendous damage inflicted by weapons the Allies were totally unprepared for—which use of Tabun (GA) and Soman (GD) would have provided—were lost forever in the final analysis.

To say that the discovery by Allied forces at war's end of over 12,000 tons of stockpiled Tabun was a very disconcerting surprise, is an understatement.[2] More disconcerting still was the fact that the Allies utterly lacked any detection capability against the nerve agents, nor did they possess adequate overall defenses against its use. It is sobering to reflect on the fact that use of the new gases at several critical points during the Allied advance into Germany, in the final campaign, could have radically effected the outcome of the war. Many feel it was a missed opportunity for Germany equivalent to that which occurred when the new German chlorine gas agent surprised the Allies completely during the famous attack on Ypres in April of 1915.

The new gases were of immediate interest to the U.S. Chemical Warfare Service in the latter part of 1945, as they were to the English chemical research establishment at Porton Down, and chemical warfare entered a whole new era of more formidable development than before. Of added significance was the fact that great volumes of technical information and samples of the new agents disappeared behind the Soviet lines as well, as all of the victorious allies scrambled to perform intelligence analyses of captured German military and scientific advancements in war technology. It must be remembered that the Soviet Union already possessed substantial expertise in CW warfare technology when it absorbed the captured wartime German materiel and research.

With the dropping of the new atomic bombs on two Japanese cities in 1945, the world suddenly entered a very new and even more frightening era. The prospect of a new need for protection from particulate nuclear fallout was evident and provided additional incentive, along with the discovery of the new nerve agents, to review the state of U.S. chemical defensive developments.

Prior to the use of nuclear weapons against Japan, the option of using chemical weapons to hasten the war's end (in the event the anticipated suicidal resistance to surrender was encountered by Allied armies) had been briefly considered by the U.S., and Professor Yoshaiki Yoshimi (Chair of the Department of History, Chuo University, Tokyo) recently stated that he had recovered detailed plans for use of phosgene and mustard agents on Japanese civilian population centers from the U.S. National Archives. Dr. Yoshimi's research also revealed that Japan had produced and stockpiled large quantities of chemical agents (in 1946 British occupying forces had discovered and destroyed over 18,000 tons of such agents, which had been stockpiled in a chemical plant just outside of Hiroshima, according to an official English document).

Earlier in the war President Roosevelt had promised that the U.S. would consider use of chemical weapons if evidence was found that Japan had used CBW agents and it has been suggested that the discovery that Japan had used mustard on a limited basis against the Chinese in Manchuria during the 1930s might have provided justification for a review of the "retaliation only" policy previously declared. In the final outcome, it appears that the sentiment prevalent in the U.S. among War Department planners was that chemical weapons were neither a wise nor expedient option for active consideration in the invasion of the Japanese homeland. This was apparently further encouraged by a Japanese decision to dismantle most of their chemical warfare preparations when the waves of American bombers began their final bombardments of the home islands, a fact which they widely publicized, and which was intended to discourage U.S. CW 'first strike' options (Intelligence assessments of their chemical warfare capabilities, conducted immediately after the war, revealed that they were rather poorly prepared for modern, large-scale gas warfare—either offensive or defensive—in the final outcome. Evidence also suggests that Roosevelt's declaration of U.S. chemical warfare policy, earlier in the war, had been taken at face value by Japanese strategic planners in the military government—further lessening the urgency of Japanese CBW defense policy).

Subsequent to the renaming of the U.S. Army Chemical Warfare Service in 1946 (to "U.S. Army Chemical Corps," with attendant full acceptance as an important branch of the Army), existence of the new nerve agents and an identified need for respiratory protection from airborne nuclear fallout contamination prompted renewed efforts to further develop the military respirator.

At war's end, the last expression of the state-of-the-art in U.S. military respirators had taken the form of hastily improvised stopgap measures. With the failure of the neoprene fabricated Assault Gas Mask design in 1944, one other effort was made to produce a mask which would take the M11 filter canister. This was the M8-11-10 snout-type mask, which was put together from reconditioned M2/M4 type molded rubber facepieces fitted with an adapter connection that would allow the M11 filter to be fastened directly to the inlet port of the facepiece.

As an advancement in respirator design, the M8 hardly qualified, and it was clear that the earlier M5 *concept*, featuring a cheek mounted filter, was not only obviously superior, but an indicator of future design efforts. Consequently, a serious effort was made by Aberdeen and the U.S. Army MIT laboratory to produce a satisfactory molded natural rubber facepiece, based on the M5 design, which would yield the desired product.

The result, introduced for the first time in 1947 after plentiful supplies of natural rubber were again accessible with the war's conclusion, was the M9 series of U.S. military protective masks. Destined to become one of those archetypes of design excellence which would be emulated throughout the world in the following decades, the M9 mask was essentially a refined, somewhat reconfigured expression of the earlier M5 design produced in gray-green natural rubber. Produced in substantial quantities throughout the 1950s, the American M9 *ABC* Field Protective Mask would be copied by at least 5 other nations, and contribute to foreign respirator designs which were developed from its basic concepts and parameters.

The M9 mask, which took the lightweight aluminum M11 drum filter (based substantially on, as we will recall, the German FE-42 filter canister) fitted to a cheek inlet port, would remain in use among U.S. military forces for many decades; even with the advent of a new design which was supposedly to replace it altogether (the M17 NBC mask) in the 60s, the venerable M9 mask would continue to serve as protection for special requirements well into the early 80s.

By 1955, several types of respirators were in use among U.S. military forces. These included a new type of armored vehicle protective mask, the M14 Tank Mask, the M13 Headwound Protective mask (an earlier type was known as the M7 Headwound Protective Mask), and older types such as the M3A1-10A1-6, the M3A2-10A1-6, the M4-10A1-6, the M4A1-10A1-6 (all four of the foregoing masks of the WWII "Lightweight" type), the M8-11-10 (snout-type), and the M2-10A1-6 (optical mask). The M14 Tank Mask was the predecessor of the later M25 type Armored Vehicle Mask and resembled it in both design and fabrication.

Also adopted for use by this time was a series of special purpose respirators which were intended for use against non-wargas type toxic chemicals only. These masks were essentially commercially designed and produced (i.e. Mine Safety Appliances) safety respirators, given military designations, and issued to personnel handling toxic chemicals, exotic fuels, etc., in non-combat, rear-echelon areas. Included in this group were the M10, M11, M11A1, and M12 models, each provided with a specific rectangular box filter for use with a designated type of toxic gas. Another series of masks, using WWII style M2 type rubber service mask facepiece assemblies, were M2A1, M2A2 and M2A3 *special purpose* models, intended for use against chemical oil vapors, ammonia and gases having acid-properties (these respirators, essentially the early WWII style "Heavyweight" gas masks fitted with special filters—similar in shape to the WWII MIXA1 filter—were carried in old MIVA1 style canvas carrying satchels). One further type of mask, which is not strictly an air-purification-only mask, was designated the M13 Oxygen Breathing Mask (this is *not* related to the aviation-type A-13 aviator's pressure-demand oxygen breathing mask, which was used in high-performance, high altitude aircraft).

The primary U.S. service respirator of the M9 series type was standardized in December of 1947, as previously referenced. With the introduction of this mask, a change was made in the old-style Army designation nomenclature. Whereas previously all military respirators had been designated with an identifying number consisting of three parts (mask-filter-carrier), from that date forward all masks would be identified only by the model of the facepiece used. For example, under the old style system (September 1940 through December 1947), the new M9 mask would have been the M9-11-7A1 gas mask. Under the new system the designation was simply M9 Gas Mask [For a review of the U.S. Chemical Corps designation nomenclature system, and an explanation of the major changes that took place in 1940 and 1947, refer to the proper appendix at the end of the text.]

In the late 1950s, the Army Chemical System Laboratory at Edgewood (Aberdeen Proving Grounds, Maryland) produced a proposed replacement for the M9 series of masks. This was the new M17 mask, a somewhat radical departure from the original cheek-filter M9 style concept. The M17 mask was standardized in the early 1960s and production runs began in 1961. The M17 series, in three subsequent modified variants (M17, M17A1 and M17A2), would continue to serve as the primary U.S. military CBW respirator for almost three decades, despite some very controversial features, which shall be described later.

The U.S. Army M9 Field Protective Mask:
A redefinition of the WWII M5 Assault Gas Mask, the M9-11-7A1 Gas Mask was standardized in December of 1947 as the M9 Field Protective Mask. This new expression of the assault or combat gas mask concept used a facepiece made of gray-green natural rubber that was produced in three sizes (small, medium and large). Extensive anthropomorphic studies done on 3,075 soldiers (representing every state in the USA) at Camp Siebert, Alabama, during the war years, had provided statistical data which allowed the three sizes of M9 mask to satisfactorily fit all American faces (these studies would continue to be the basis for all subsequent U.S. military NBC respirators up through the latest models).

The C8 elasticized black head-harness was used, which featured 6 straps joined to the faceblank via adjustable buckles fitted to short woven canvas attachment straps that were secured by rivets. The standard C15 rubber shrouded expiratory valve was fitted to the lower front of the facepiece, and the facepiece used the conventional inner oronasal nosecup, fitted with one-way check valves, for positive air flow deflection as a demisting aid. A neck strap, for further securing was used as a component of the head-harness. In a congruent manner to all previous masks from the M2 onwards, transparent, semi-triangular safety-glass lenses were fitted to metal lens frames that were clamped in place. The facepiece was manufactured in both left cheek and right cheek filter mount models to accommodate right and left handed individuals, and was produced in three sizes (small, medium and large). The filter mounting screw-ring fitting was made of lightweight aluminum, and featured a circular rubber disc serving as a one-way check valve. The standard filter used was the M11 combat filter canister, painted slate gray, and composed of a mechanical aerosol element and an ASC type charcoal absorbent component. The M9 mask was carried in the M7A1 OD colored canvas duck carrier satchel, which was proofed on the inner side with a butyl rubber, and worn in the standard side carry (under arm) position through use of a shoulder and waist strap.

The U.S. Marine Corps used the C15R1 carrier (very similar to the M7A1 carrier), after the M9A1 mask assembly became standard for the U.S. Army, with its new M11 carrier.

The U.S. Army M9A1 Field Protective Mask:
In about 1950, the Army substituted the new, reshaped and unproofed OD canvas duck carrier satchel for the older M7A1 carrier. This

change resulted in the M9 mask being redesignated the M9A1 mask. Except for use of the new carrier, the facepiece assembly of the M9A1 mask was absolutely identical to the M9 facepiece—there were no other changes in any of the mask's components. When this change occurred, the U.S. Marine Corps retained the older M7A1 proofed carry satchel for use by its troops (based upon a requirement for proofed protection for its masks during amphibious operations) but under the C15R1 designator.

Several features of the M9/M9A1 respirator are worthy of closer examination and analysis. First among these was the cheek-mounted lightweight filter configuration. Recognized almost universally as a major advancement (just as the inner oronasal cup for air flow control had been similarly regarded), the cheek-mount filter has proven to be one of those archetypes of respirator design.[3] It should be again observed here, that the *British "Light Type Respirator"* of late 1943 was the original inspiration for this approach, but it has been the American M9 respirator which has seen subsequent translation in almost half a dozen masks produced by other nations. Almost all of the copies were license produced, with a few exceptions. Included among the M9 inspired copies are the Korean KM9A1 (still in production), the Finnish M61 (production completed), the Norwegian NM-16 (made for that country by Sweden's Forsheda AB firm; production completed), the Swedish Skyddsmask 51 (production completed), and the Serbian M1 (formerly the Yugoslavian M-59, and still in production). Still other respirators, such as the Serbian M2, owe a substantial debt to the primary design parameters and concepts featured in the American M9.

Of interest are the textured (pebble-grain) inner face-seal of the M9 mask and the through-the-mask riveted web harness retention strap features. The non-smooth inner face seal feature has remained the same in almost all the foreign made-copies, despite the fact that it contradicts the sweat-seal theory described earlier in the text. Additionally, the penetration of the facepiece by mask head-harness retention rivets, as found in the U.S. M9 and most foreign copies, poses a potential weakness in that agents might possibly enter the mask after repeated or heavy exposure to agents (The Swedes, in their Skyddsmask 51 copy of the M9, corrected that error in designing a non-penetrating strap fastening system).

Furthermore, the innovative Finnish M61 mask featured a type of reversed peripheral lip for enhanced facial-seal—something that is today almost universal, but was not found in use on any other CBW masks (with the exception of a special U.S. Navy protective mask design of 1944 and a Dräger manufactured version of the GM-38 gas mask made entirely from molded synthetic rubber in the early 40s) before 1960. American Army NBC masks did not feature the reversed peripheral seal as a routine component until the advent of the XM-29 silicone experimental model developed in the late 70s.

With regard to the M11 type drum filter (concept originated with the WWII German FE 42 filter, after which the M11 design was adapted, in which a mechanical/particulate filter element was combined with an absorbing ingredient), the early versions carried the designation E3 prior to standardization as M11. WWII issued versions, intended for use with the M5 Assault Gas Mask and later issued with the 1950s Civilian defense mask (M16) CD V-800, used asbestos in combination with the mechanical aerosol filter element. The deleterious potential health hazard of this was not immediately noted until somewhat later, but the asbestos was eliminated in subsequent versions. The M11 filter canisters produced during the 50s were also a different color than the dark gray WWII produced version, appearing in a green-gray hue. Packed for storage in a hermetically sealed can, the M11 filter was provided with a removable rubber stopper on the filter inlet end, and was protected with a screw-cap on the outlet end.

A butyl-proofed fabric hood was initially used with the M9 for complete protection from vessicants and biologicals; the hood enclosed the entire head, fitting around the eyepieces of the M9 or M8 masks, and could be used with either. Gathered about the neck with a draw-cord when used with the M9, it entirely enclosed the M11 type drum filter, leaving only the M11's inlet orifice open. The hood could also be used with the snout-attached M11 filter as found on the old style M8 gas mask. The first version was designated the *Chemical Protective Hood*, although a later version was designated the M4 Chemical Protective Hood. The hood rendered more complete protection from spray/droplet dispersal agents, blistering agents, and biologicals, and was worn either with protective clothing, or with the mask alone (depending upon the type of threat anticipated).

The U.S. M9/M9A1 has been in continuous service for almost 40 years with the U.S. military, as well as civilian police units, and it was only after the current '4th Generation' type M40 mask came into production that the last M9s were declared no longer needed surplus by the U.S. Army.[4] The various foreign versions of this respirator are still in use, and the Serbian (M59) M1 was procured and used extensively by Iraq in the 1980s, while the Korean KM9A1 has been procured and used by Saudi Arabia, among other nations.

The U.S. Army Tank Gas Mask M14:
Fabricated from molded rubber, and using the same C8 head harness assembly as the M9 series, the M14 mask featured an oblong, transparent, flexible, single eyepiece measuring 7 by 5 inches. A C15 expiratory exhaust valve assembly is situated under the chin of the facepiece, directly behind the wire-reinforced M8 hose and inlet ferrule. The M10A2 tank filter canister is the standard M10A1 gray metal cylindrical filter canister to which an M1 canister coupling assembly has been added and the filter may be used either discretely or connected to the standard tank collection protection filter. An OD colored M13 Tank Mask carrier satchel is used with the M14 Tank Mask; it is fabricated from water-resistant (not proofed) canvas duck material and features an opening in the end through which the filter connector coupling port protrudes. The M14 facepiece is fitted with a microphone and cord so that the unit may be used with a standard armored vehicle communications system. The M14 tank mask, as mentioned, was the forebear of the later M25/M25A1 tank mask and as such bears a striking resemblance to the later 60s M25 series armored vehicle mask.[5]

The M13 Hospital Collective Protector Headpiece:
The M13 'headwound' CBW protector assembly was intended for use by patients who had sustained wounds of the head or neck

thereby rendering them unable to use the standard service gas mask. The facepiece was made from transparent flexible plastic material (similar to the earlier M7 Headwound Gas Mask), except that purified air was entrained into the mask under pressure via a hose connected to a common collective filter system.

The U.S. Army M2-10A1-6 Lightweight Optical Gas Mask: This mask, following the earlier versions of the optical mask incorporated a slightly more advanced diaphragm/expiratory valve (C11) design than the WWII (MI Optical Mask) predecessor, but used a single hose fed black rubber facepiece not entirely dissimilar in certain respects to the earlier style, and featured the same small circular optical quality glass eyepieces of the former model. Also used was the M10A1 gray metal cylindrical filter connected to the mask via an M3 rubber hose. The facepiece used the C7 head harness assembly, and was carried in the canvas duck OD colored M6 carrier satchel. Although not a 'new' mask, this unit was retained for use well into the 50s. Certain variants of this mask used a special slide adjustment unit for setting intraocular distance, as opposed to the adjustable screw version normally used.

The U.S. Army Mask, Gas, M10, M11, M11A1 and M12: Coming into use in the late 50s, all four of these respirators were intended for use only with non-war agent toxic chemicals. Each used a common black rubber facepiece of commercial design (MSA), which was used with interchangeable rectangular filters specifically designated for use with a particular type of hazardous gas (or chemical). The masks and filter canisters themselves were MSA manufactured safety respirators, originally developed for civilian business applications concerned with toxic chemicals and unsafe atmospheres (mining, fire fighting, chemical manufacturing, etc.), and had been accepted without significant change for use in non-combat roles within the military.

The M10 respirator filter was used as protection against acidic and other organic vapors; the M11 and M11A1 respirator canisters, similar in shape to earlier standard Army service respirator filters, although with slightly smaller dimensions, were specifically used for protection against carbon monoxide concentrations of 2% or less alone, or in combination with other gases (except acid vapors). The M12 respirator, again with an identical facepiece and hose assembly as that used with the M10, and M11 type units, was provided with a special filter used for and limited to protection against ammonia vapors.

The common facepiece was molded of black rubber, had molded-in Tissot type air deflecting tubes for lens demisting, twin large, metal framed eye lenses with bilateral outboard screw locking devices (of safety glass or plastic material, providing excellent vision), and a lower, frontally located expiratory valve of the old flapper type protected by a metal cage assembly directly over the air hose's inlet. An adjustable rubber head-harness featuring radial straps enabled quick donning and fitting. The hose joined the box-like canister and was carried on the lower chest or waist through use of a canvas securing device equipped with straps, and screwed onto the filter. The entire issue of M10, M11, M11A1 and M12 respirator systems were provided in a fiberboard case fitted with hinges and a latch [A later version of the common commercial type facepiece featured an improved expiratory valve of a more contemporary type. It is worth observing that the Japanese produced a mask bearing a striking similarity—at first glance—to this U.S. Army model in the early 1950s. It used a snout-type circular filter, a side located exhalation valve, and featured a set of twin, bilaterally screw-secured lenses quite like those on the U.S. Army/MSA M10-M11 and M-12 masks.]

CHAPTER ELEVEN: New Departures in Design The 1960s and 1970s

The 60s could be looked upon as a period in which innovative searching began for new answers to old problems in chemical and biological protection, and several new designs would be later introduced which were characteristic of this time; one or two of them would prove useful and well-conceived, but others would be subject to contention and controversy among NBC specialists. Considered in retrospect, the unspectacular developments of the 60s prompted a renewed need for advanced proposals a decade later.

In the very late 1950s, the U.S. Army Chemical Corps' Chemical System Laboratory at the Edgewood facility, Aberdeen, introduced an entirely new protective NBC respirator design. The new mask was innovative in that it did away with the externally screwed-on filter canister, relying instead on a pair of internally fitted filters shaped somewhat like 'pork chops.' The new mask was finally standardized as the M17 NBC Field Protective Mask, and the soldier wearing the new mask presented a rather unusual appearance due to the built-up bilateral cheek areas containing the new filtering elements.

This intended replacement for the conventional M9 series mask incorporated several of the preceding mask's tried and tested features, such as the oronasal cup for air flow control, the twin semi-triangular safety glass lenses (which provided a fairly good field of vision), and a head-harness of unremarkable if proven convention (elasticized straps). Still lacking a full circumference reversed peripheral face seal (something that many civilian toxic chemical safety masks had by then incorporated), the mask's central interest lay in its internally fitted twin filter elements, and therein would lie the controversy about this design which would remain in contention for nearly two decades.

The M17 mask's filters, one of which was fitted internally into each side of the facepiece, required that the mask be removed from the face in order to replace them. This mandated, of course, either an agent free environment or a safely protected collective gas shelter in which to accomplish the task. The filters themselves would provide a substantial level of protection against all known war agents, but as may be imagined, there might possibly be battlefield situations in which a severely sustained chemical or biological attack would require that the filters be exchanged for fresh units during the attack—something impossible to do without removing the mask entirely for a significant period of time.

Although providing a high level of protection (assuming a perfect face-seal and perfectly functioning faceblank components such as expiratory valve, etc.) against most reasonably anticipated chemical/biological agent threat situations, there would always be the question of how the mask would protect against extraordinarily high-concentration, long-duration CBW attacks due to the tricky, internally fitted filter design.

Fortunately, the M17 respirator, relied upon for primary NBC protection in all U.S. military forces for more than two decades, would never have to prove itself in this 'worst-case' scenario. During the 60s, 70s, and 80s, the M17 was used in limited service against riot agents (CS/CN) and has also been used by police and law enforcement units for crowd control, but the mask has never been tested in actual war-time CBW agent situations. Therefore, this single but potentially rather serious design oversight shall always remain in contention—just like the question concerning Germany's avoidance of CB warfare during the Second World War.

Owing to the filter replacement problem, the older M9 mask was retained by the U.S. Army as a special purpose mask, rather than being retired as had been intended, and much as had the older M2, M3 and M4 (WWII) gas masks been retained for special purpose use, the M9 mask continued to fulfill similar requirements (Critics could *conceivably* point to this as evidence of the M17's basic design shortcomings).

When the M17 mask was introduced (early 60s), it had no provision for enabling the wearer to drink liquids while masked. A subsequent modification (M17A1), appearing in the late 60s, incorporated a drinking tube system. The new M17A1 version also featured a novel innovation: a resuscitation valve component which enabled the expiratory valve to be attached to a resuscitation tube so that emergency respiratory support could be provided to a soldier wearing the mask by another soldier similarly masked. The short length of corrugated resuscitation tubing could be screwed to the mask's exhalation valve for use, but was normally kept in the M17A1 mask's carrier when not needed.

The drinking tube component of the M17A1 was quite well thought out, but the resuscitation assembly, aside from being un-

versions feature three. The additional connection point helps stabilize the visor in place on the faceblank and serves to help prevent distortion of the inner reversed peripheral seal during storage, something occasionally noted on older masks fitted with the two point attachment feature. As noted before, all MCU type masks now serve as protection for ground personnel only, and have been replaced in aircraft applications by modern specialized respirator developments.

One last accessory peculiar to the MCU series masks is a special, tan-colored fabric anti-flash hood that is flame retardant. It fits the mask in a manner identical to the standard, OD colored, proofed butyl hood that is more commonly used with the MCU series.

The U.S. Army Protective Mask, Aircraft/Helicopter, M43 (new designation M48):

The M43 Aircraft NBC respirator system, by initial intent, was specially developed for use by U.S. Army helicopter aircrews. The actual production has resulted in two models of the M43, known as Types I and II. The Type I version, visually distinctive owing to its ellipsoid shaped eye lenses, is specifically fabricated for use in the AH-64 helicopter and is equipped with components that are compatible with the Honeywell integrated Helmet and Display Sighting System (HADSS) used in that aircraft. The Type II version uses circular lenses and is issued to all U.S. Army air crew except those flying the AH-64 helicopter. Both feature a black, form-fitting bromobutyl/natural rubber facepiece to which an OD butyl proofed chemical hood has been permanently attached. A visual characteristic of these masks are their small, close-to-the-eye lenses, necessitated by the HADSS and other aids such as night vision systems. The facepiece is secured by straps to the head, over which the hood is drawn (worn under the aircrew protective helmet). An inlet attachment on the left cheek connects a reinforced hose to the twin-filter/blower unit which helps ventilate the mask while providing CBW agent protection. The system was developed in cooperation with the ILC Company, and a modified version designated M43A1 was produced and flight tested in AH-64 prototypes. A drink system is incorporated in the design that is similar to that used in the M40/M42 masks. The primary liability of the M43 system is that it uses an actively blown filtering system, requiring an elaborate set of accessories and a complex electronic support system; this has resulted in an unusually high per unit cost factor—not a favorable characteristic in the new budget-conscious defense spending era. The M43 mask is produced in 4 sizes (S, M, L, and XL). It has been a desire to replace the costly and complicated M43 type system with a less costly alternative that has served to spur development of the latest, much less expensive XM-45 helicopter crew protective mask, discussed briefly in the next chapter. Due to substantial modifications made to the M43 design (as of February 1997), the mask has now been redesignated *Protective Mask, Aircraft/Helicopter, M48*.

The U.S. Army Protective Mask, Aircraft/Helicopter, M43A1 (new designation M49):

An upgraded version of the M43, the M43A1, is also produced in two types, corresponding to the M43 versions (Type I & II). Among the enhancements of the M43A1 version are visual correction outserts for aircrewmen with refractive index variations; also incorporated is what has been termed a "double-skirted" hood, which increases protection capabilities. Additionally, an auxiliary blower has been incorporated into the forced ventilation system which provides back-up in the event of an aircraft power failure or emergency egress, and the main blower has been reconfigured to accept standard U.S. Army batteries. Type I and Type II masks use M171/AIC and M133/U microphones respectively, following the same pattern as the M43 Type I and Type II masks. Donning time for these masks is claimed to be less than 9 seconds. Reference is made in literature describing the M43A1 hood as having an enhanced 'nuclear protective' function. As of February of 1997 the M43A1 protective mask has been redesignated the *Protective Mask, Aircraft/Helicopter, M49* , owing to substantial modifications made to the original design.

CHAPTER THIRTEEN: Into the Future

With the American expression of the so-called "Fourth Generation" NBC respirators complete and in production, it is certain that the search is continuing at the U.S. Army's research and development laboratories at Edgewood for the definition of tomorrow's protective NBC technological concepts.[1] Spurred on by the untimely and lackluster efforts of the 80s, and further encouraged by a resolve not to repeat the costly mistakes of that decade, this renewed awareness of the importance of maintaining our NBC posture (brought about in part by the momentary scare posed by the Gulf War of 1991) is being nurtured amidst a great period of budgetary restraint and emphasis on cost-cutting as the U.S. military copes with a dire need to down-size. Influences such as these rarely bode good for specialized areas of defense research, such as is NBC protection technology, which are frequently regarded by traditionalists as exotic, expendable 'prize pigs' that are among the first candidates for sacrifice when budgetary considerations predominate.

One very recent development has just been publicized. This is the new U.S. Army XM-45 Aircrew Chemical/Biological Mask, which was engineered as a replacement for the M43A1 (M49) helicopter respirator system. The newly standardized M45 uses a discrete facepiece made from black silicone rubber, retained by a conventional 6 strap head-harness.[2] A reversed peripheral seal is integrated into the facepiece, and a separate proofed hood is used with the mask. Again, the eyepieces are relatively small and placed close to the eye plane for use with optical sighting systems, night vision equipment, etc. A primary voicemitter is located in the front of the mask and inlet ports are situated on each cheek. From the left side inlet fitting, a low-profile interoperability hose runs to a filter canister component in the manner of previous aircraft and tank respirators, but unlike the M43A1 (M49), there is no integrated forced air blower in the circuit. A secondary voicemitter disc may be used to secure the unused inlet port and a conventional expiratory valve is sited under the primary voicemitter. It is assumed that a microphone is fitted to the mask for use with helicopter communications systems and the mask has a drink tube assembly, as well. One of the overwhelming motivations behind the development of the M45 is the very costly nature of the M43A1(M49) system. With advances in materials and fabrication techniques, it is presumed that the M45 mask in its final production standard will count a substantially lower unit-acquisition cost among its desirable features.

The new M45 design benefits from recently enhanced CAD/CAM capabilities found in the Edgewood "Rapid Prototyping Facility" at Aberdeen Proving Grounds and at a anticipated procurement cost of about $350 per unit (compare this to over $1200 per unit for the M43A1/M49), the new system is expected to be in standard service by 1998. A call for potential contracting manufacturers was recently made (1996) by the U.S. Army Chemical and Biological Defense Agency (Edgewood) to orient prospective producers of the new respirator, and as of February 1997 final contractual negotiations are in process for the first production run of the newly standardized M45 mask.

There is no indication that there are programs underway to develop a replacement for the MCU-2A/P mask, and it is likely that that respirator will stay in service into the foreseeable future. The M40 and M42 series masks, controversial as they may be, shall likely continue to evolve slightly and remain in service as well. Evidence of this, with regard to the latter mask (the newer M40A1 version) is found in the development of the new EPDM 'second skin' & "quick-doff" butyl rubber proofed hood assembly (consisting of two discretely separated component items) which *theoretically* makes the mask less vulnerable to penetration agents and permits quicker and less complicated doffing of the respirator. The M40A1 is admittedly much improved, because of this new hood and skin assembly, over the original M40 with its one-piece hood and EPDM faceblank protector component.

At present there are a number of very specialized aeronautical NBC protection designs either in late development testing phases or ready for production (an example is the USAF MBU-19/P), and work continues in the Air Force for better aircrew NBC equipment integrated into overall high-altitude life support systems. Several of these are the result of work being done by the ILC Company in cooperation with Air Force human factors labs. One (non-aircrew application) in particular, for which USAF procurement contracts have been issued (USAF F08635-93-C-0067), is a design cooperatively produced by the Kemira Safety Company of Finland, and the U.S. Interspiro Company. The Interspiro Spirolite 9030 High Performance Breathing Apparatus (SCBA)—for which the Kemira Company manufactures the rubber facepiece—has been modified with a chemical warfare accessory kit, which allows the unit to be used for chemical threat as well as conventional hazardous environments (fire-fighting, etc.). The kit includes a specially modified facemask assembly, butyl proofed hood, carrier bag and standard metal bodied C-2 filter. The unit has been approved for use as of September 1994 under NSN 4240-01-359-5641.

A relatively recent development is the new C2A1 filter canister which is currently replacing the older C2 filter. Although both utilize a metal shell instead of one of the newer polymeric materials, the chief difference between the two filters is the type of carbon they employ. The C2 uses ASC type carbon whereas the C2A1 filter is fabricated with ASZM-TEDA type carbon (Canada's C2A1 standard filter uses TEDA treated ASC carbon). Performance specifications are virtually identical. The U.S. standard C-2 is also differentiated from the newer C2A1 by its black metallic color (the C2A1 is a dark green metallic color).

Racal Filter Technologies has approached the U.S. Government about possible adoption of the C-7 type filter, but the idea was rejected, 'compatibility' concerns with U.S. systems designed to use the existing C-2 filter design being identified as a possible problem area. A further argument was made that since two U.S. companies are currently capable of making the U.S. version C-2 filter, standardization of a plastic-bodied filter would offset favorable competition elements in the existing contracting process.

Also at this stage of development are several civilian NBC protective designs, although whether or not they end up being accepted and produced—especially in the cost-constrained 90s—is open to speculation (some of these are joint ILC/Edgewood projects).

As regards future directions for respirator design research, one identifiable trend seems to be exploration of 'whole head' respirator systems. Partly due to the persistent problem of obtaining adequate face-seal in conventional face-only masks and the inherent limitations in attempting to engineer discrete face-protection for a wide range of human facial configurations, new emphasis is being directed towards development of hood-type respirators which will fit a wide range of head sizes and accommodate considerations such as facial hair, gender, age differences, etc. A good example of this is the ILC *DERP* (Disposable Eye Respiratory Protection), which was originally produced in response to a U.S. Army specification requirement. The *DERP* was not procured in quantity by the U.S. military, despite the original anticipated need for a civilian NBC protective respirator design such as this, but it remains a very cost-effective, functionally sound and well conceived design for emergency NBC protection.

The 1991 Gulf War served admirably to remind the United States military establishment that chemical warfare threats are just as much a concern now than before—possibly more so now, in view of the lack of moral restraint which certain nations have demonstrated in the past several years (Iraq, notably). It is reasonable to hope that these reminders will keep U.S. NBC protection programs operative at least, if not flourishing, as a new era of finite resources, funding and materiel procurement capability is encountered in the 90s.

One hope is that the functional advantages and cost-effective benefits to be found in civilian protection designs such as the ILC *DERP* are not overlooked as NBC protection for the civilian population of the United States is given reduced priority due to fiscal realities America faces in the years ahead. The *possibility* of substantial quantities of such protective civilian NBC protection designs being needed in the immediate future, as the reality of cheaply developed and produced biological agents in the hands of terrorist groups and partisan extremist groups becomes the next great world concern, ought *not* to be completely overlooked or dismissed out of hand.

Spurred by both the harsh reality of future defense funding constraints and the need for continuing CBW protection development, a new task force has recently (1994) come into being within the U.S. Defense Department. This is the JSMG (Joint Service Material Group), established by the 1994 U.S. National Defense Authorization Act (Public Law 103-160: Title 17), which brings all the various existing CBW programs among the U.S. Armed Forces under a single DoD budget line, with the U.S. Army as executor. This will serve to assure continued development of CBW individual protection for all future military applications while trimming or eliminating costly duplications and redundancies.

Regarding the future of U.S. respirator development, it is to be hoped that new U.S. mask proposals will take advantage of the latest advances in polymer materials research and that materials selected for facepiece, lenses and component assemblies will be chosen with great and studied care. With the increasing costs of scientific technology forcing a new and unpleasant encounter with reality (vis-à-vis R&D costs), tolerance for expensively flawed and inordinately protracted respirator development programs will no longer be forthcoming.

These words of caution should not be misconstrued as denigrating the excellent individual efforts of those involved in our NBC protection programs; *they should, however, make it clear that better coordination and control of such complex and costly projects is a requisite for future success*. This will now hopefully be more of a reality with the new JSMG structure in place, despite the unfortunate likelihood that military funding excesses in non-essential areas and cutbacks in areas of demonstrated, practical need shall continue—to a certain degree—as they always have.

Conceivably, systems such as state-of-the-art CAD/CAM facilities will help forecast and eliminate potential problems, leading to less costly resolutions and more efficient development. CAD/CAM has been increasingly incorporated into all areas of military and civil research and development; excellent examples of CAD/CAM applications are to be found in the Canadian C-4 and Swedish F2 military respirator designs, which profited greatly through their use.[3] CAD/CAM has, of course, been used for years in aircraft and space research, so it is appropriate that such benefits may finally be routinely accessed in NBC protection development work as well.

State of the art technology remains merely a tool, regardless of how valuable a tool it is, and it should never be forgotten that advanced scientific know how is not a substitute for basic soundness in planning, coordination and carry-through of thoughtfully conceived and efficiently organized projects. Without philosophical integrity and careful management, technology can be a costly and monstrous liability, potentially outweighing the anticipated benefits implicit in its utility.

PHOTO SECTION
British Small Box Respirator

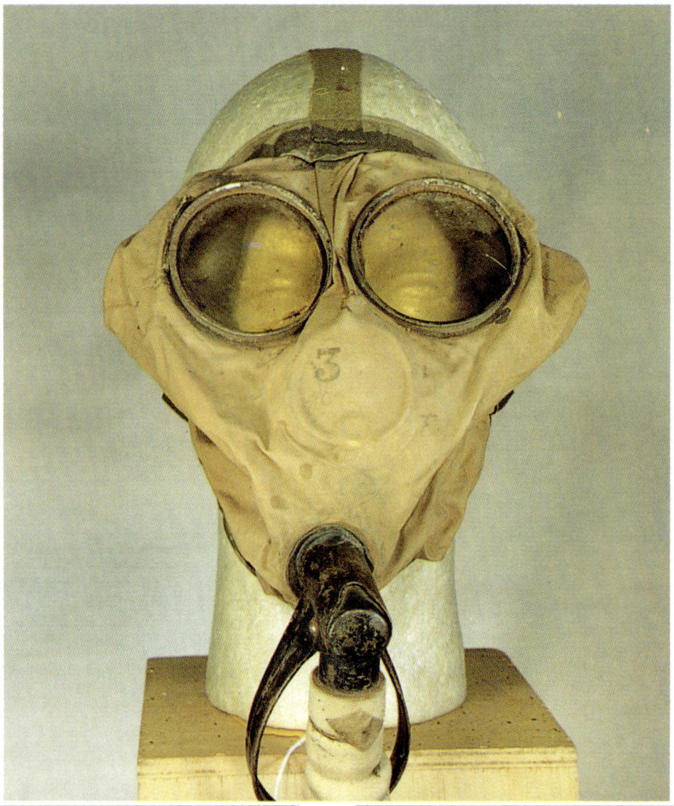

British Small Box Respirator (BSBR), example no. 1. Size is indicated by numeral 3 on facepiece. The rubber flapper exhalation valve is missing.

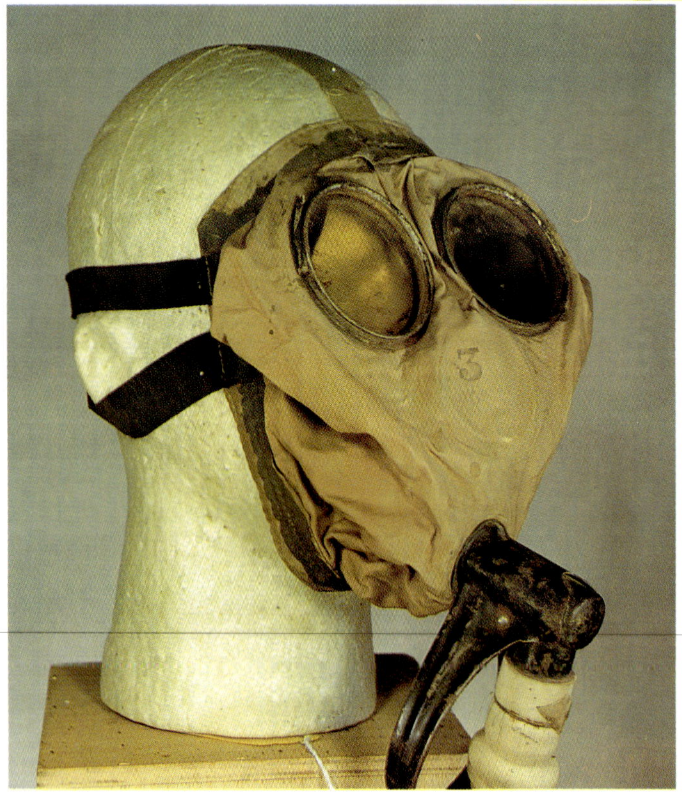

British Small Box Respirator (BSBR), example no. 1. Note string used to secure lenses to frames.

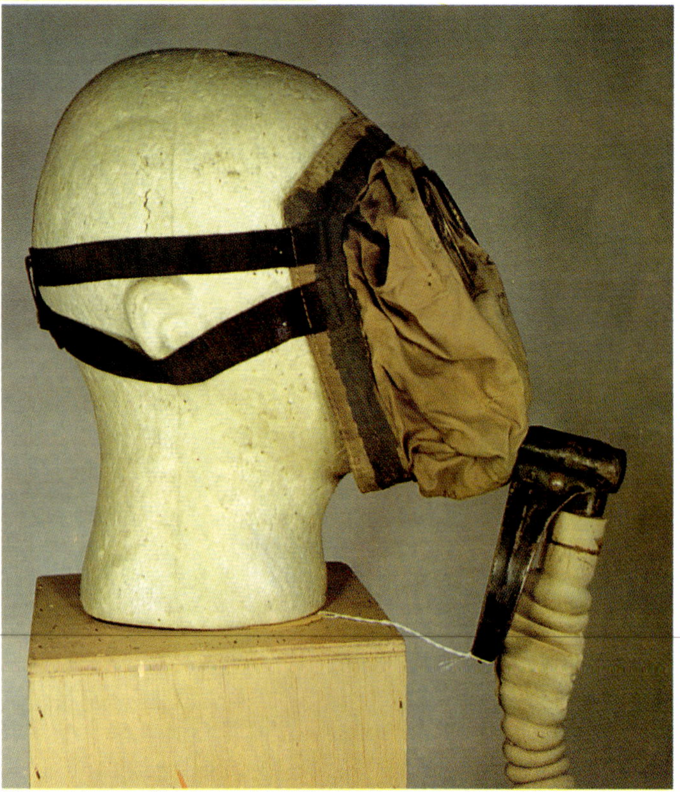

British Small Box Respirator (BSBR), example no. 1.

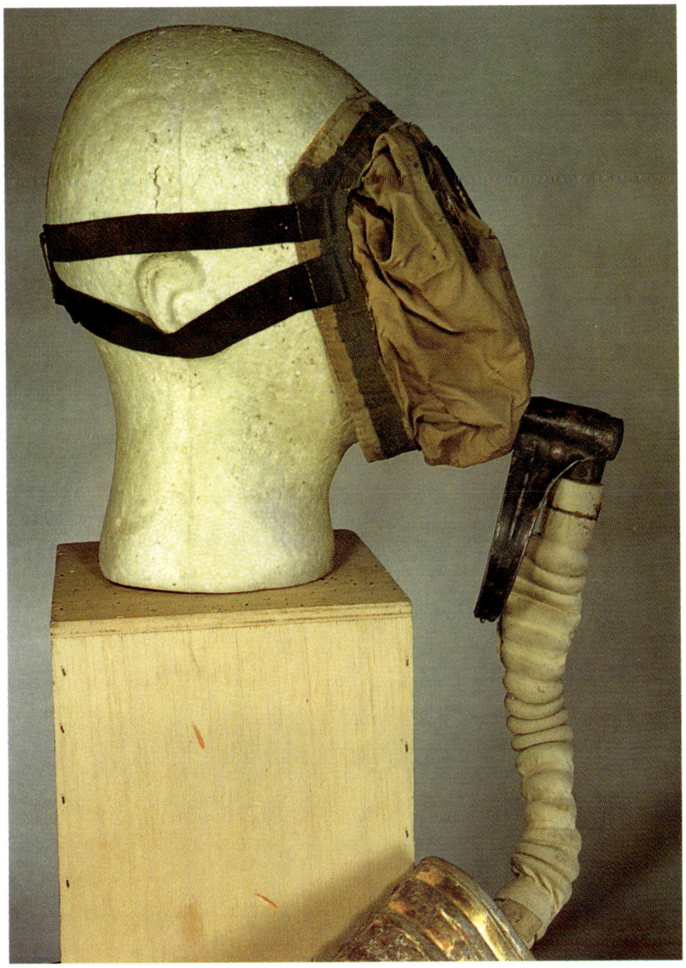

British Small Box Respirator (BSBR), example no. 1. Note distinctive yellow tinge of lacquered sheen on natural metal filter canister, a feature quite different from U.S. filters patterned on the BSBR.

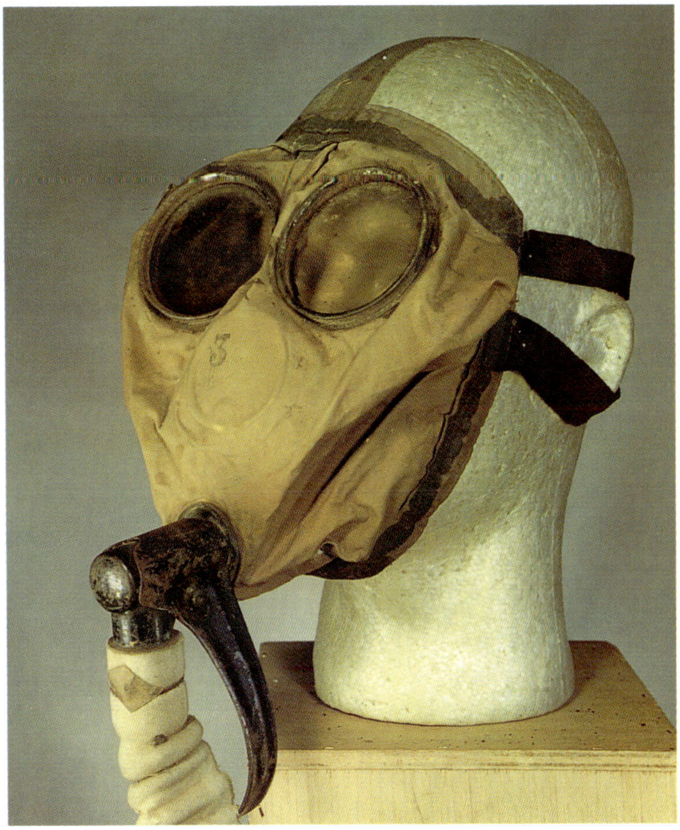

British Small Box Respirator (BSBR), example no. 1. Semi-circular exhaust valve guard shape was characteristic of BSBR.

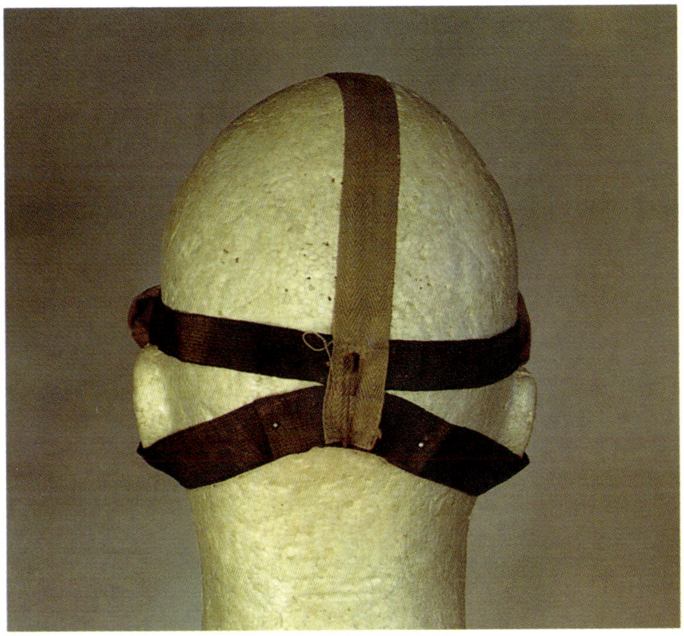

British Small Box Respirator (BSBR), example no. 1. Five strap harness included a safety pin for sizing; lateral straps were elasticized, while the top strap was made of non-stretching fabric.

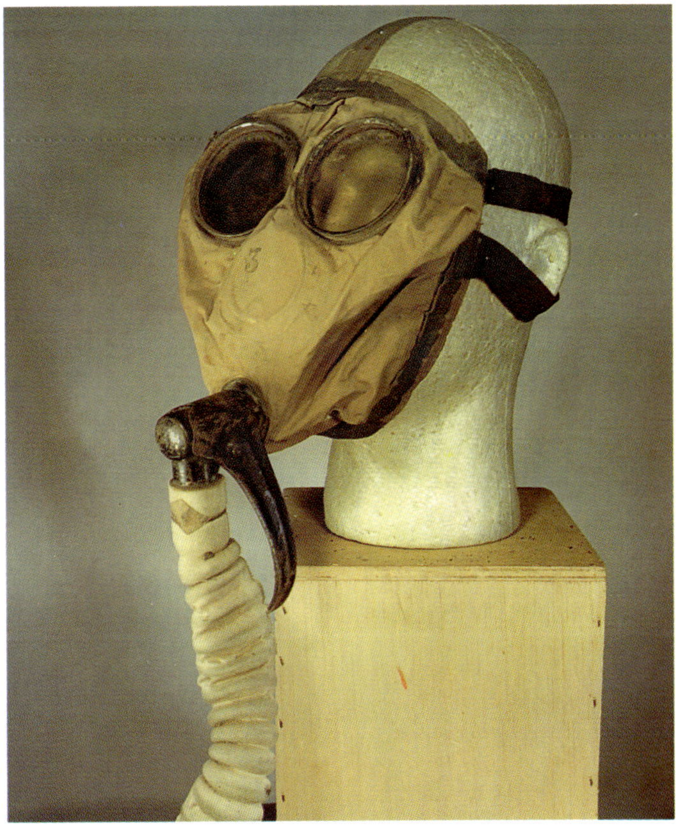

British Small Box Respirator (BSBR), example no. 1.

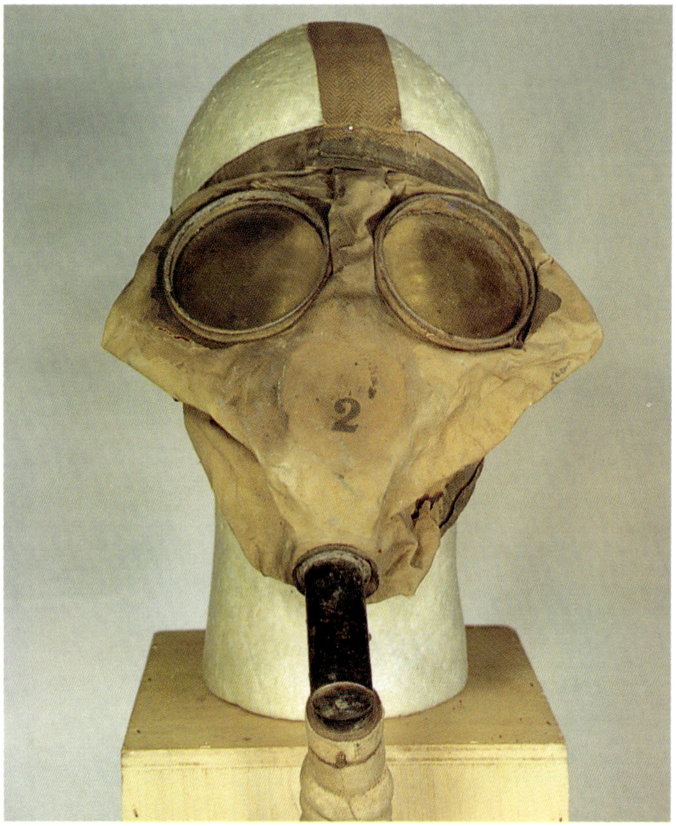

British Small Box Respirator (BSBR), example no. 2. Size indicated as "2" by numeral.

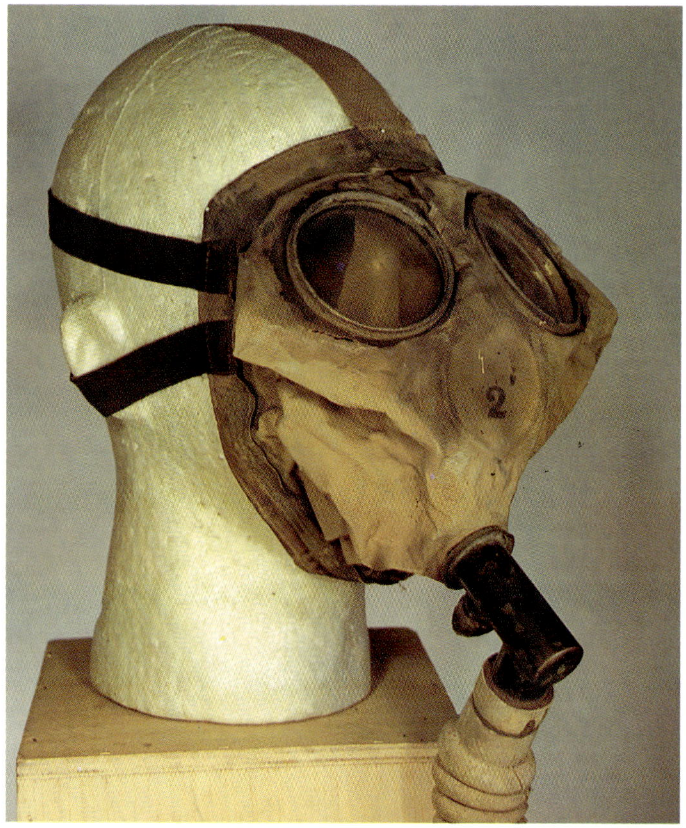

British Small Box Respirator (BSBR), example no. 2. This specimen lacks the metal exhalation valve guard, having been manufactured without it attached (the rubber exhalation valve is missing).

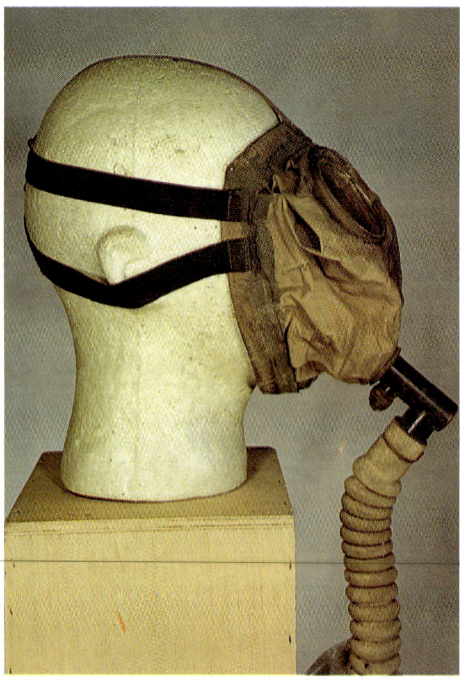

British Small Box Respirator (BSBR), example no. 2.

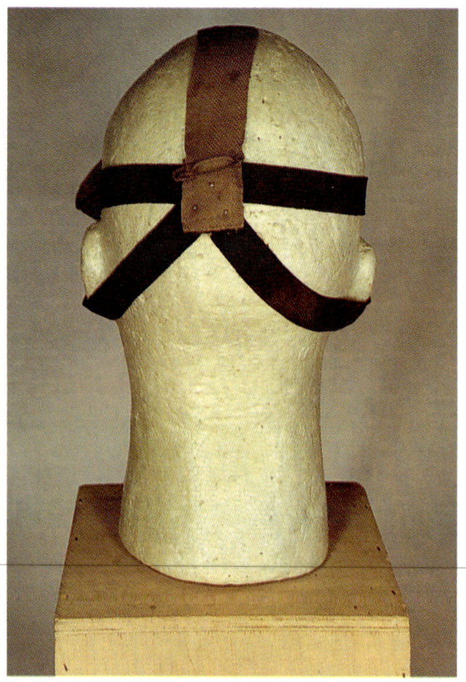

British Small Box Respirator (BSBR), example no. 2. This specimen had a slightly reinforced fabric strap juncture at the rear of the head, but featured the ubiquitous safety pin.

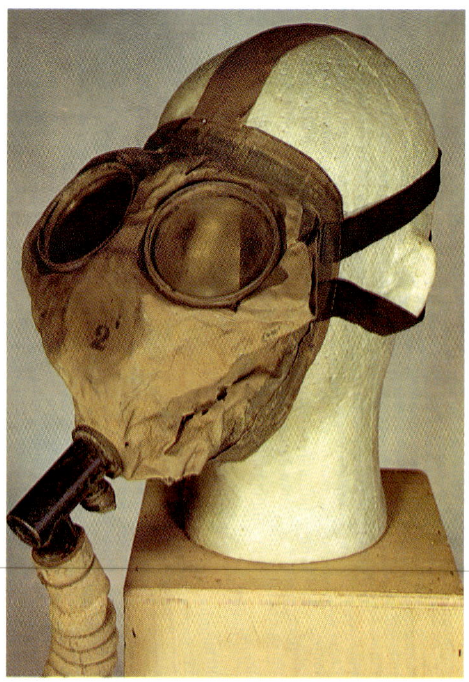

British Small Box Respirator (BSBR), example no. 2. Left side of the facepiece is in very obvious state of disrepair, typical of the effects of time and exposure on these old masks.

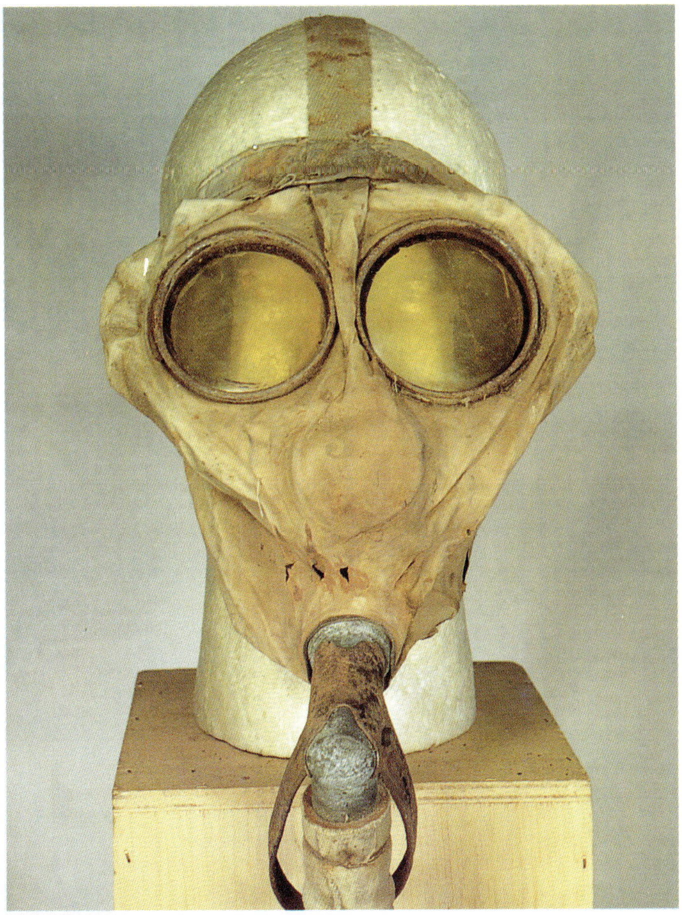

British Small Box Respirator (BSBR), example no. 3. Sizing numeral is barely visible.

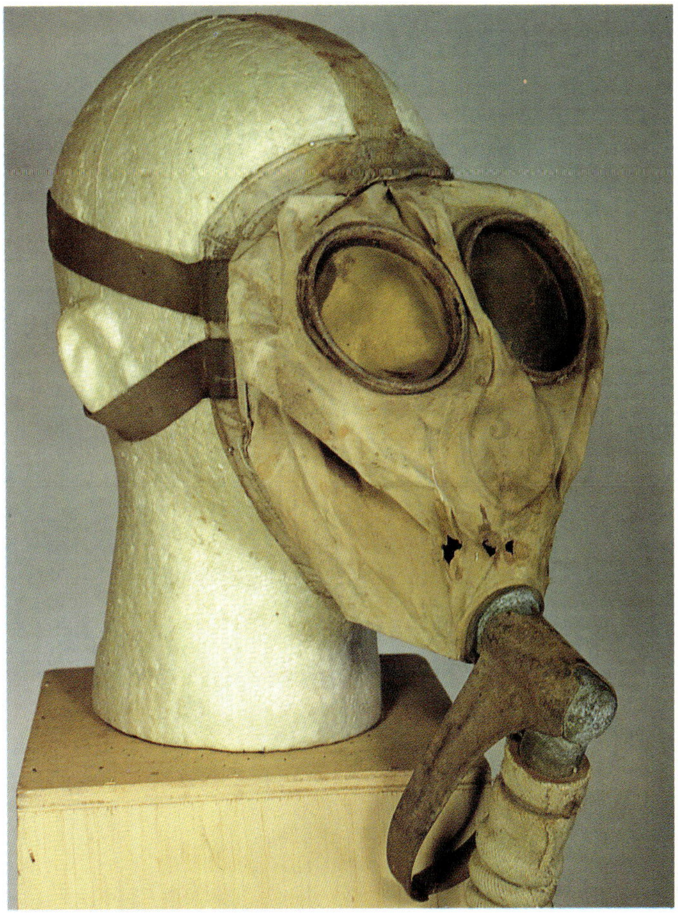

British Small Box Respirator (BSBR), example no. 3. Some detail of the eye lens string may be seen, and the poor state of the fabric facepiece is apparent.

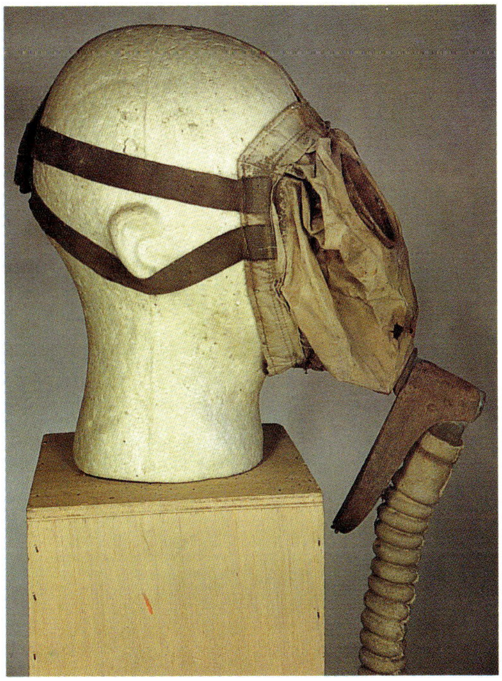

British Small Box Respirator (BSBR), example no. 3.

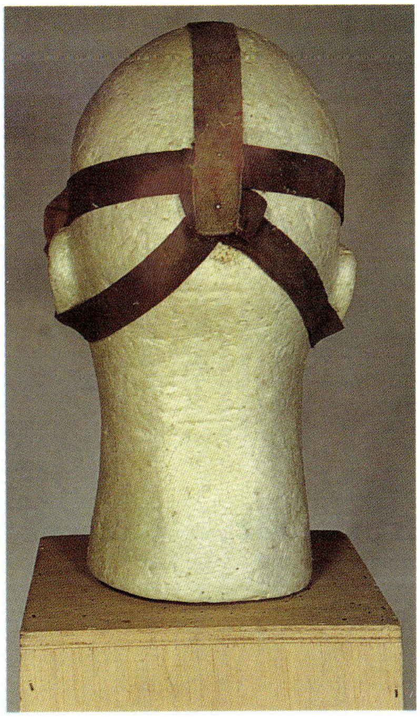

British Small Box Respirator (BSBR), example no. 3. The elasticized harness straps have been tucked and pinned, due to stretching effects. The safety pin is missing.

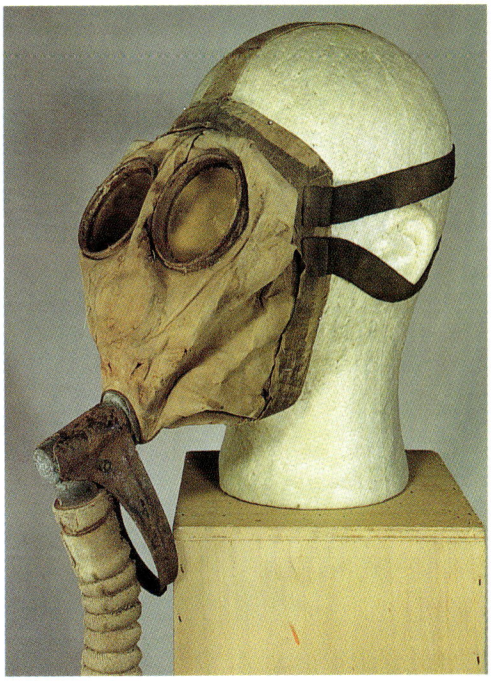

British Small Box Respirator (BSBR), example no. 3. The shape of the exhalation valve guard is easily discerned, due to the differing oxidation on it (as compared to the 'angle-tube' it is fitted to).

American Small Box Respirator ("Training Mask")

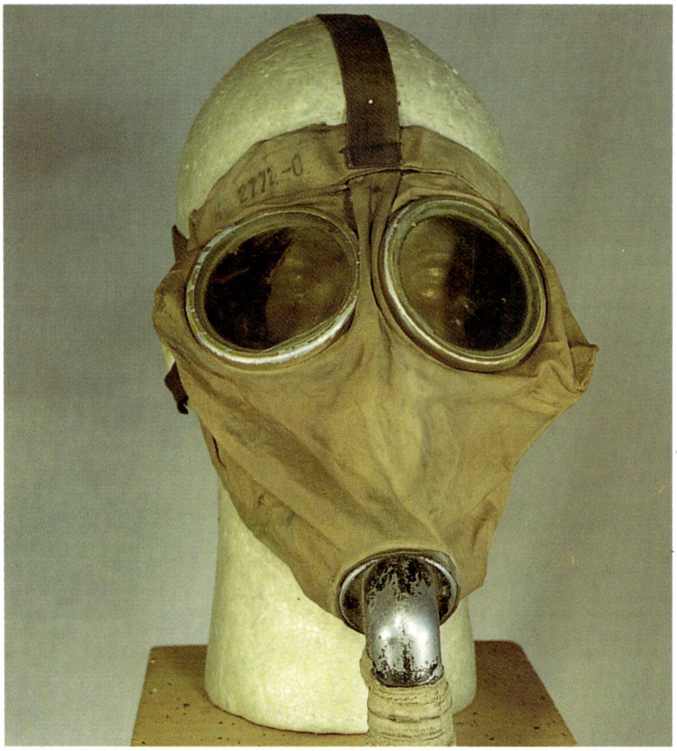

American Small Box Respirator (ASBR, also called 'the Training Mask'). A poorly conceived copy of the BSBR, there was no exhalation valve guard. Khaki colored metal eye frames are press-fitted. Aluminum 'angle tube' was painted black.

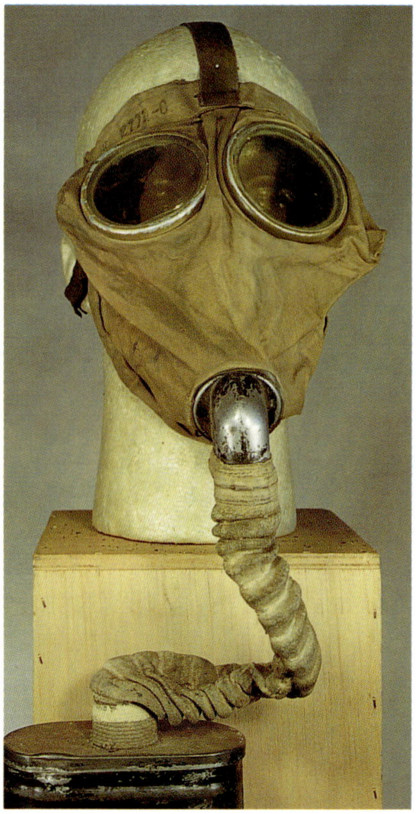

American Small Box Respirator (ASBR, also called 'the Training Mask'). Poor state of the fabric covered, corrugated rubber hose is typical of almost all surviving examples. Black painted filter canister is characteristic of ASBR; it was taller than the subsequent 'H' and 'J' canisters. Red painted top of filter indicates "training purposes only—do not use against gas," an easily seen indicator when the filter is stowed in place in the carrying satchel.

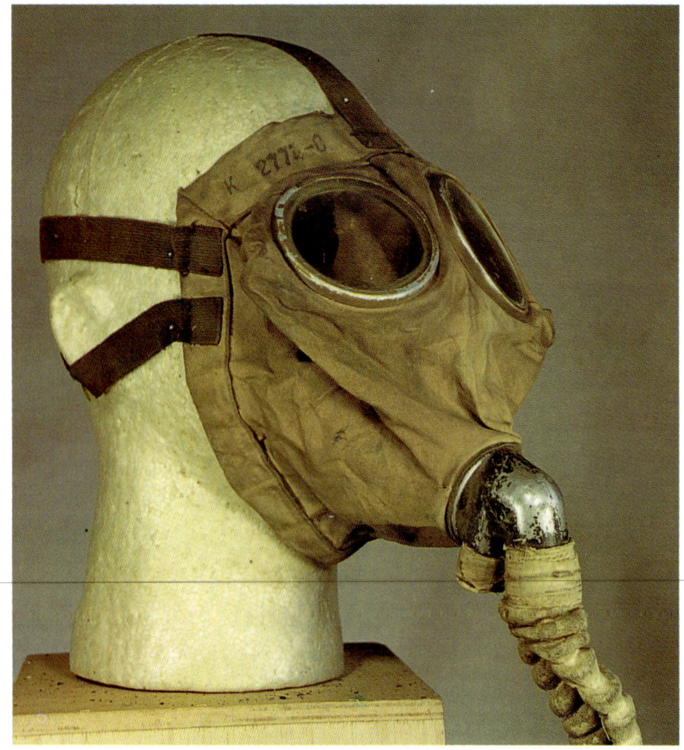

American Small Box Respirator (ASBR, also called 'the Training Mask'). Rubber MI exhalation valve is missing from 'angle tube'.

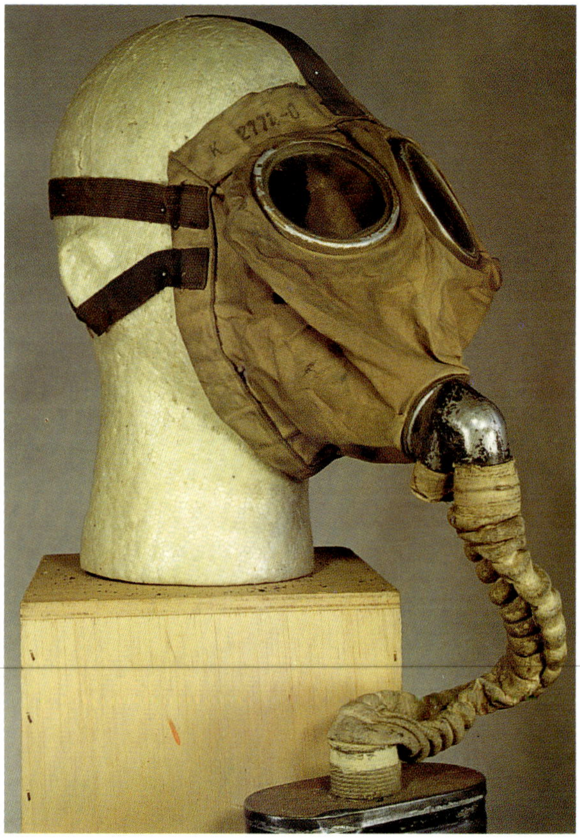

American Small Box Respirator (ASBR, also called 'the Training Mask').

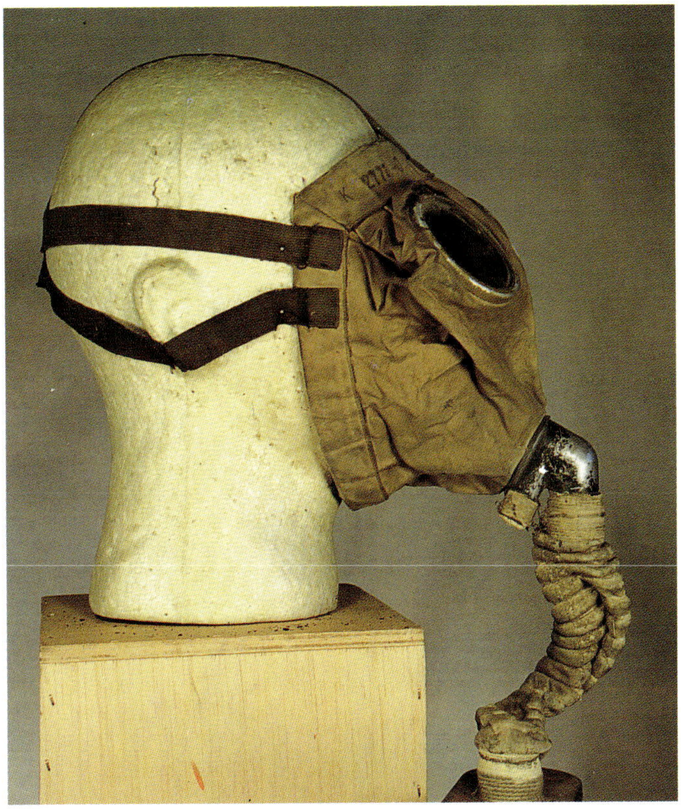

American Small Box Respirator (ASBR, also called 'the Training Mask').

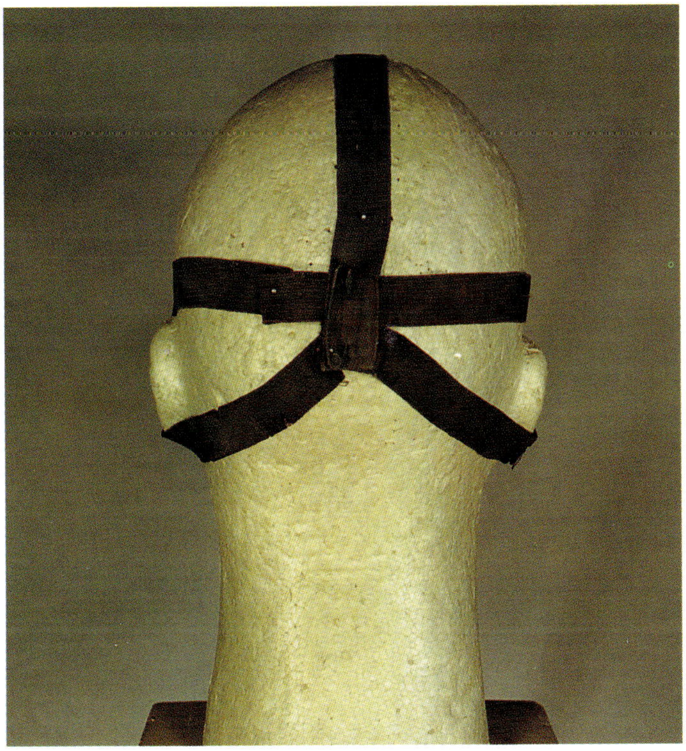

American Small Box Respirator (ASBR, also called 'the Training Mask'). Lateral head harness straps were elasticized; central (forehead) strap was made of non-elastic, black fabric. Straps have been pinned, due to stretching effects of time and exposure. Safety pin is standard, as with BSBR.

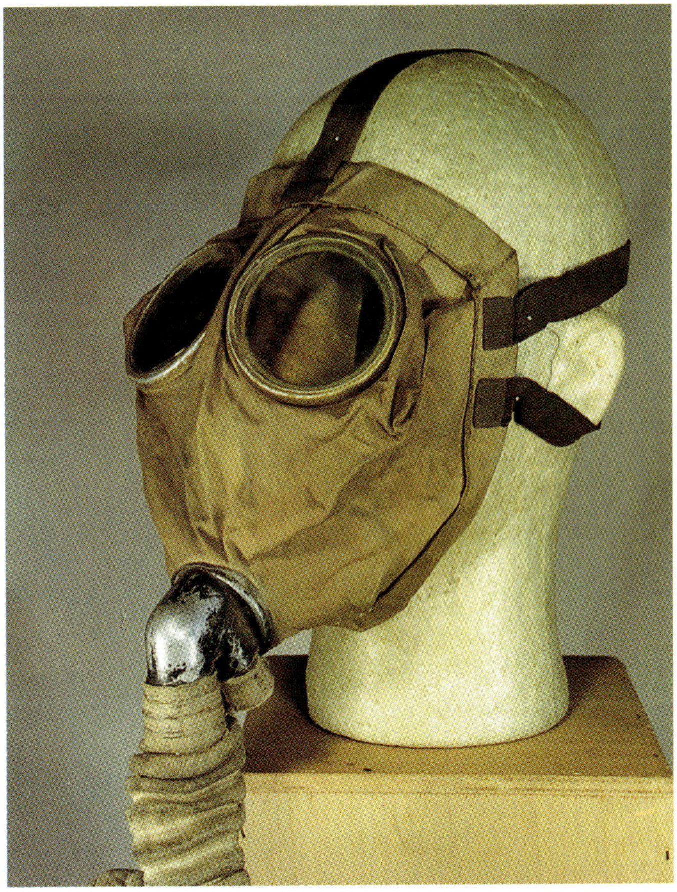

American Small Box Respirator (ASBR, also called 'the Training Mask').

Corrected English Model

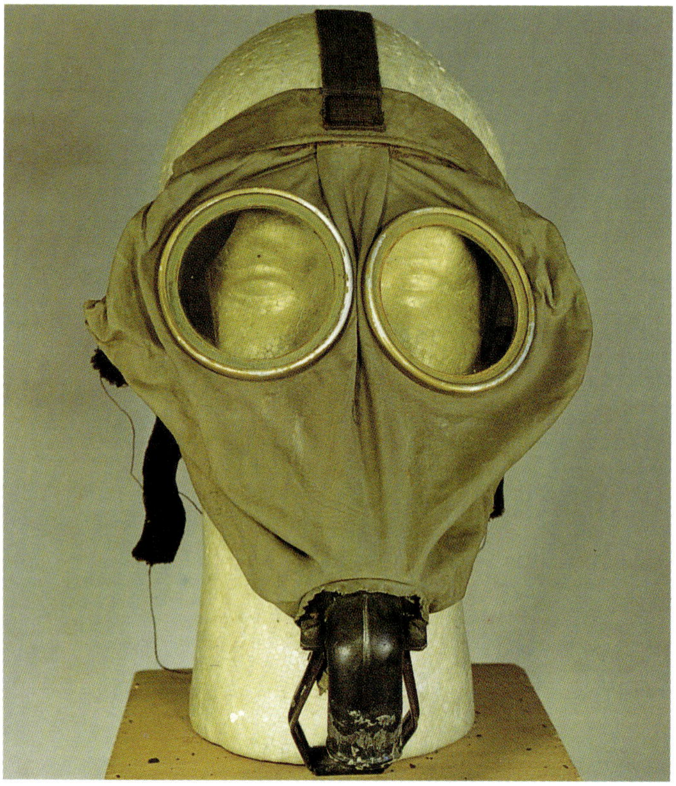

Corrected English Model (C.E.M.), shown without hose attached to 'angle tube' for clarity. A total of 1,864,000 C.E.M. masks were produced.

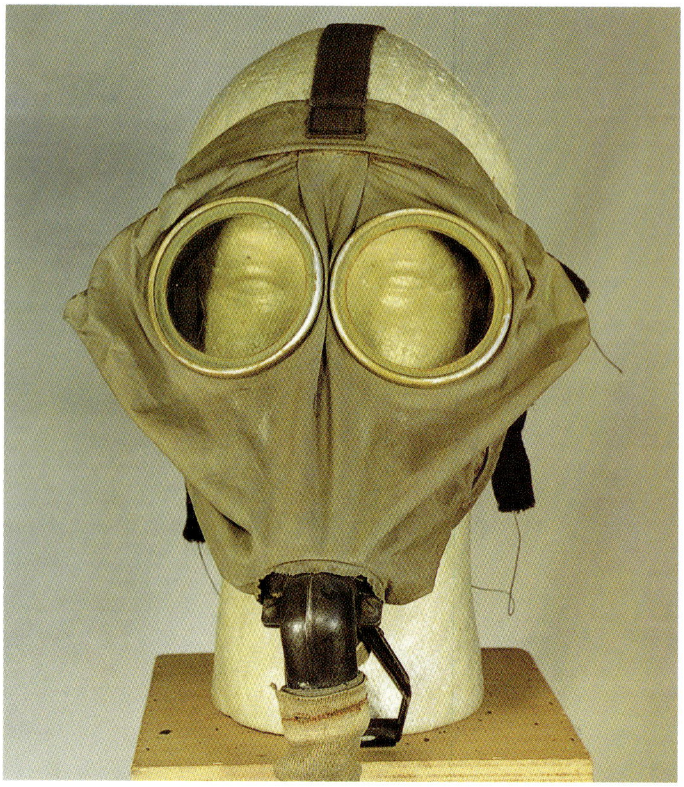

Corrected English Model (C.E.M.), example no. 1, with stockinet-covered, corrugated rubber hose attached.

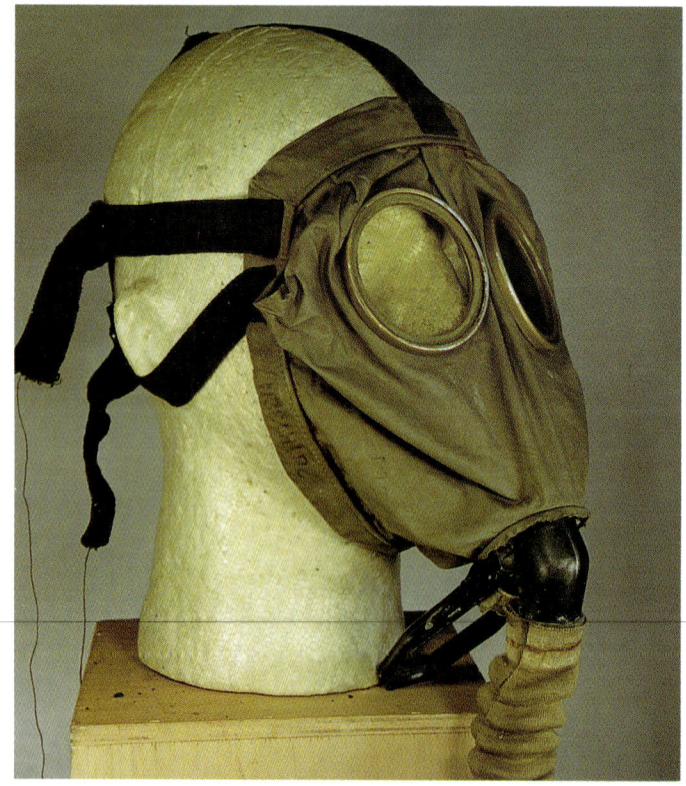

Corrected English Model (C.E.M.), example no. 1. Rubber MI style exhalation valve is missing.

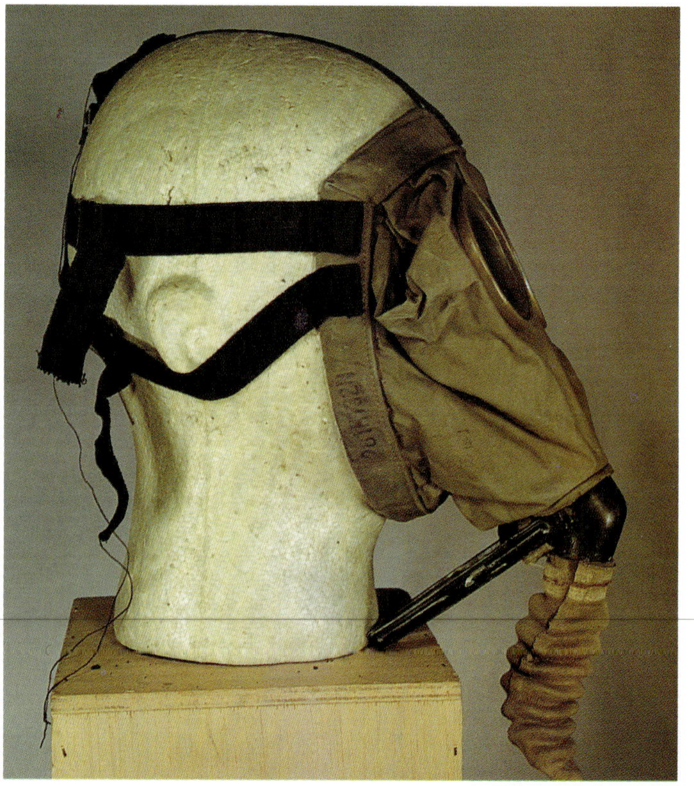

Corrected English Model (C.E.M.), example no. 1. Some details of exhalation valve (missing) guard and its attachment to 'angle tube' may be observed.

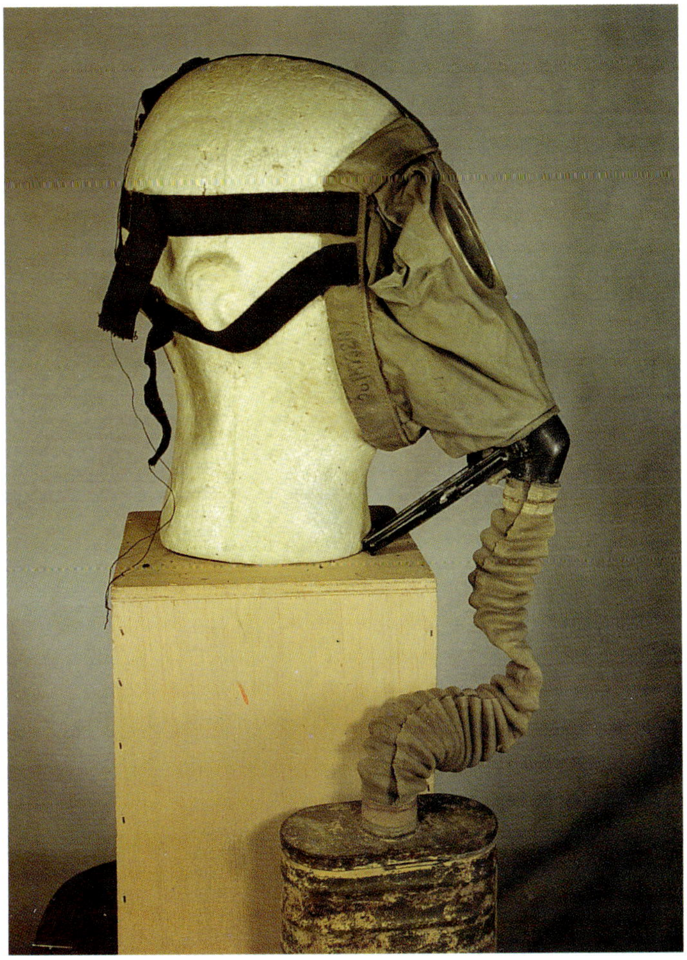

Corrected English Model (C.E.M.), example no. 1. The C.E.M. was typically issued with the yellow painted "H" filter canister attached, which is slightly shorter than the black ASBR filter canister. Much of the paint on this example has worn away.

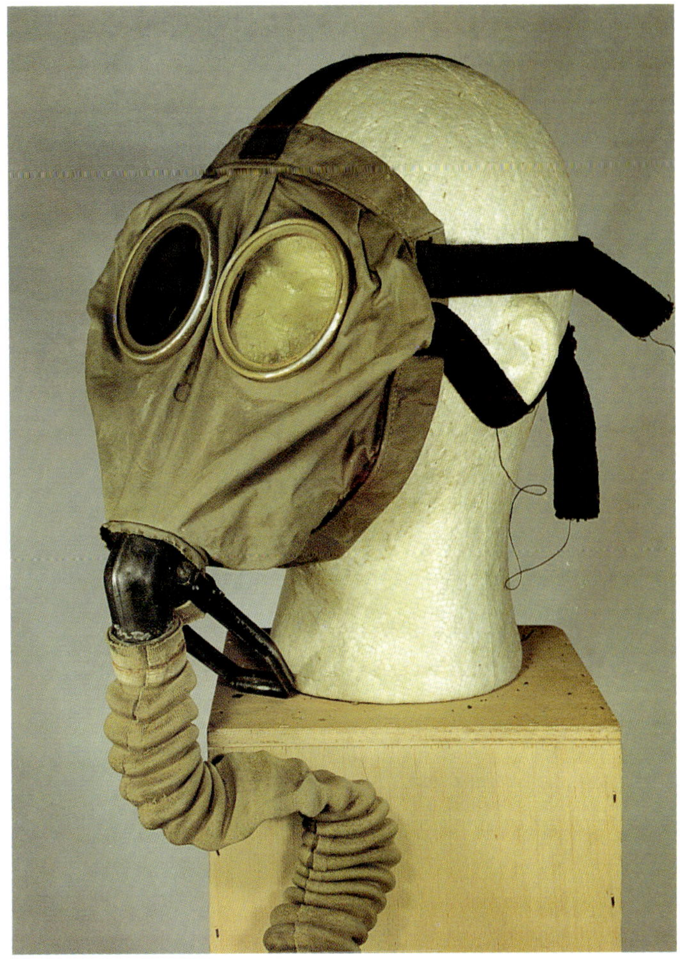

Corrected English Model (C.E.M.), example no. 1. Face sizing numeral is barely visible in central crease of facepiece (between and slightly below eyes).

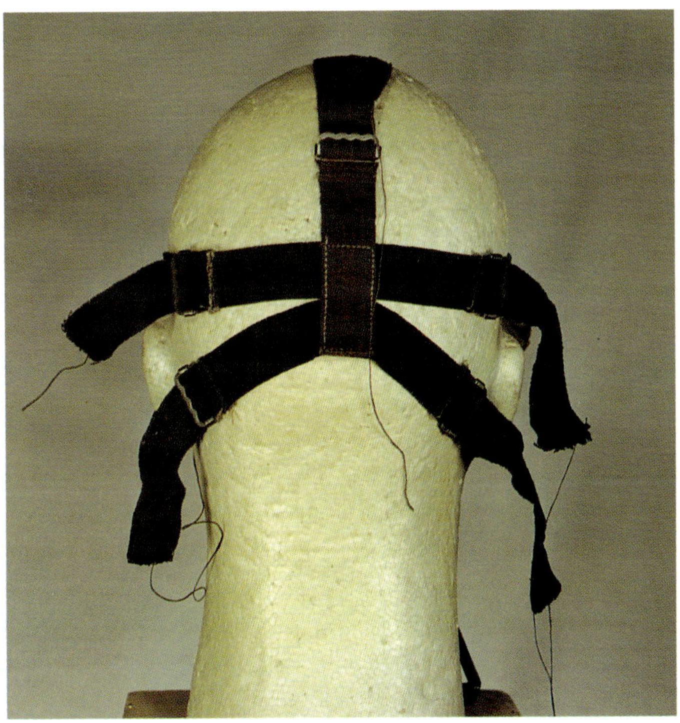

Corrected English Model (C.E.M.), example no. 1. Unusual is the fully adjustable head harness, with 5 buckles—a feature most C.E.M.s did not have. Lateral straps are elasticized, top strap is not.

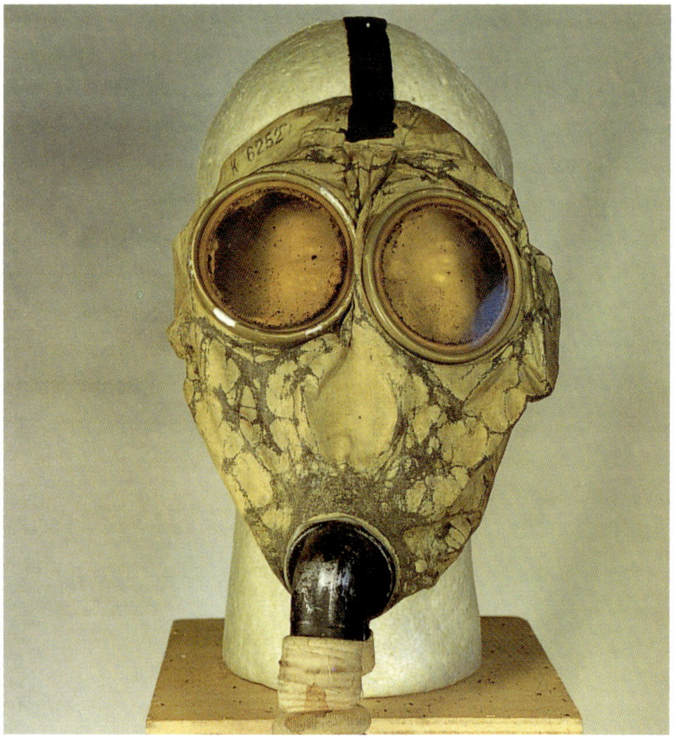

Corrected English Mask (C.E.M.), example no 2. Stiff facepiece fabric is typical of many surviving examples of WWI masks.

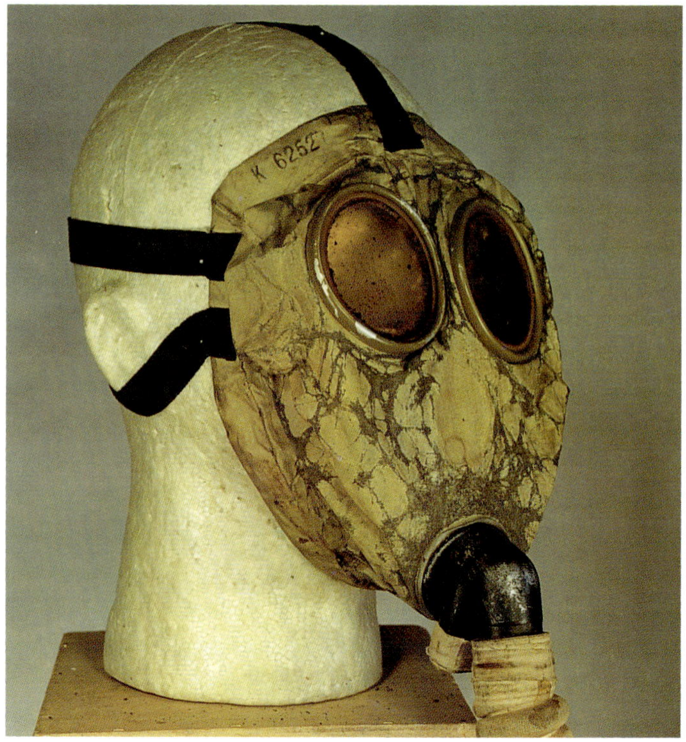

Corrected English Model (C.E.M.), example no. 2. Rubber MI exhalation valve is missing; there is no guard fitted.

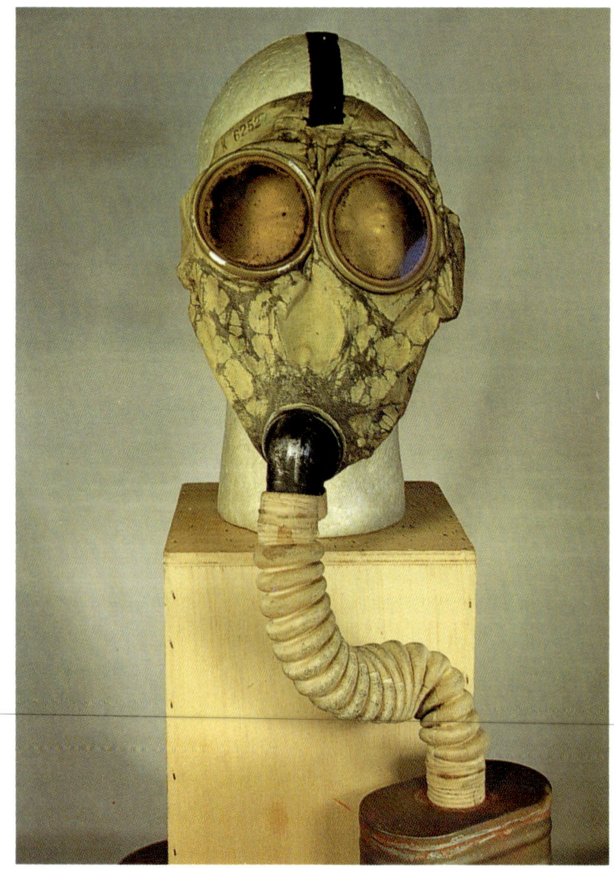

Corrected English Mask (C.E.M.), example no 2. Filter canister has been painted red for training use only, although most of the color has worn off.

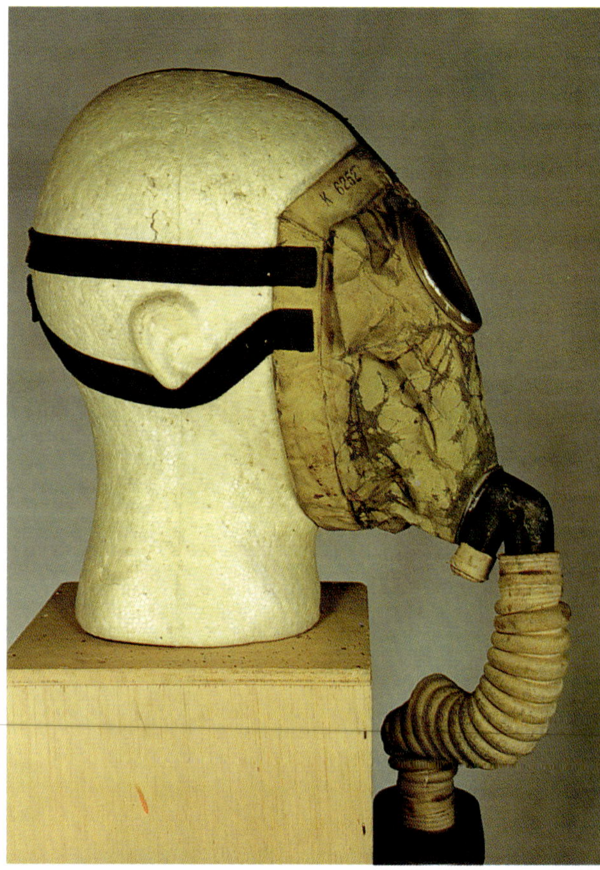

Corrected English Model (C.E.M.), example no. 2. Good view of aluminum 'angle tube' and production control number stamped on right upper exterior of facepiece.

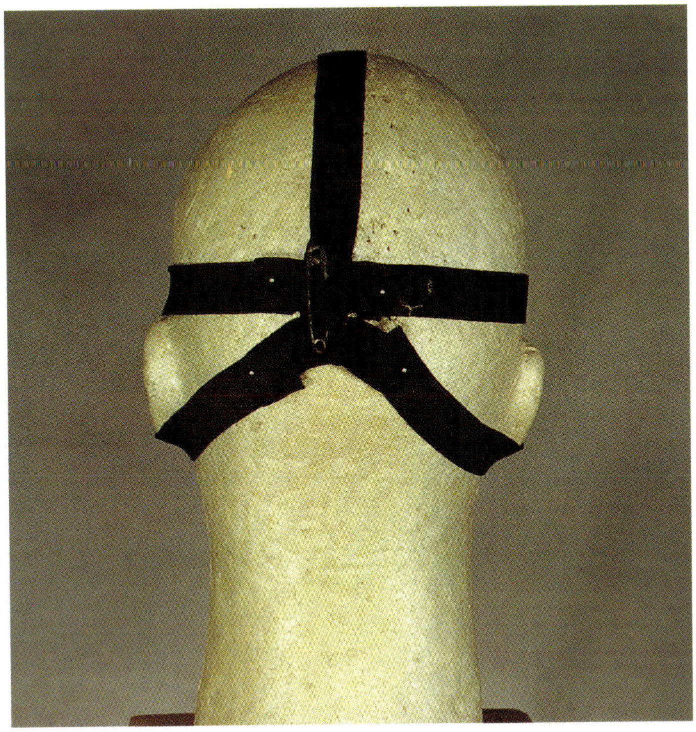

Corrected English Model (C.E.M.), example no 2. Typical 5 strap C.E.M. head harness (non adjustable), with two later elasticized straps and a non-stretching fabric top-strap.

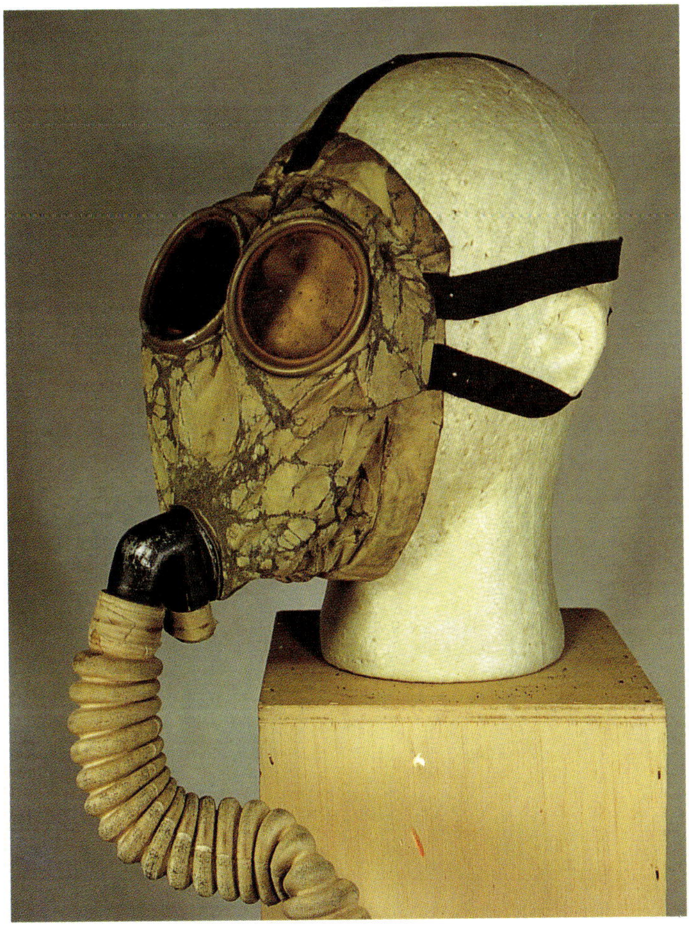

Corrected English Model (C.E.M.), example no. 2.

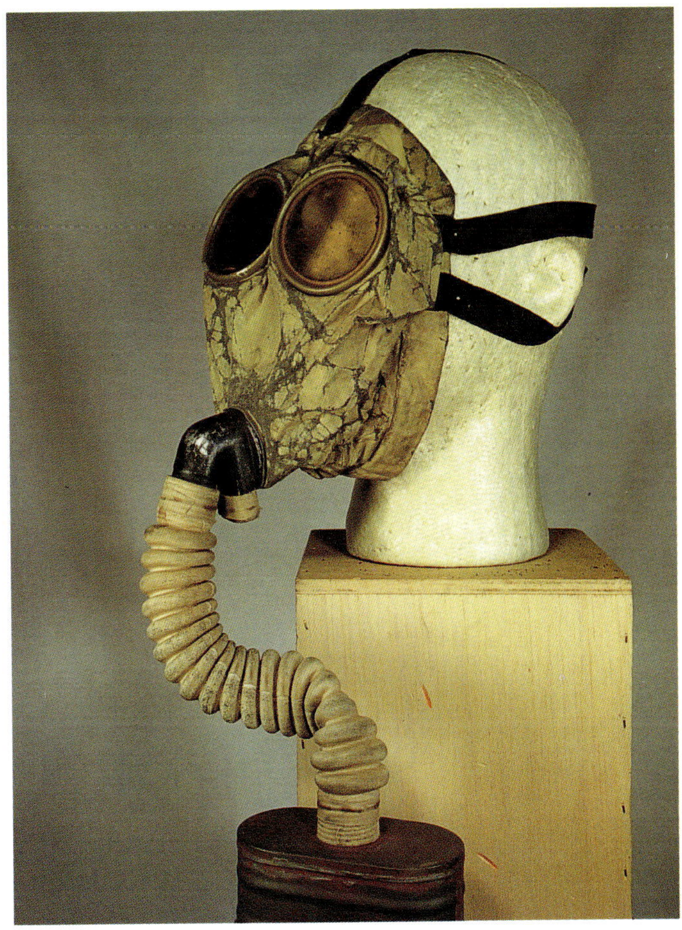

Corrected English Model (C.E.M.), example no. 2.

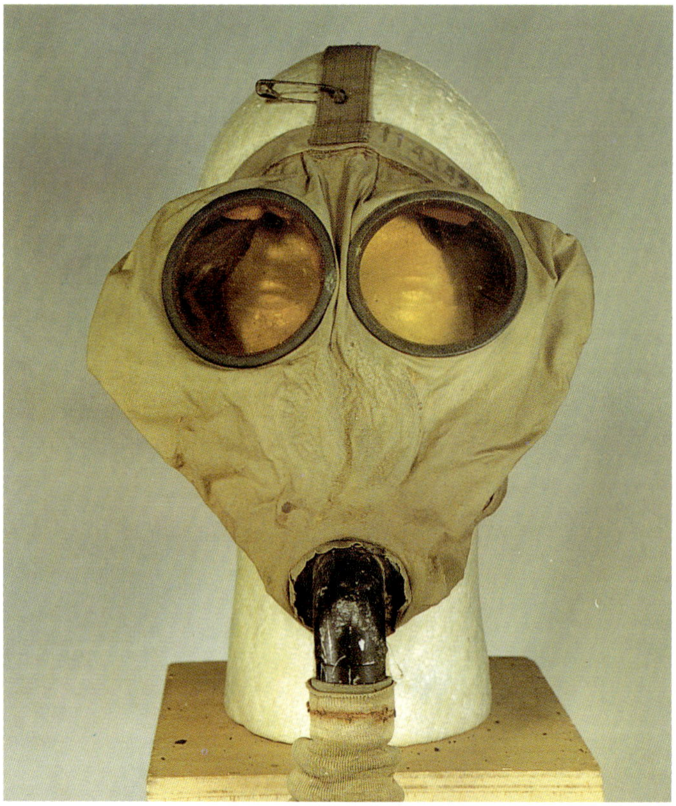

Corrected English Model (C.E.M.), example no. 3. Eye frames are an earlier C.E.M. type.

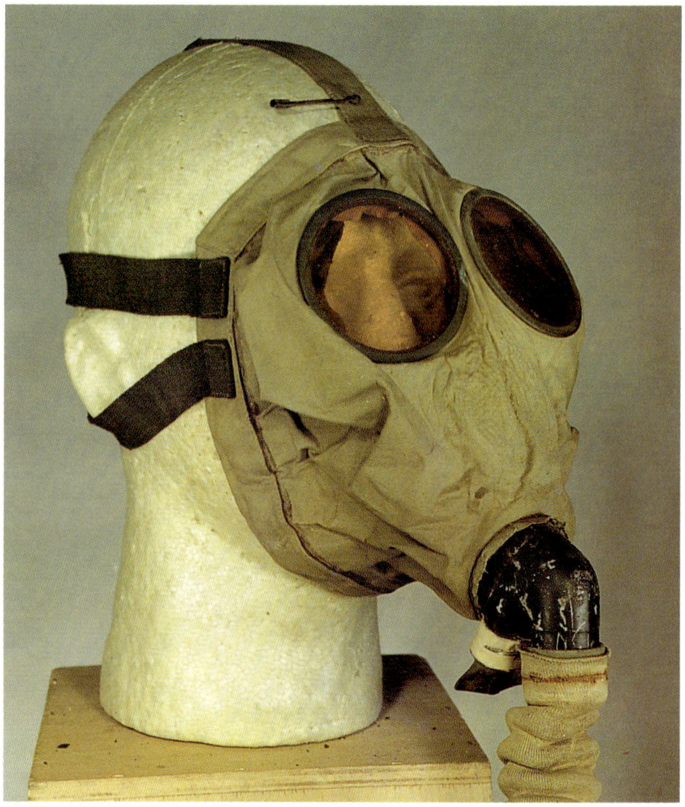

Corrected English Model (C.E.M.), example no. 3. Most of the rubber exhalation valve is missing but the facepiece is in exceptionally good condition (very soft and pliable). Top of yellow "H" filter canister is visible, connected to typically distorted stockinet-covered rubber hose.

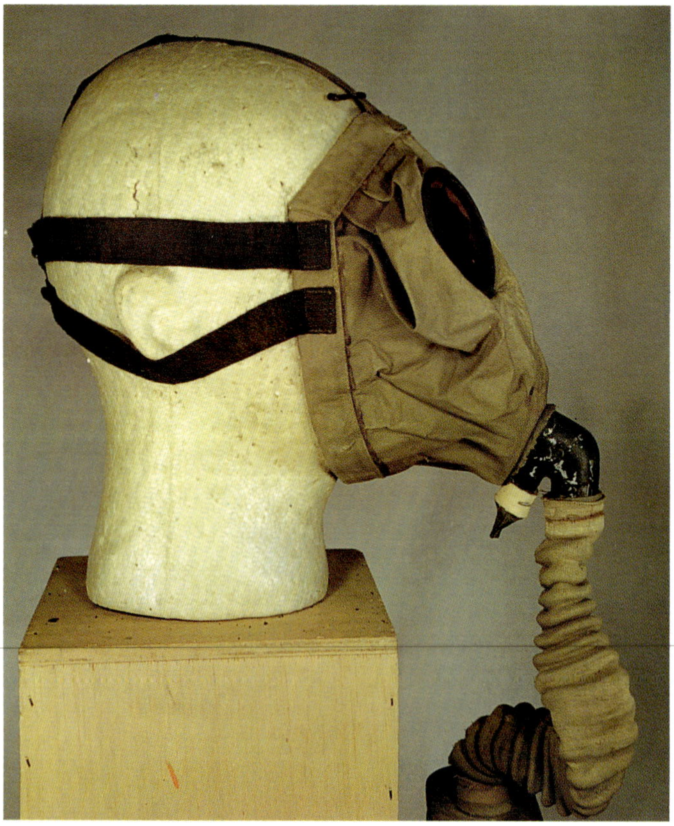

Corrected English Model (C.E.M.), example no. 3, side view detail.

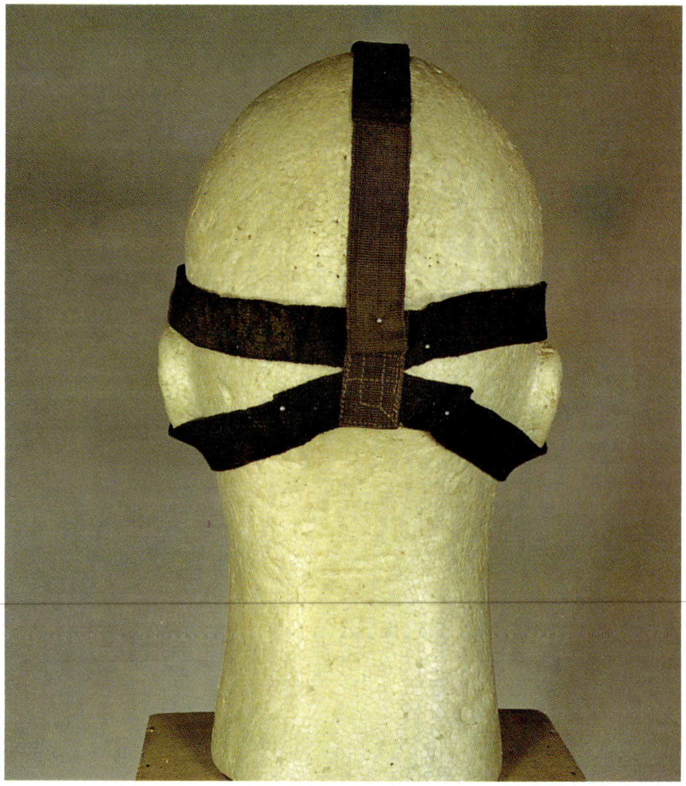

Corrected English Model (C.E.M.), example no. 3. Typical C.E.M. 5-strap harness (although top strap, made of non-stretching fabric, is dark khaki color).

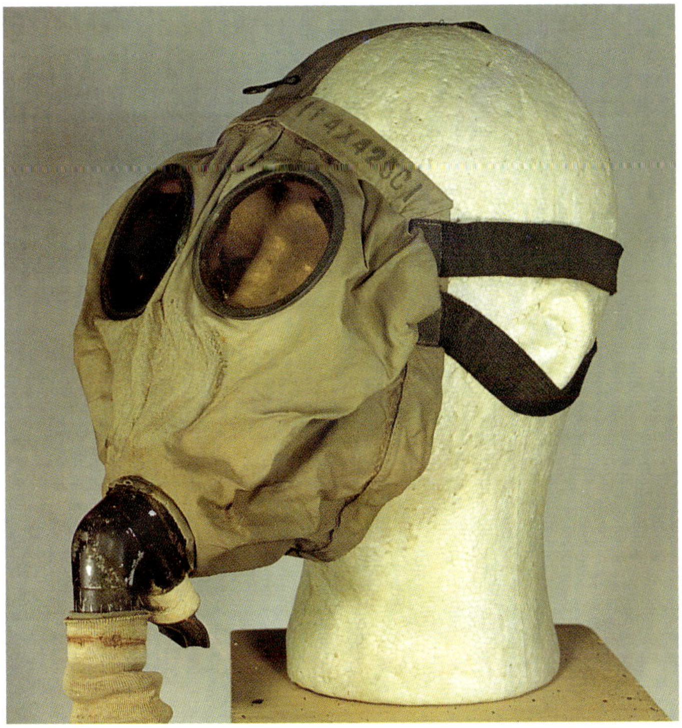

Corrected English Mask (C.E.M.), example no. 3. Hose was secured to 'angle tube' by a single strand of wire, covered by wound adhesive cloth tape.

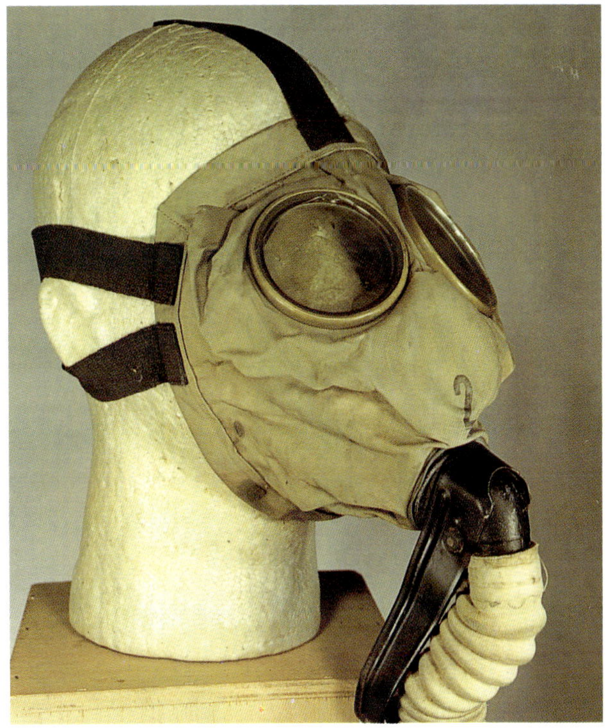

Corrected English Model (C.E.M.), example no. 4. Facepiece is well-preserved, soft and pliable, with intact inner rubberized layer. The rubber MI style exhalation 'flapper' valve, which is missing on this mask, has the later metal guard fitted in place on the 'angle tube.'

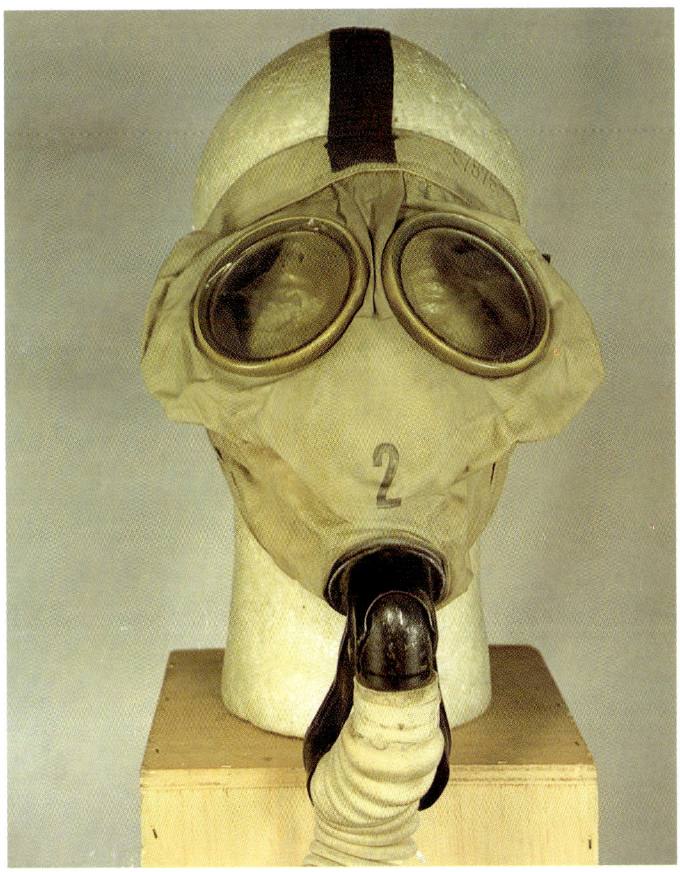

Corrected English Model (C.E.M.), example no. 4. Sizing numeral is clear and distinct.

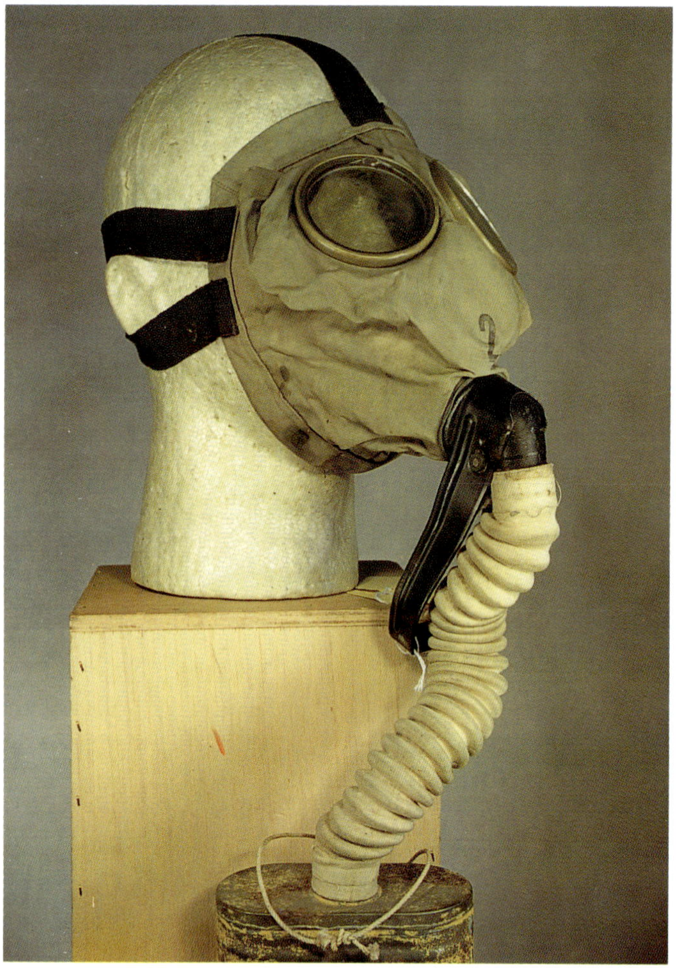

Corrected English Model (C.E.M.), example no. 4. Yellow "H" filter canister may be seen attached to the well-preserved stockinet-covered rubber hose. The cord visible secures the 'use and maintenance record,' which was provided with each mask to monitor filter exposure (to gases) status.

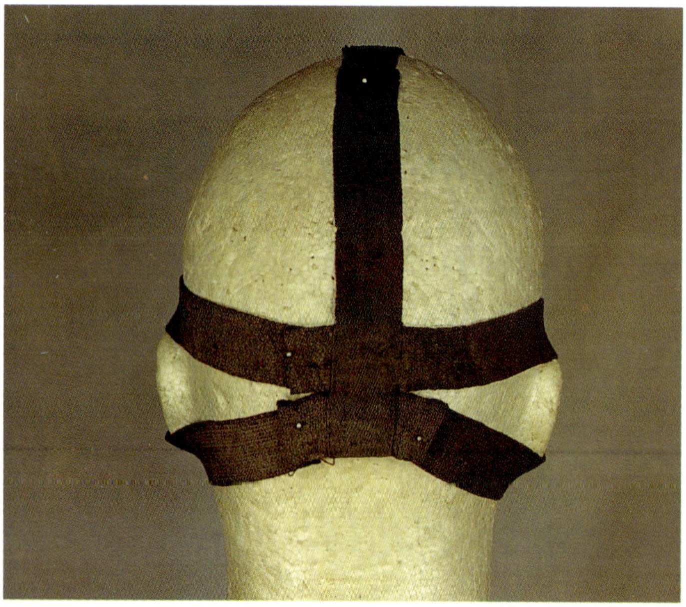

Corrected English Model (C.E.M.), example no. 4. Unusually, the top strap on this C.E.M. is also elastic (straps have been tucked and pinned, due to over stretching).

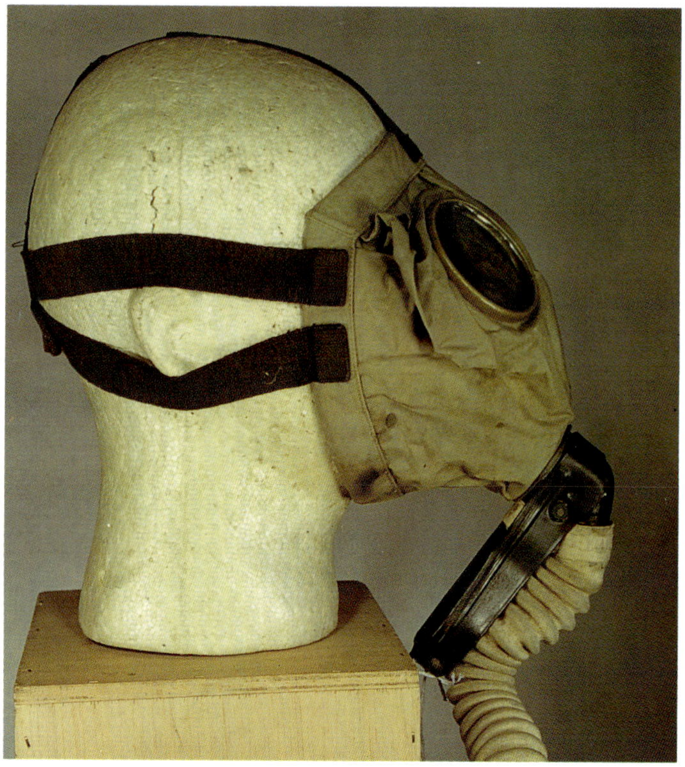

Corrected English Model (C.E.M.), example no. 4. When properly sized, lateral straps went over and under ears.

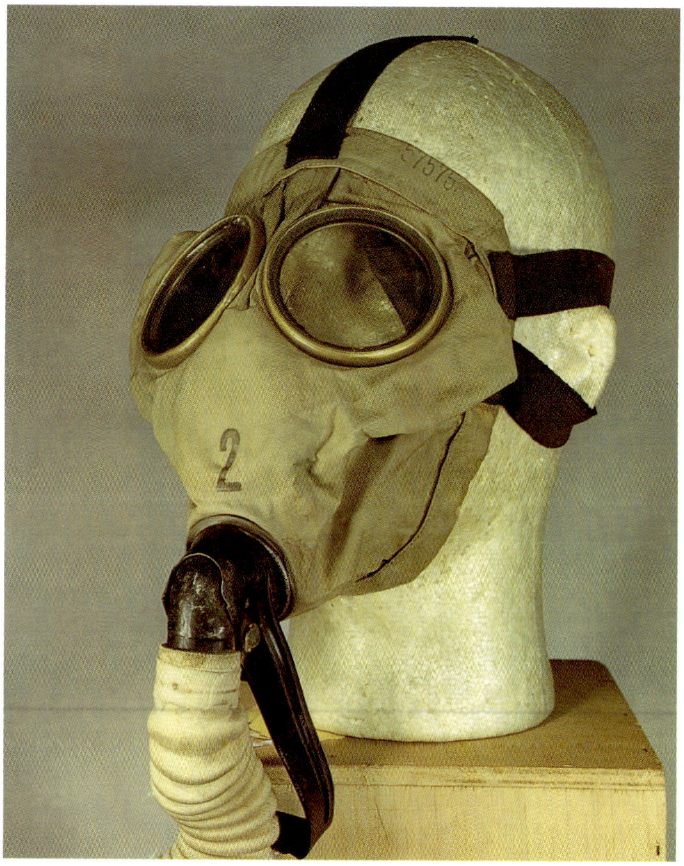

Corrected English Model (C.E.M.), example no. 4. This example has glass/celluloid sandwich lenses

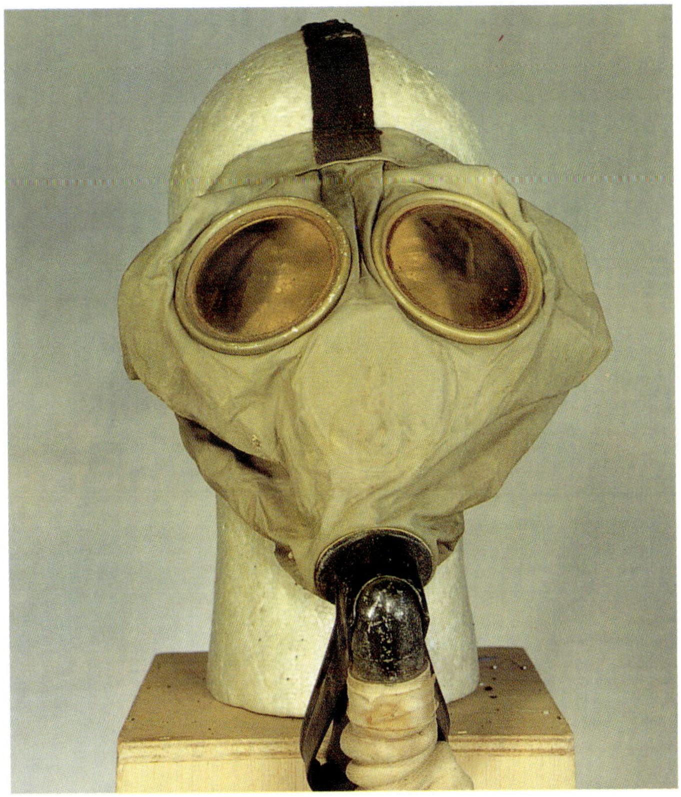

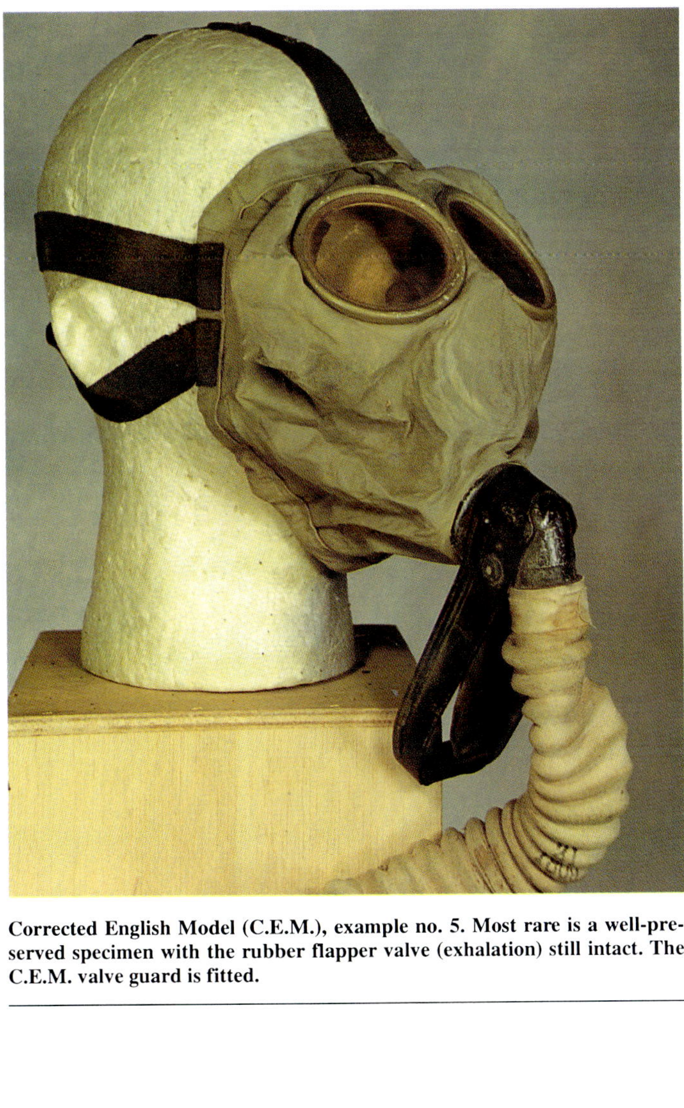

Corrected English Model (C.E.M.), example no. 5. Most rare is a well-preserved specimen with the rubber flapper valve (exhalation) still intact. The C.E.M. valve guard is fitted.

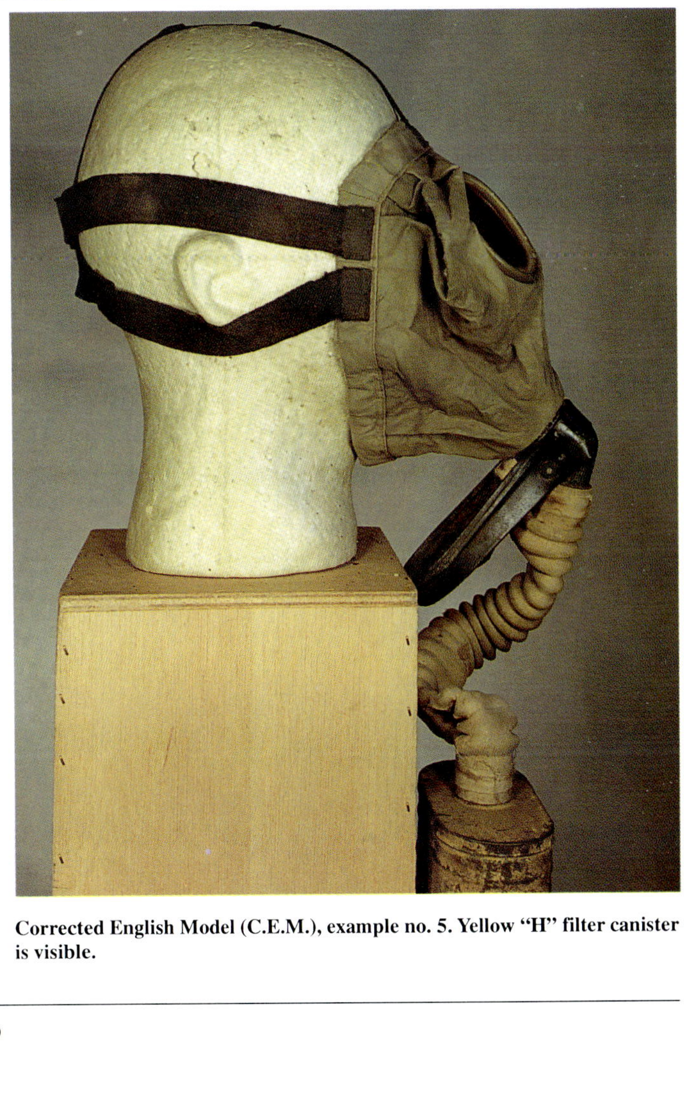

Corrected English Model (C.E.M.), example no. 5. Yellow "H" filter canister is visible.

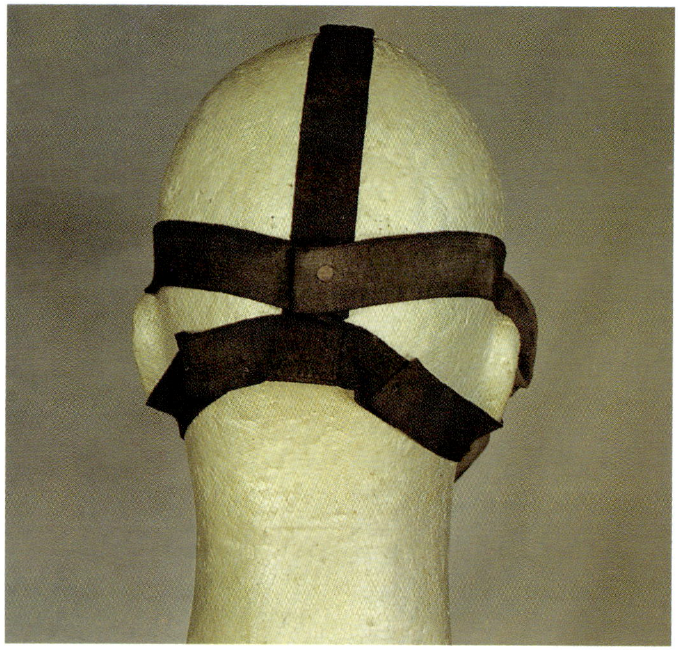

Corrected English Model (C.E.M.), example no. 5. Typical C.E.M. strap harness (tucked and pinned, due to age).

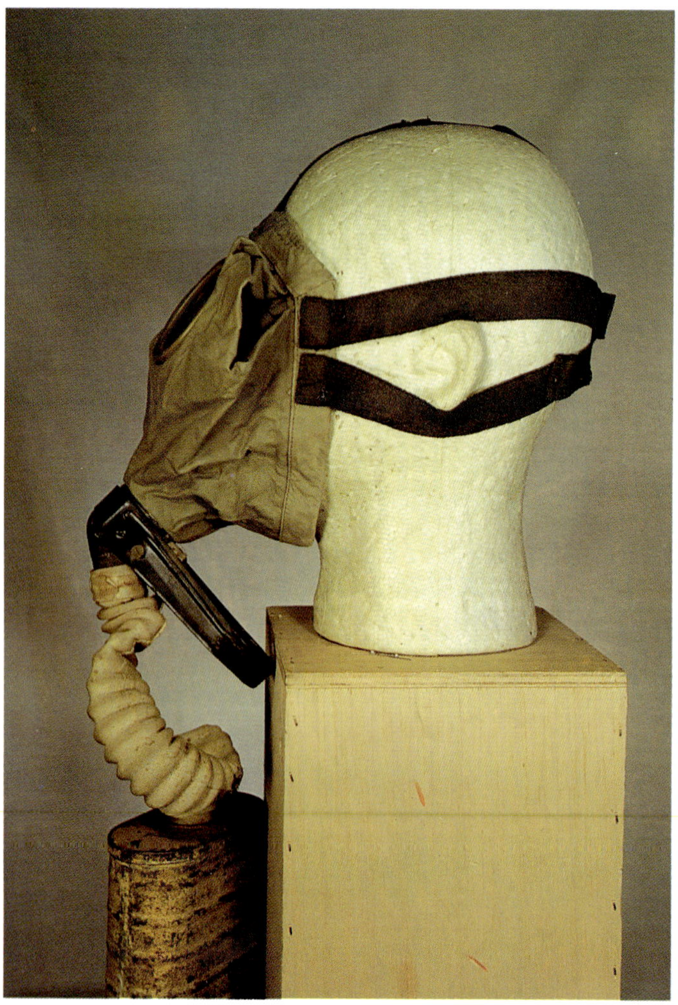

Corrected English Model (C.E.M.), example no. 5.

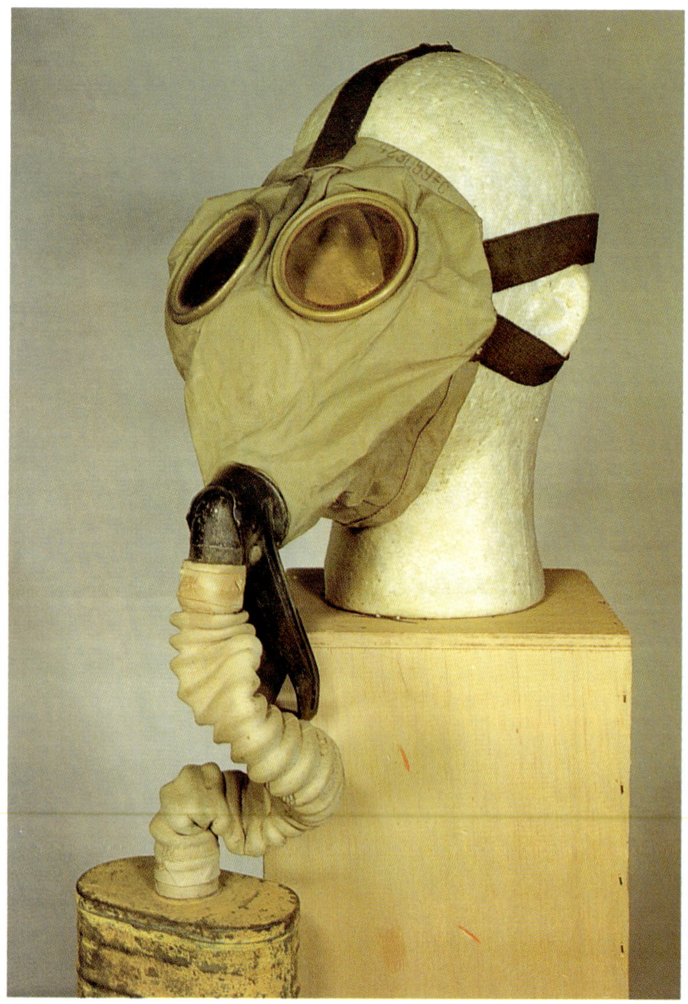

Corrected English Model (C.E.M.), example no. 5.

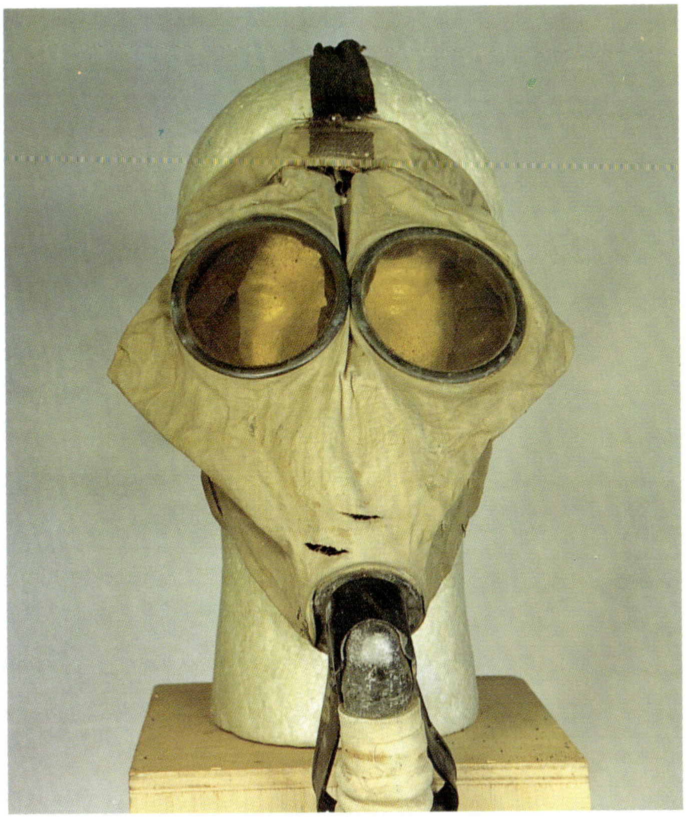

Corrected English Model (C.E.M.), example no. 6. Fabric facepiece in poor condition (rips), but hose well-preserved. Eye lens frames are early type, lenses themselves are celluloid.

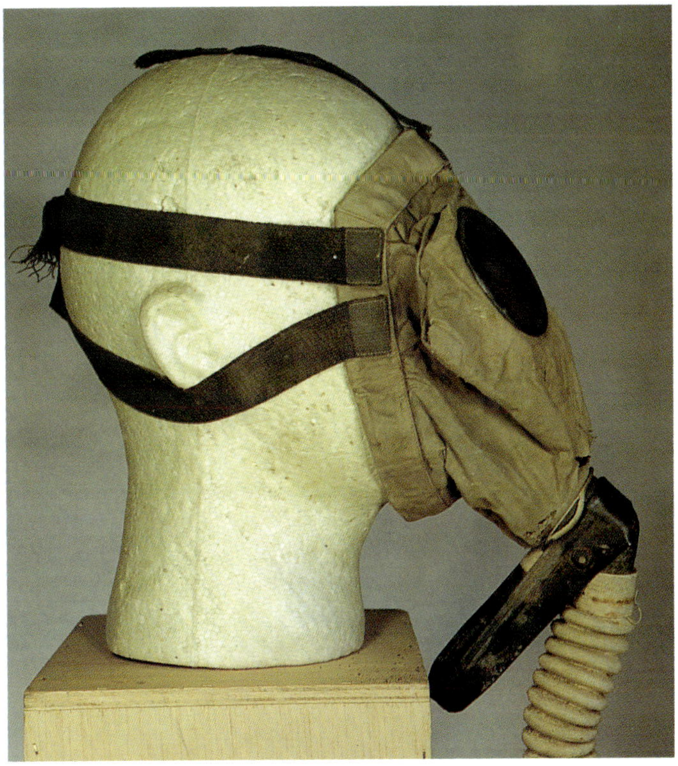

Corrected English Model (C.E.M.), example no. 6. Harness is in poor condition (missing part of top strap).

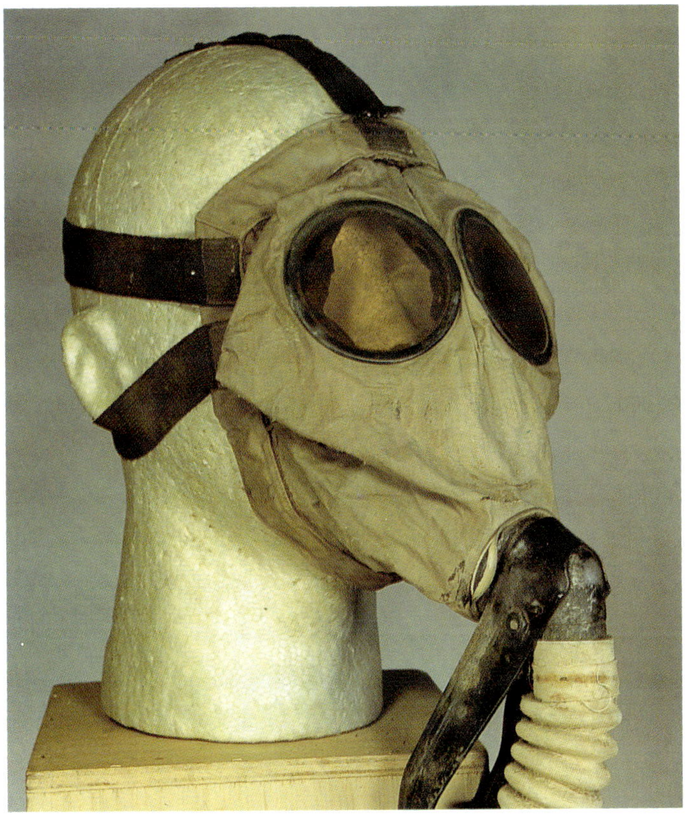

Corrected English Model (C.E.M.), example no. 6. MI valve (exhalation) missing, as is circular spring nose-clip (not visible—inside facepiece).

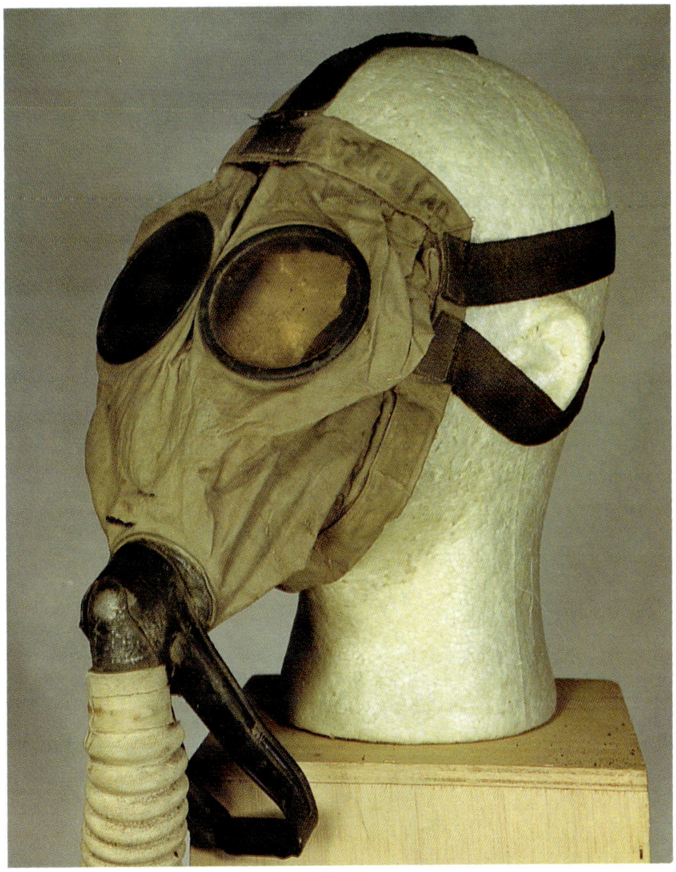

Corrected English Model (C.E.M.), example no. 6.

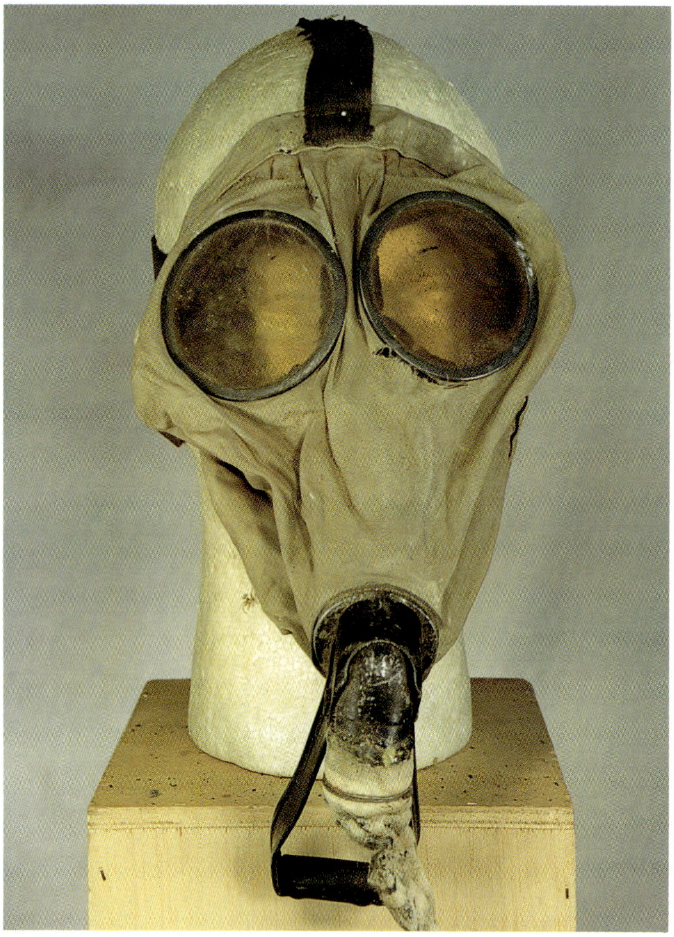

Corrected English Model (C.E.M.), example no. 7. Specimen in overall poor condition, early style lens frames (celluloid lens), rips in facepiece fabric, internal spring nose-clip missing, rubber MI exhalation valve missing. Metal exhalation valve guard is fitted. Hose is typically distorted by effects of age.

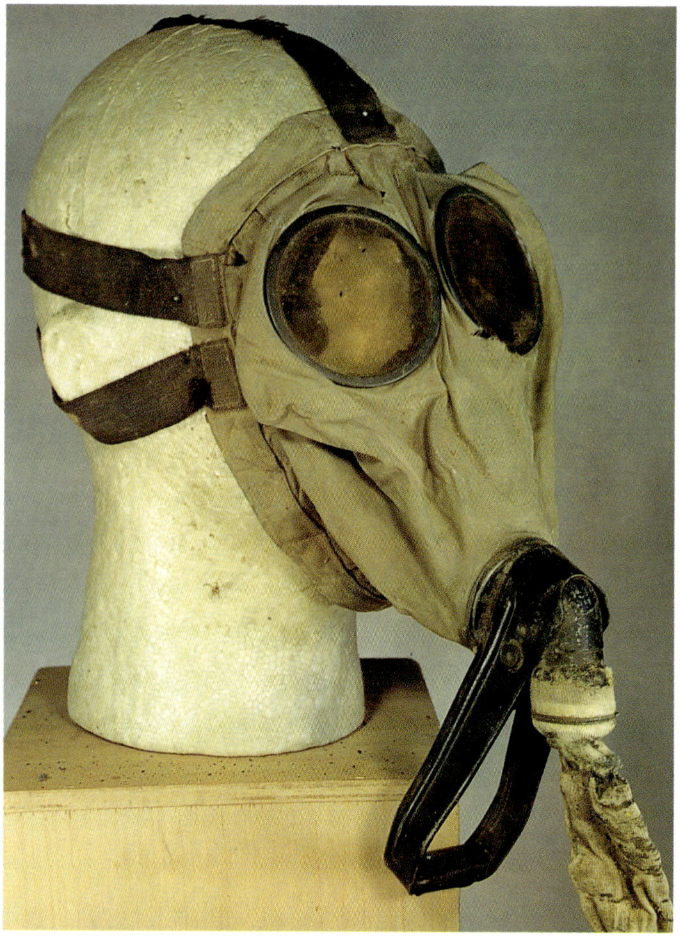

Corrected English Model (C.E.M.), example no. 7.

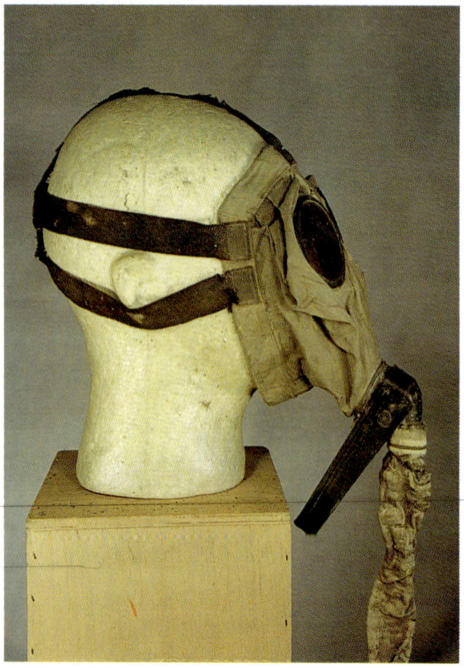

Corrected English Model (C.E.M.), example no. 7.

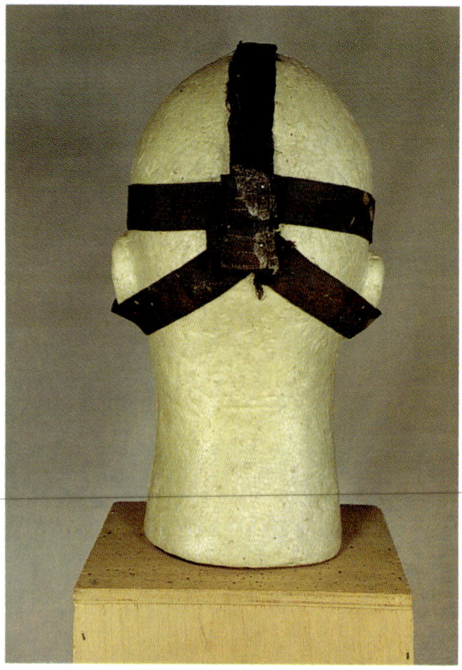

Corrected English Model (C.E.M.), example no. 7. Harness in poor condition (tucked & pinned).

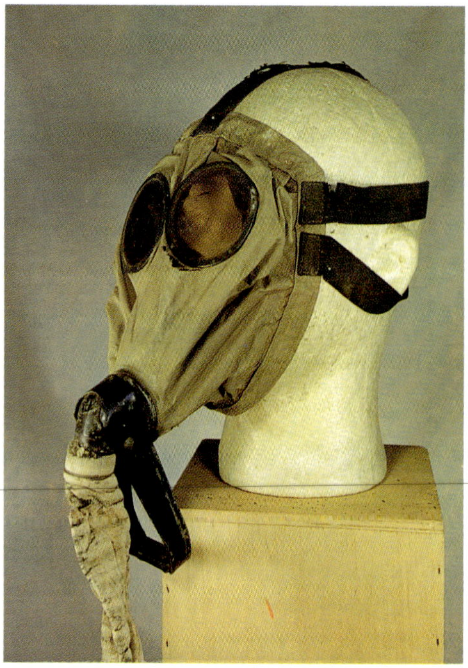

Corrected English Model (C.E.M.), example no. 7.

U.S. Navy 'Head Canister' (Old Mk.II)

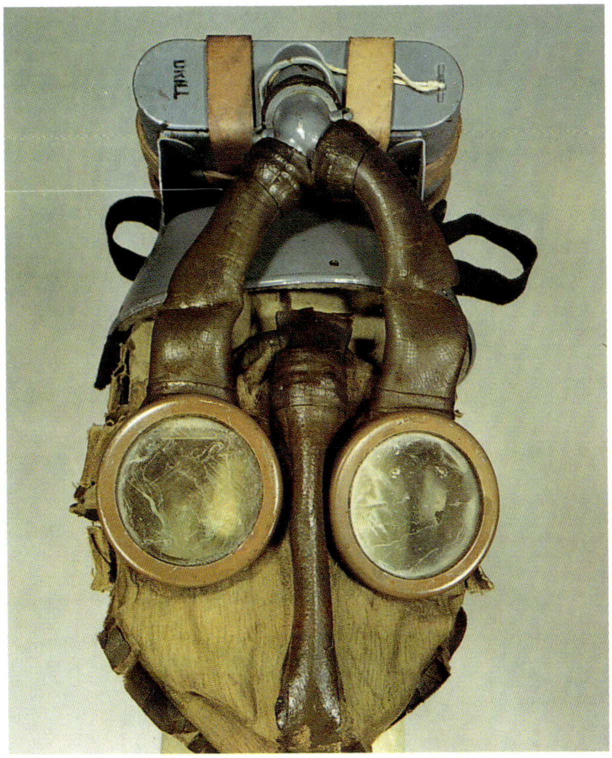

U.S. Navy 'Head Canister' mask (old Mk. II), WWI. One of the more bizarre styles to emerge from the First World War, the effects of age, heat and exposure have taken their toll on this specimen. Still, it is entirely intact, minus only the bilateral smoke filter elements that flanked the top metal filter compartment.

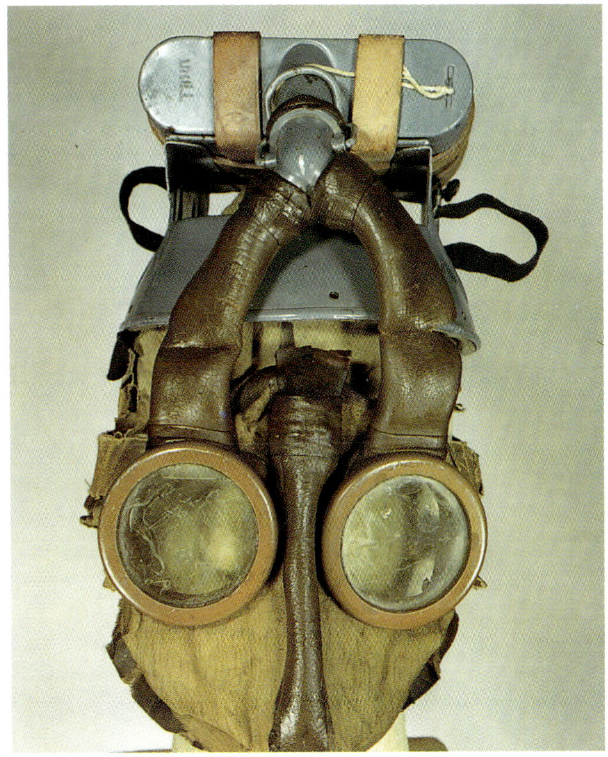

U.S. Navy 'Head Canister' mask (old Mk. II), WWI. From a slightly different angulation, the top-mounted filter container may be better viewed. Air was drawn in from the rear of the filter and distributed to the eye lens area via bifurcated rubber tube (shown over each eye). The rubber flapper type exhalation valve was situated above the nose (the upper half of the rubber valve is missing).

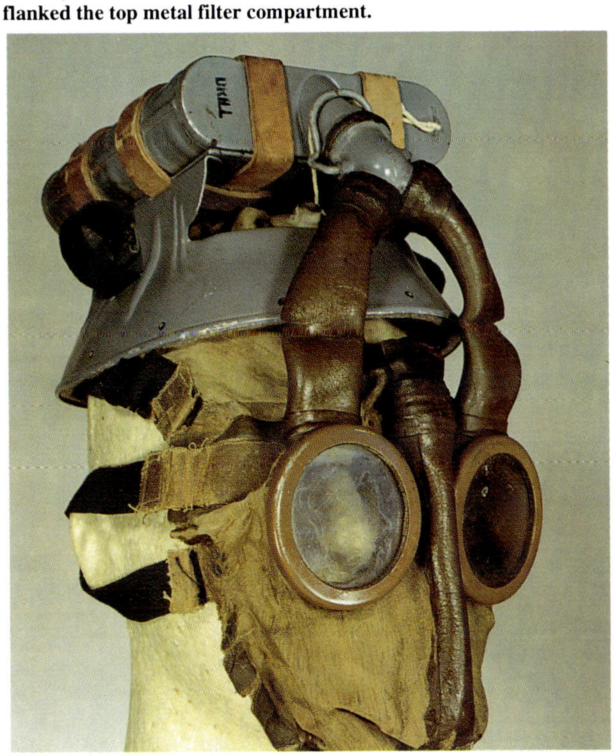

U.S. Navy 'Head Canister' mask (old Mk. II), WWI. The rubber-backed fabric facepiece was secured via a complex strap arrangement and a 'skull-cap' section. The upper straps secured to the bowl shaped metal assembly which supported the filter canister.

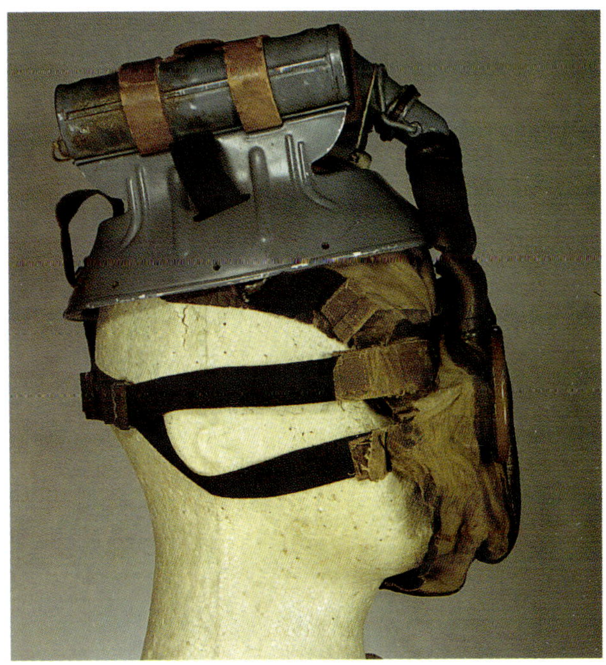

U.S. Navy 'Head Canister' mask (old Mk. II), WWI. This view shows the deteriorated condition of the fabric facepiece on this specimen, and the black straps atop the inverted bowl which were used to secure the elongated rectangular smoke filter elements (not shown) that flanked the filter canister.

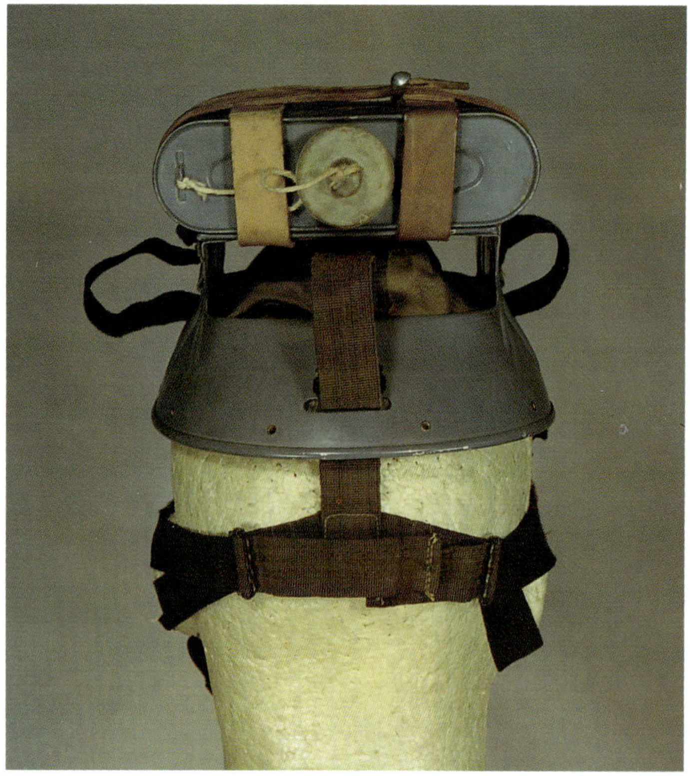

U.S. Navy 'Head Canister' mask (old Mk. II), WWI. Plug at rear of filter canister connected to another bifurcated hose which drew air through the smoke filter elements (not fitted). Side loops were for securing these smoke elements. Head harness attachment in rear is clearly shown.

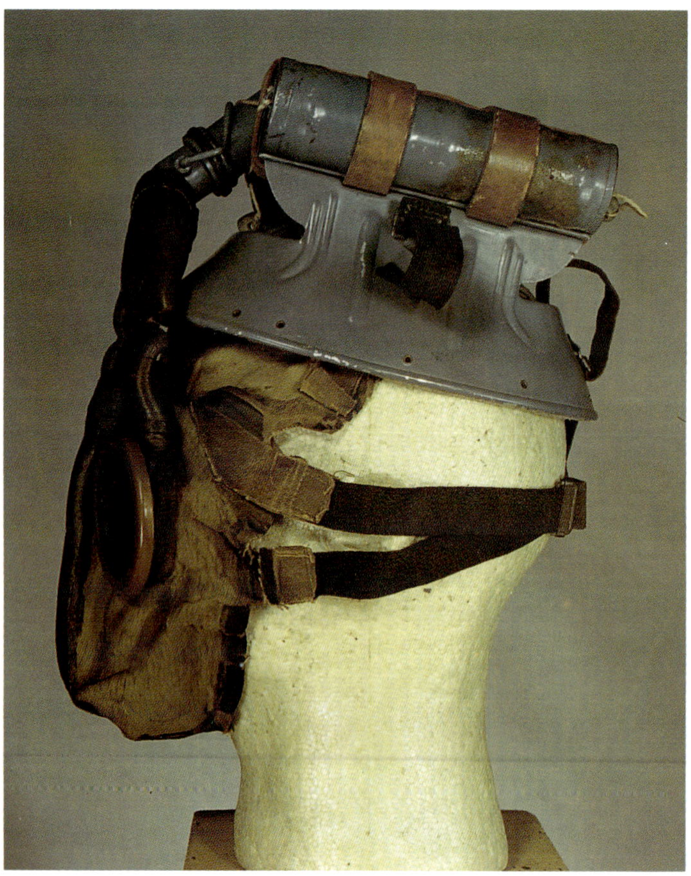

U.S. Navy 'Head Canister' mask (old Mk. II), WWI. Upper left head strap is folded up under 'bowl' and out of view. The 'Head Canister' design kept the filter from posing a 'range of motion' obstacle to the user. Filter outlet (to eye hose ducts) is clear in this view.

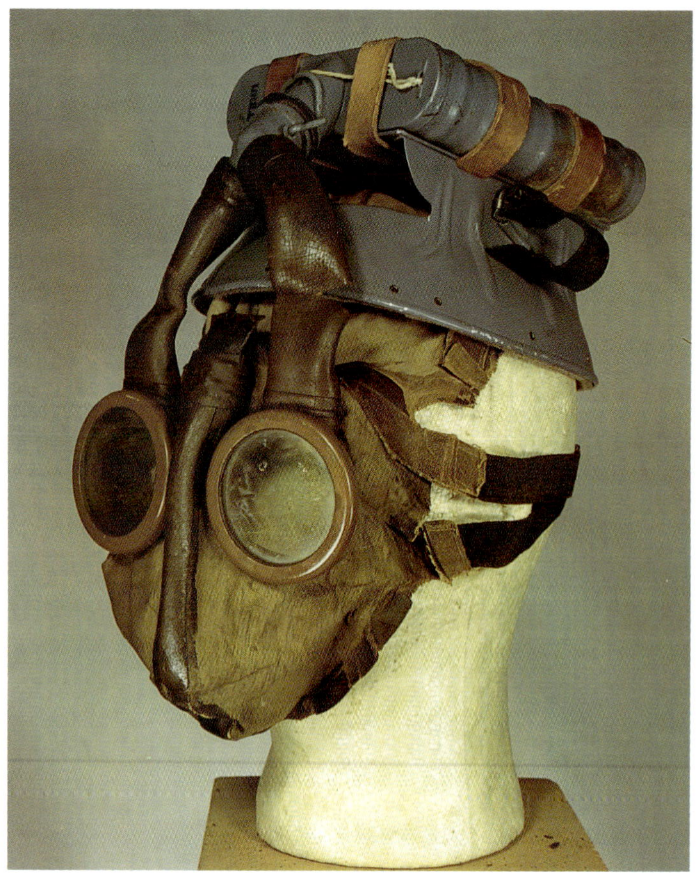

U.S. Navy 'Head Canister' mask (old Mk. II), WWI. A good general view of this mask, which is occasionally misidentified as an earlier design study of somewhat similar appearance (illustrated in the black and white photo section), confusingly designated the "Navy Head Mask and Canister."

U.S. Army MIA2

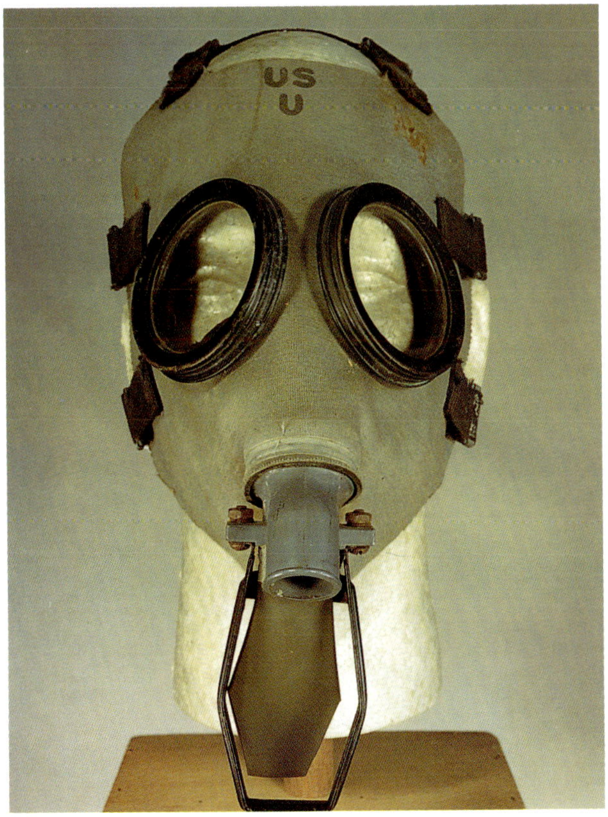

U.S. Army MIA2 mask, about 1936, example no. 1. Facepiece is immediately distinguishable from the MIA1 by "U" on forehead (the MIA1 was produced in a range of 4 individual sizes). There were practically no other differences between the MIA1 and the MIA2, and both featured screw-threaded eye lens frames. This example is in particularly good condition and has the exhalation flapper valve intact.

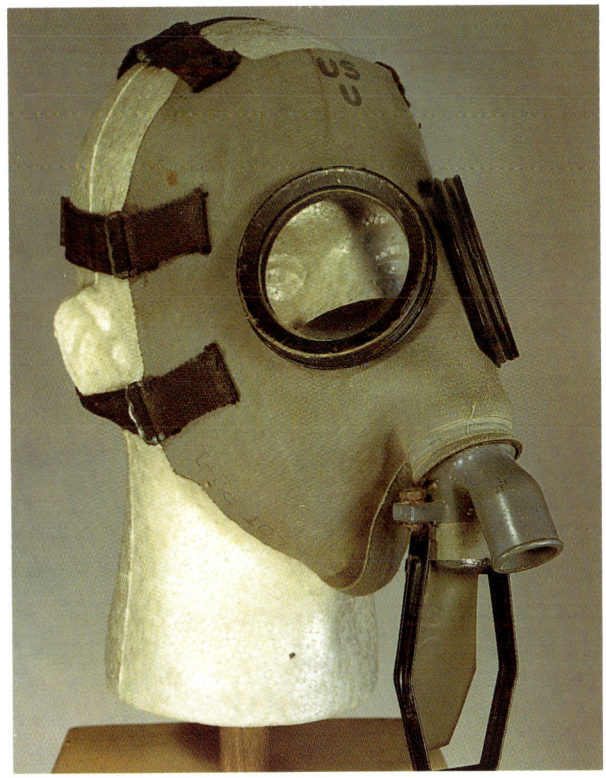

U.S. Army MIA2 mask, about 1936, example no. 1. Lot number is located on lower, outer portion of left facepiece. Chin-seam was considered most vulnerable aspect of the design. Note gray color of stockinet fabric coating rubber of facepiece.

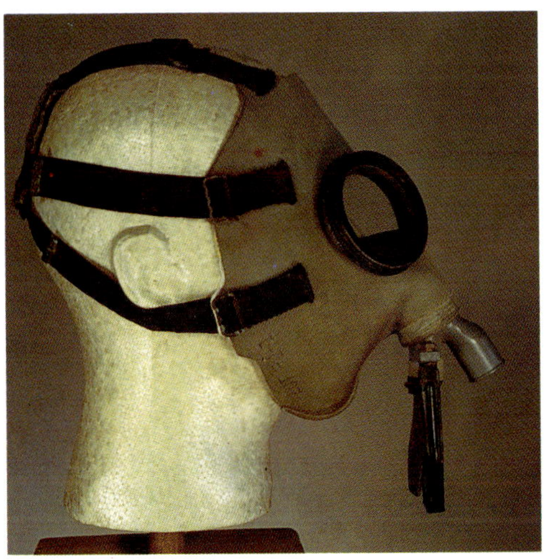

U.S. Army MIA2 mask, about 1936, example no. 1. Sizing buckles of head harness are viewable. Compare this harness with the USN version on the U.S. Navy Mk. I (new) Diaphragm Gas Mask.

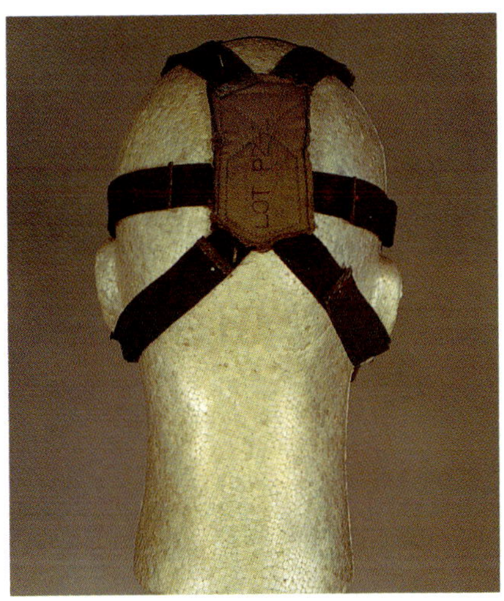

U.S. Army MIA2 mask, about 1936, example no. 1. The fully elasticized, 6-strap head harness is viewable in this image. Amazingly, this basic harness configuration would continue to be used (with minor variations) on most subsequent U.S. Army masks, up through the 1960s, and it is only an improved version of the much earlier R.F.K. mask harness!

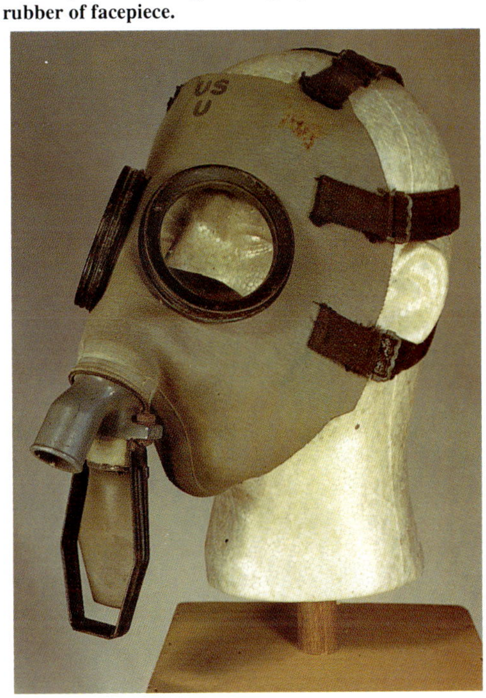

U.S. Army MIA2 mask, about 1936, example no. 1. Some rust stains mark the external, upper left side surface of this specimen, but it is in overall 'very good' condition, considering its age. The black area below the eyes, inside the mask, is part of the Tissot air distribution channel.

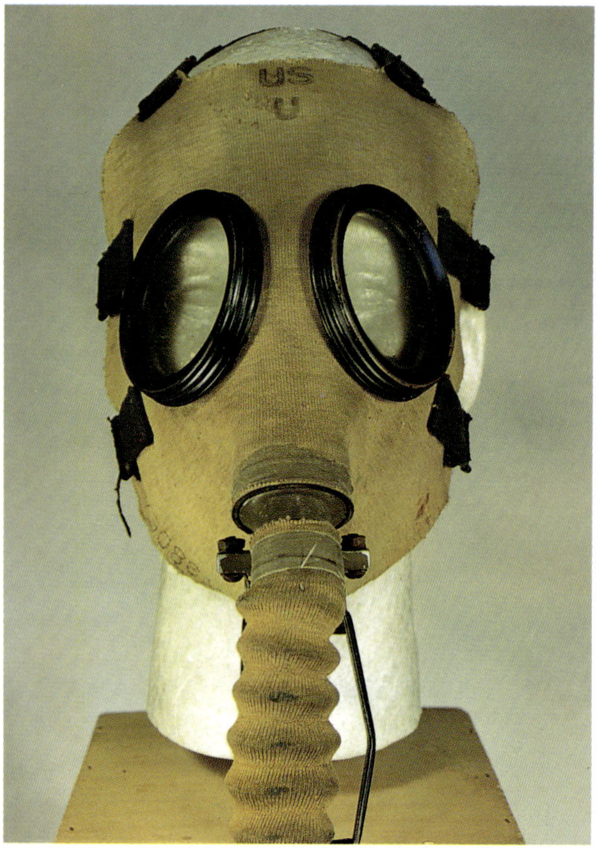

U.S. Army MIA2 mask, about 1936, example no. 2. An interesting comparison with the previous MIA2 specimen, the stockinet fabric cover on this mask's facepiece and hose is colored a light brown and is stained darker by exposure to sunlight and the elements. The rubber exhalation valve is missing.

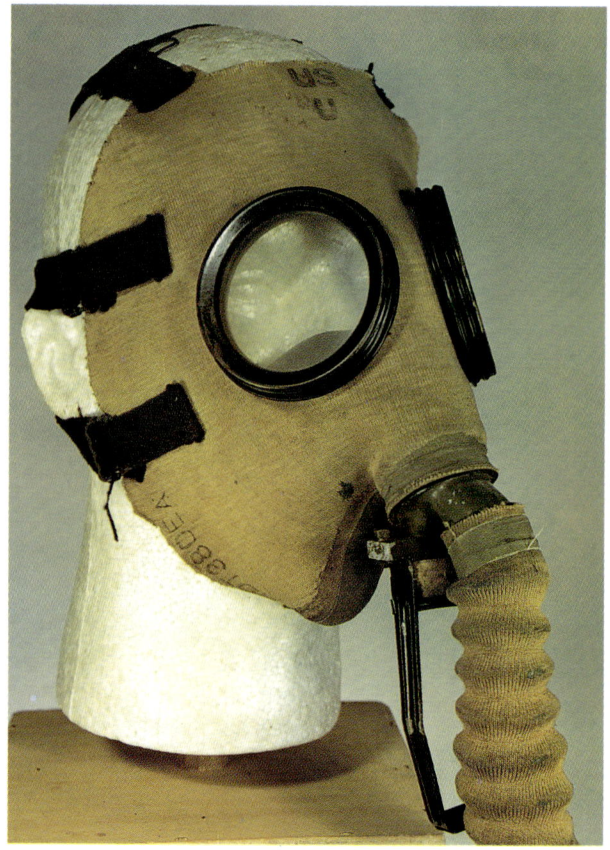

U.S. Army MIA2 mask, about 1936, example no. 2. Despite the missing rubber (MI) exhalation valve, this mask would be considered to be in 'good condition, due to the fact that it is almost entirely intact and in reasonable repair for a 61 year old mask.

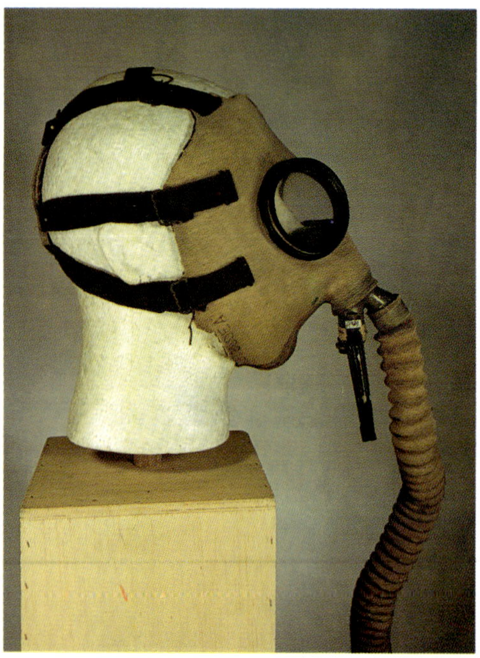

U.S. Army MIA2 mask, about 1936, example no. 2. Some minor deterioration of facepiece edge near lot number marking viewable (usually resulting from heat exposure in storage).

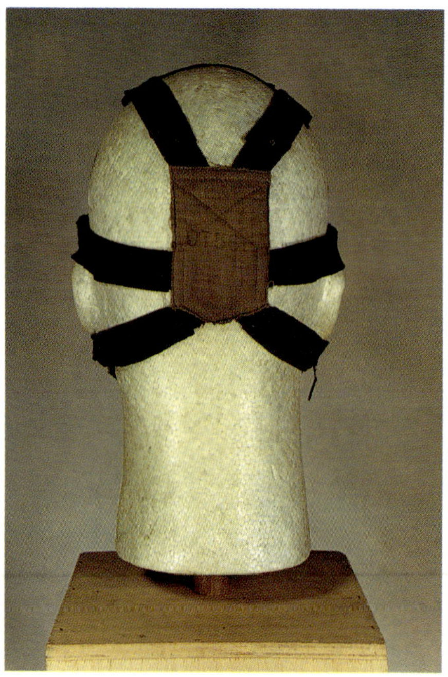

U.S. Army MIA2 mask, about 1936, example no. 2. Straps are pinned to head form for clarity.

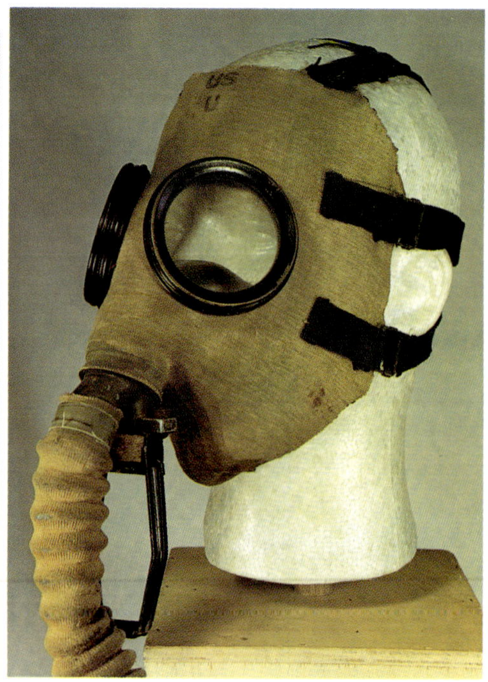

U.S. Army MIA2 mask, about 1936, example no. 2. Examples of the MIA2 mask are currently found, quite easily, still packed in their original hermetically sealed storage tins (MII tin) and theoretically in mint, unused condition.

U.S. Navy Diaphragm Gas Mask (Mark I)

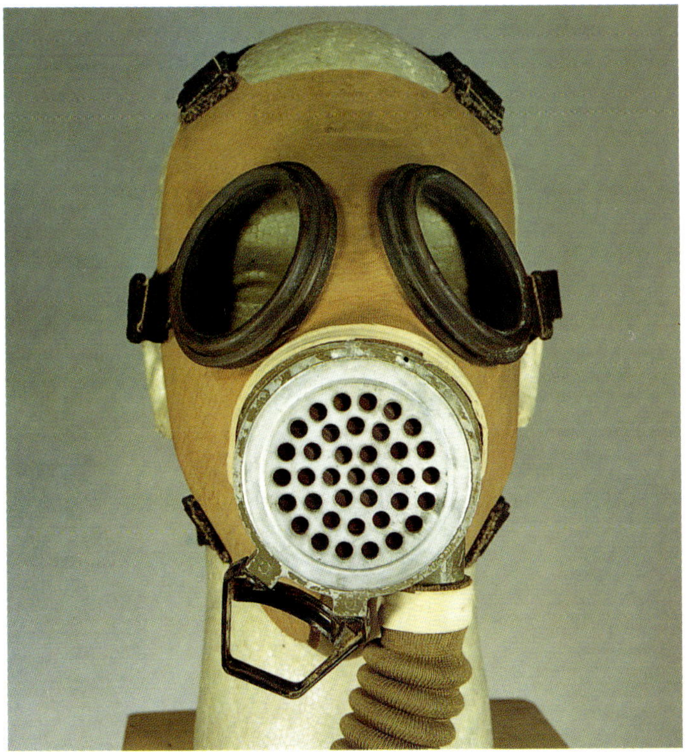

U.S. Navy Diaphragm Gas Mask, (new) Mark I, late 20s/early 30s. This is the Navy version of the U.S. Army MI Diaphragm Gas Mask. The facepieces of both masks are identical; only the head harness strap configuration is different. A rare specimen, this example is in excellent condition, missing only the rubber exhalation valve. Note the sizing numeral "2" on the forehead under the barely discernible "U.S.."

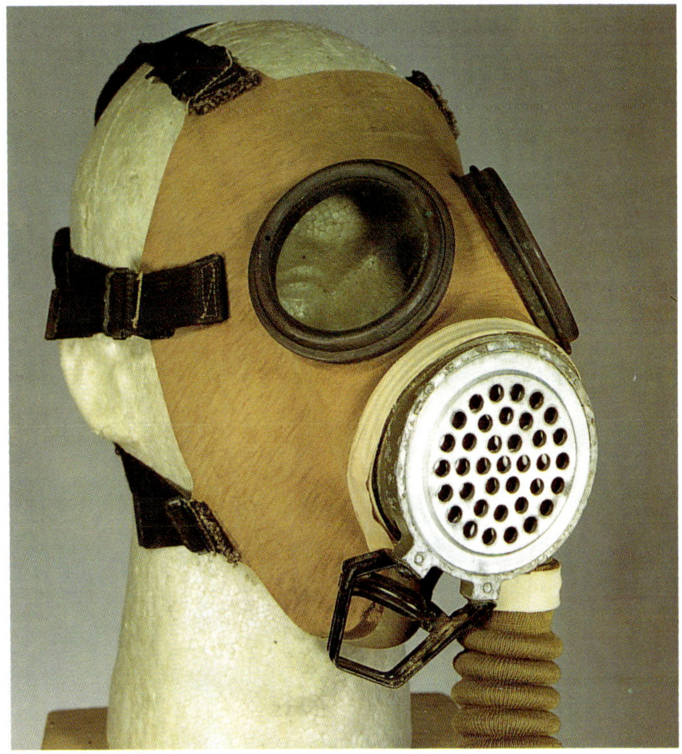

U.S. Navy Diaphragm Gas Mask, (new) Mark I, late 20s/early 30s. Note the crimped-on eye lens frames, which are unique to the MI Army mask and the USN Mk. I Diaphragm gas mask.

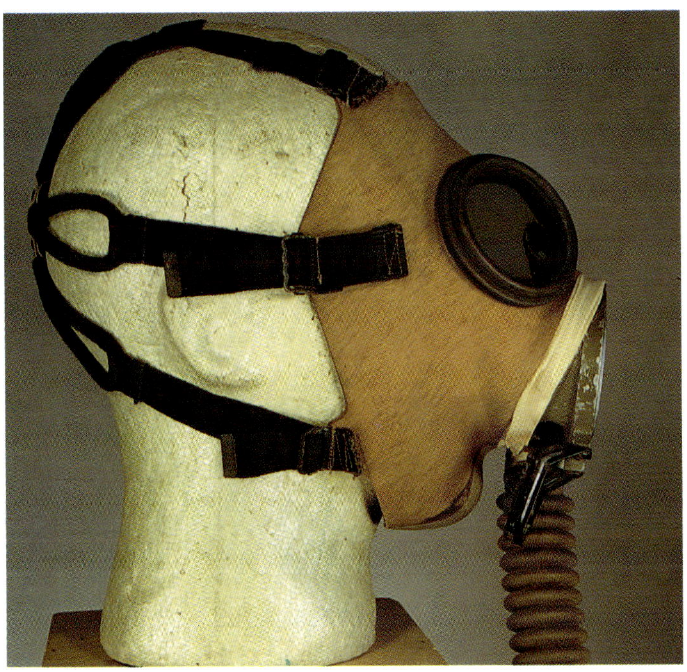

U.S. Navy Diaphragm Gas Mask, (new) Mark I, late 20s/early 30s. The Navy head harness is derived from the U.S. Army M3 head harness (used on the Army MI Optical Mask) and was subsequently used on all U.S. Navy service gas masks through the Mk.IV.

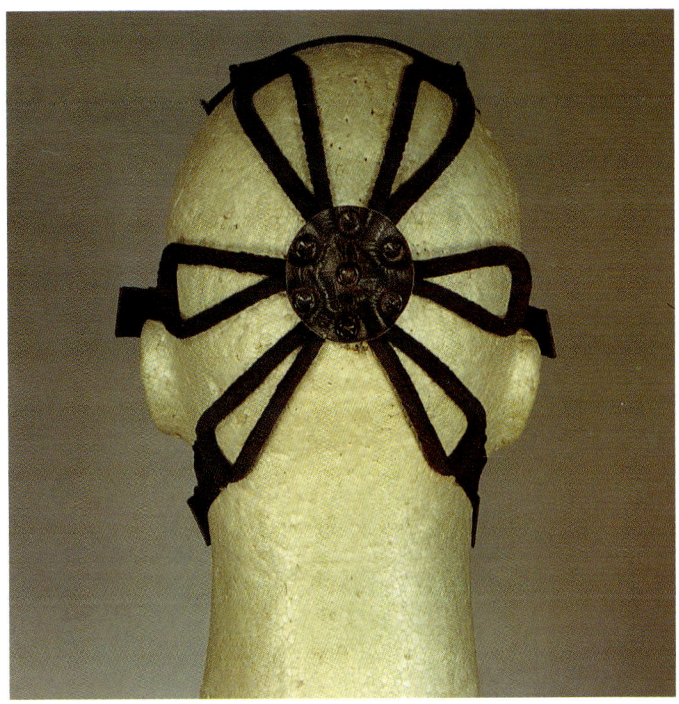

U.S. Navy Diaphragm Gas Mask, (new) Mark I, late 20s/early 30s. The distinctive U.S. Navy head harness system (adaptation of the U.S. Army M3 harness, originally used with the Army MI optical mask), which was used with some variation on all subsequent Navy masks through the Mk. IV, is clearly shown in this image. It secured the mask quite well against dislodging motion.

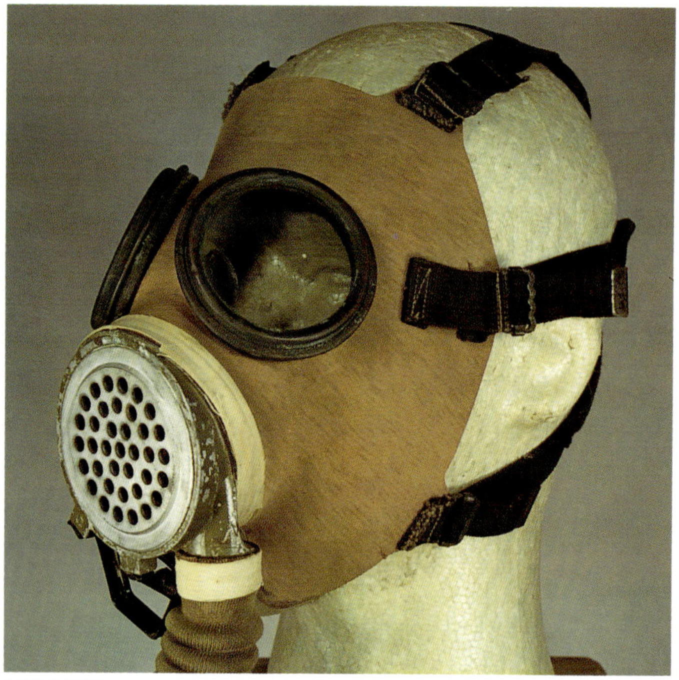

U.S. Navy Diaphragm Gas Mask, (new) Mark I, late 20s/early 30s. A good view of the inlet and outlet diaphragm housing block, made of aluminum.

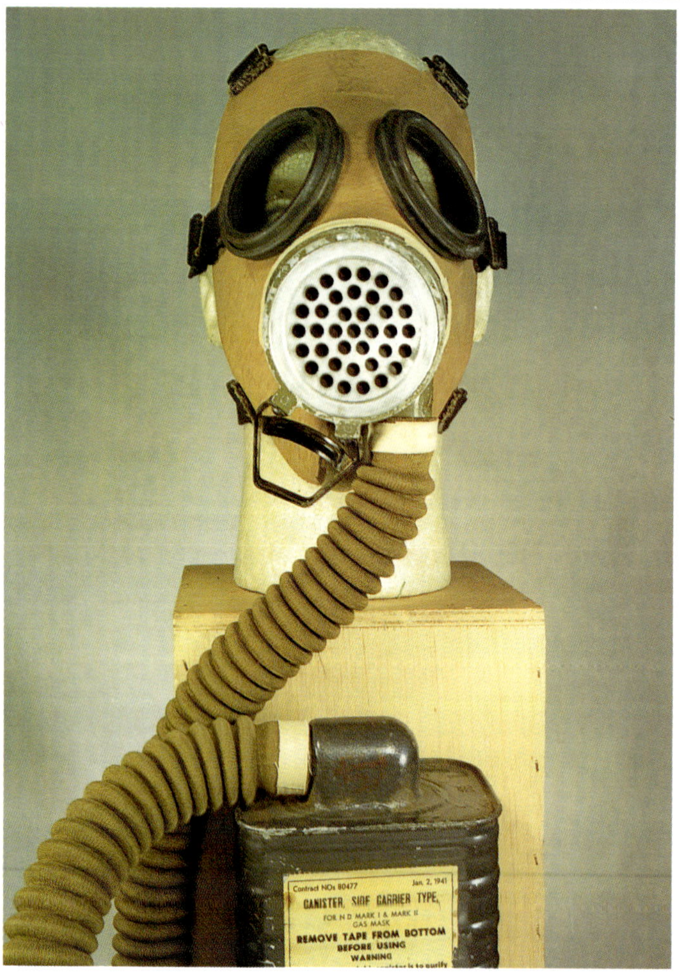

U.S. Navy Diaphragm Gas Mask, (new) Mark I, late 20s/early 30s. The Navy used its own version of the U.S. Army service filter canister, which is shown. The date on the canister is given as 2 Jan 1941, indicative of the fact that it was added somewhat after the facepiece assembly had been manufactured.

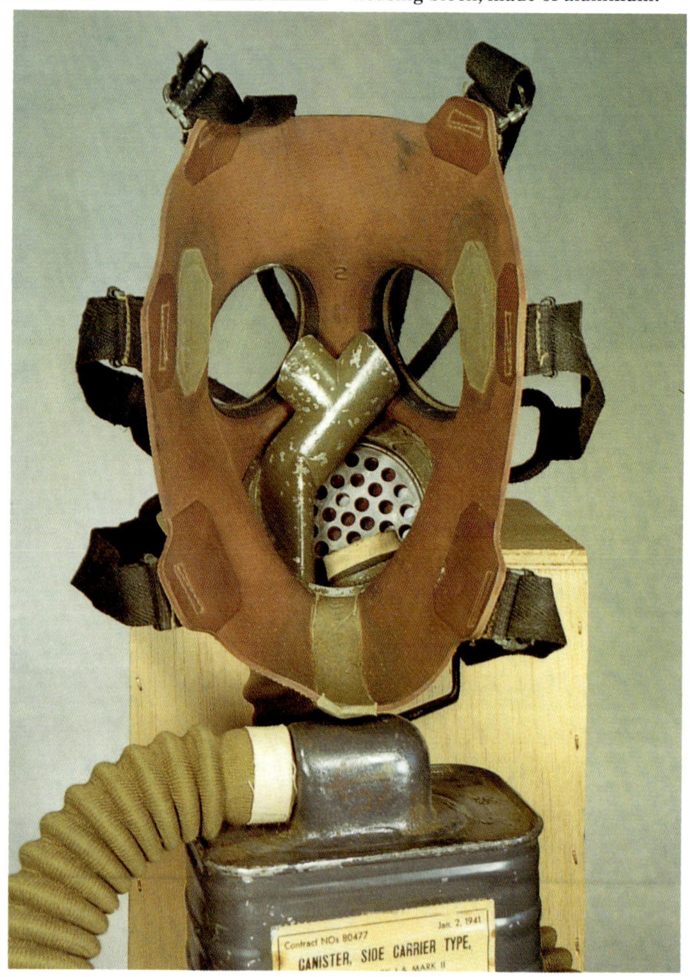

U.S. Navy Diaphragm Gas Mask, (new) Mark I, late 20s/early 30s. An interior view that serves to illustrate the internal configuration of both the U.S. Army MI Diaphragm Gas Mask and the U.S. Navy Diaphragm Gas Mask, Mark I. Metal Tissot distribution tube is bifurcated and located in front of speech diaphragm and above the exhalation valve outlet.

U.S. Navy Diaphragm Gas Mask (Mark II)

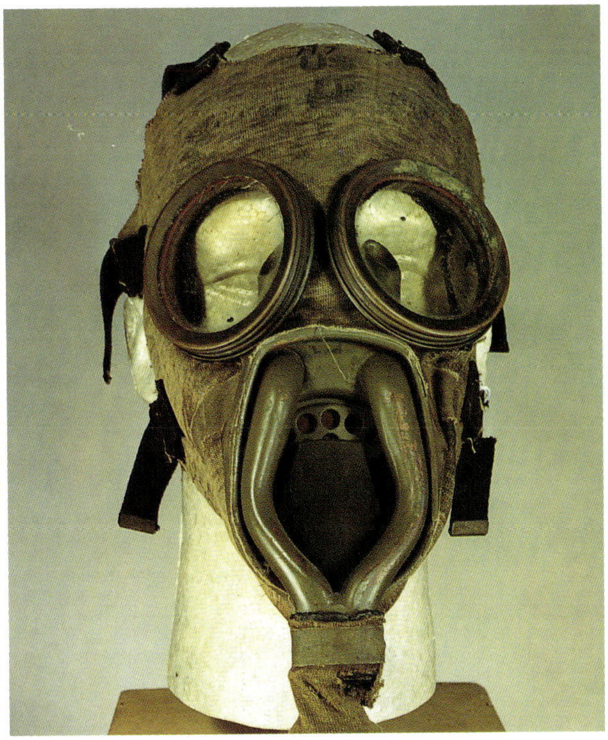

U.S. Navy Diaphragm Gas Mask, (new) Mark II, mid 30s, example no. 1. An example of the 2nd generation diaphragm mask used by both USN and U.S. Army, but one that is in "poor" condition.

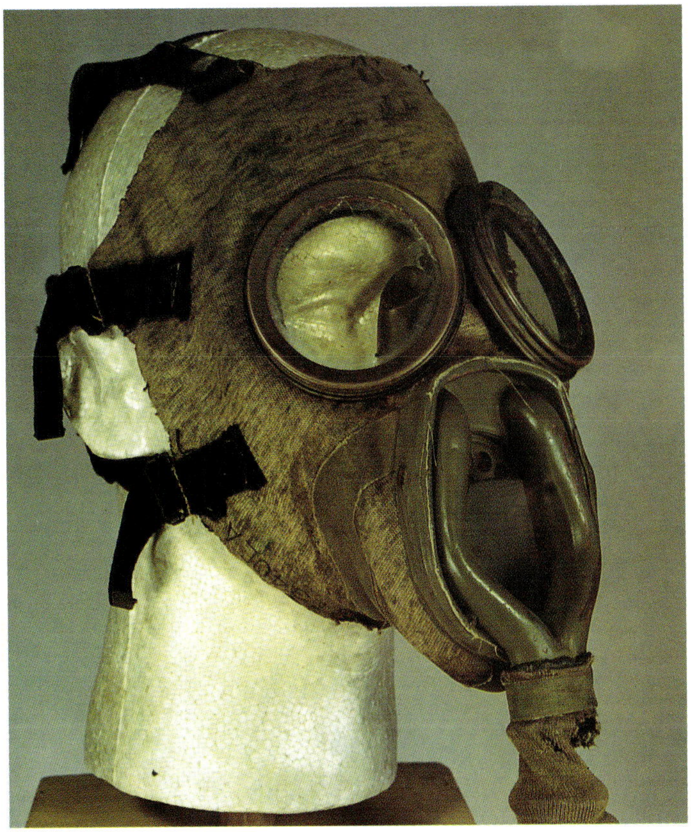

U.S. Navy Diaphragm Gas Mask, (new) Mark II, mid 30s, example no. 1. Note "U" universal sizing numeral and screw-thread lens frames (characteristic of U.S. Army MIA2 and ND Mk. II masks). The fabric of the rubber facepiece is severely discolored by effects of aging and poor storage conditions, and there are ripped areas of the facepiece around the eye lens frames.

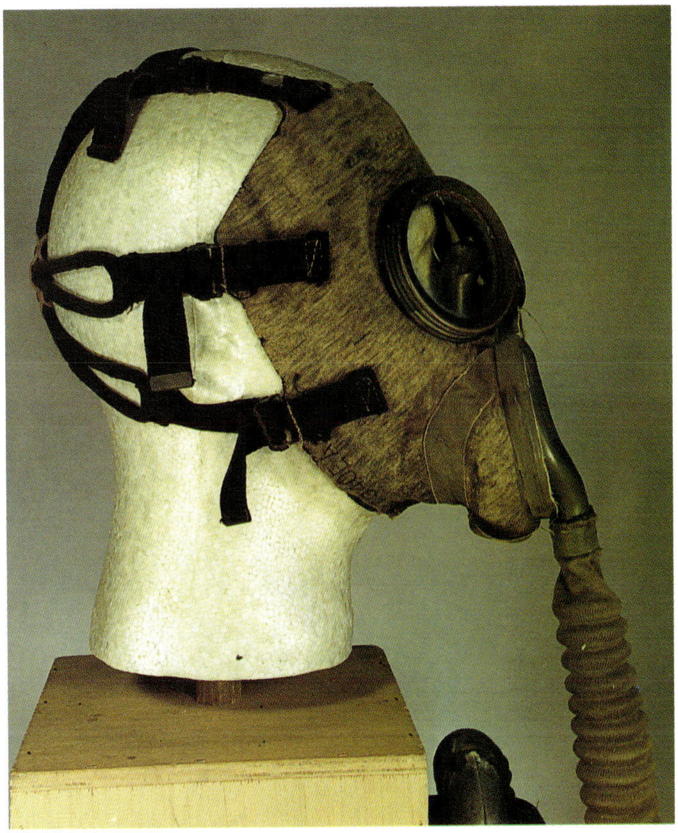

U.S. Navy Diaphragm Gas Mask, (new) Mark II, mid 30s, example no. 1. U.S. Army olive colored MVIII filter canister is in use with this example.

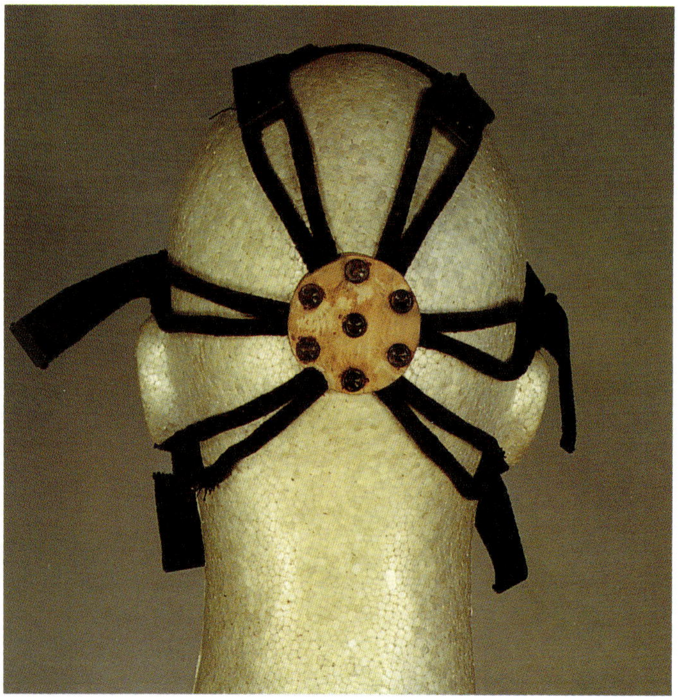

U.S. Navy Diaphragm Gas Mask, (new) Mark II, mid 30s, example no. 1. Details of Navy style (M3 type) head harness clearly seen.

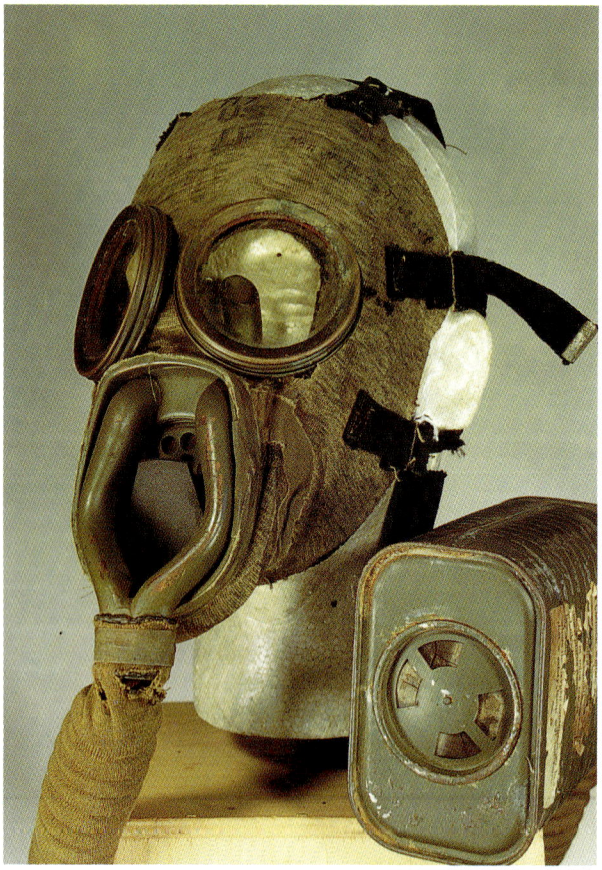

U.S. Navy Diaphragm Gas Mask, (new) Mark II, mid 30s, example no. 1. Some detail of the (MII) exhalation valve may be seen, which is flanked by twin metal inlet tubes taking air from the filter canister to a site directly below each eye. The rubber valve was thus well protected, although it presented a small obstacle to clear transmission of speech from the 'voicemitter' located directly behind it.

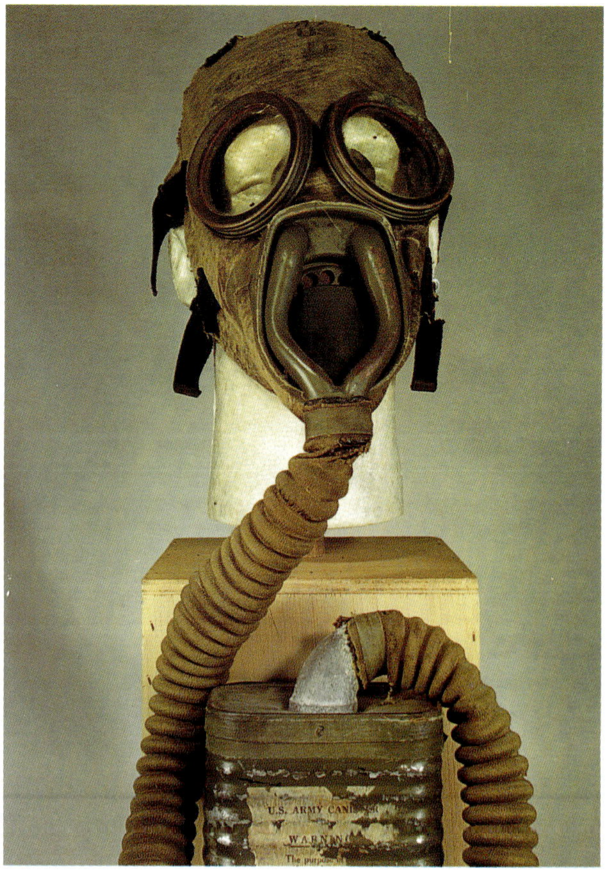

U.S. Navy Diaphragm Gas Mask, (new) Mark II, mid 30s, example no. 1. The U.S. Army MVIII filter canister may be partly seen in this view. The stockinet covered rubber hose is in generally poor condition.

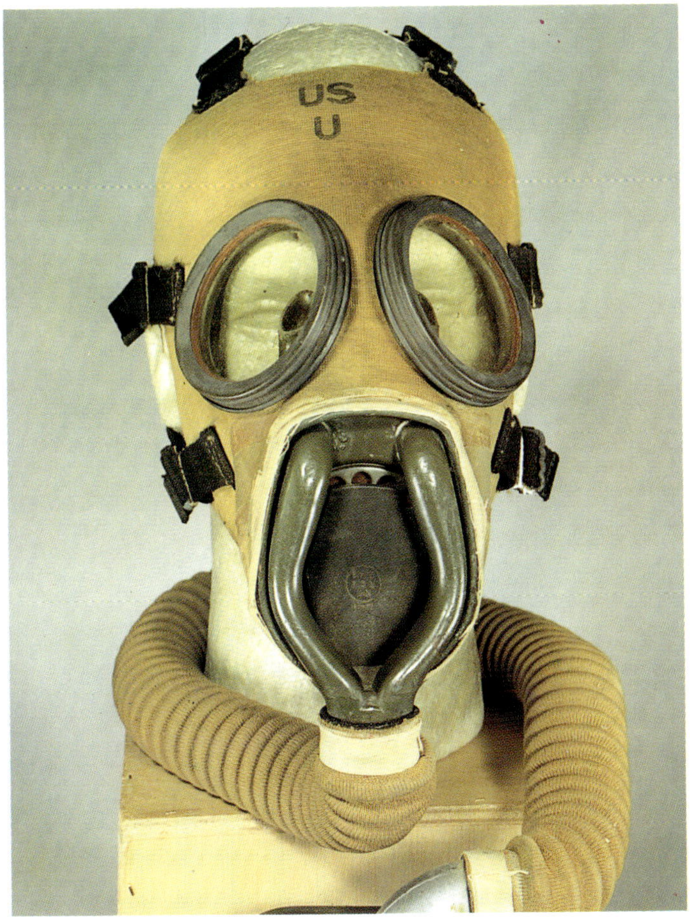

U.S. Navy Diaphragm Gas Mask, (new) Mark II, mid 30s, example no. 2. This specimen is in overall 'excellent' condition, remarkably preserved throughout. Most details may be clearly seen.

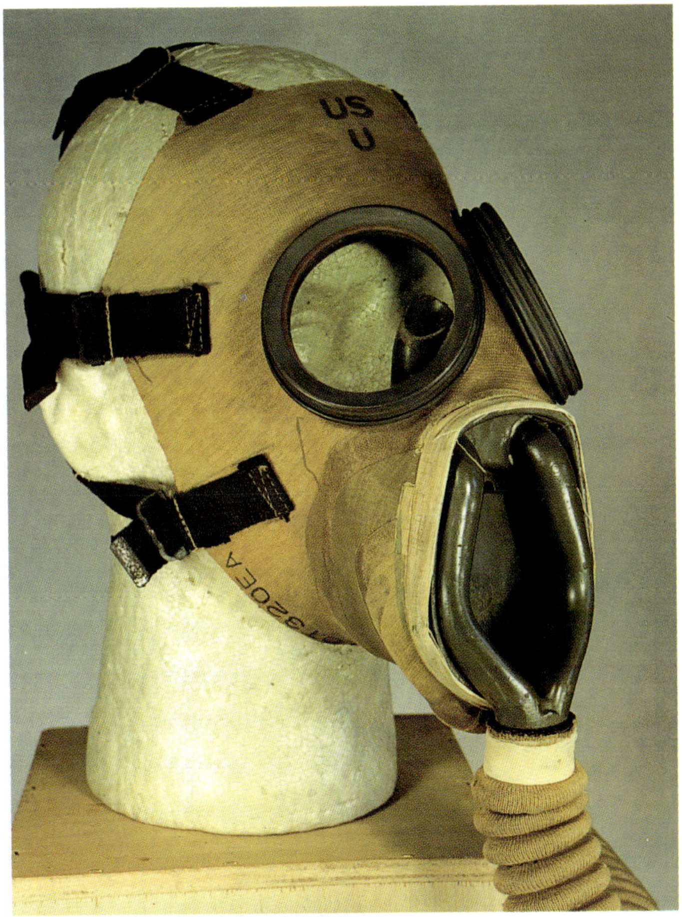

U.S. Navy Diaphragm Gas Mask, (new) Mark II, mid 30s, example no. 2. Fine details such as harness stitching, lot number and Tissot tube ducts may be visualized.

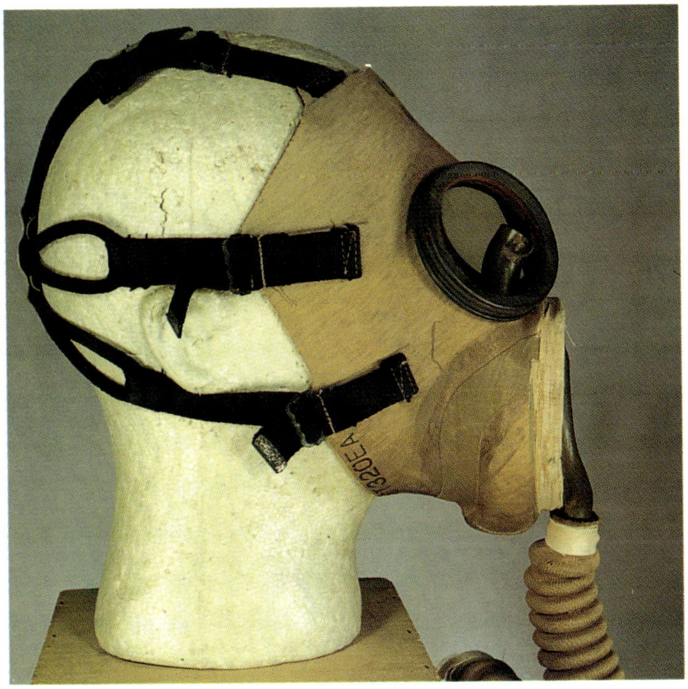

U.S. Navy Diaphragm Gas Mask, (new) Mark II, mid 30s, example no. 2. Clear view of lateral head harness straps, attachments and buckles.

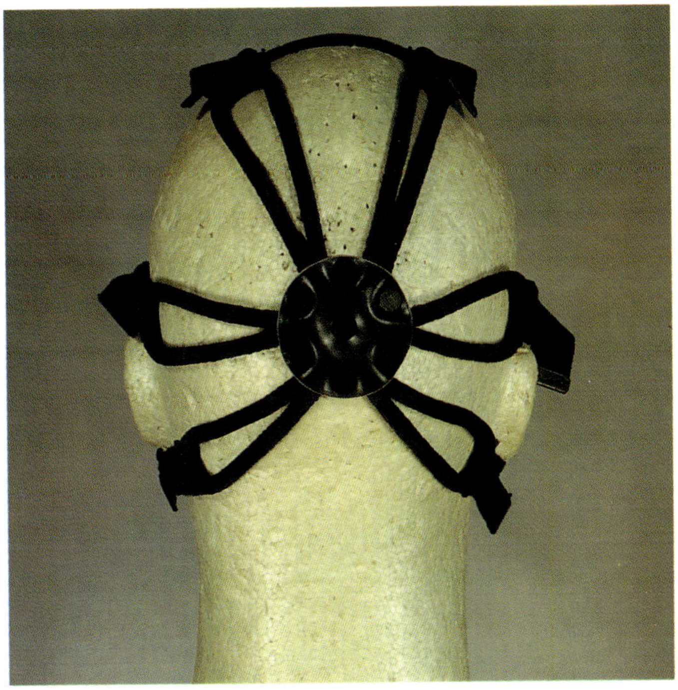

U.S. Navy Diaphragm Gas Mask, (new) Mark II, mid 30s, example no. 2. Good view of U.S. Navy style (M3 type)fabric covered looped-spring head harness, with circular central leather juncture.

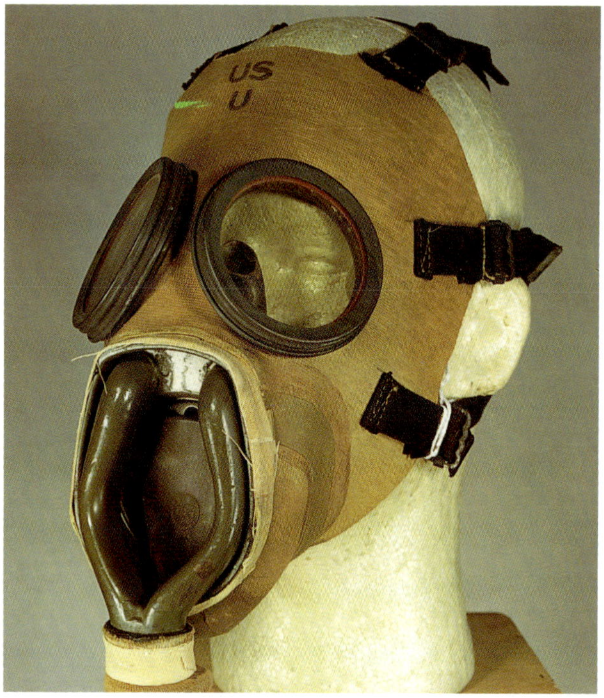

U.S. Navy Diaphragm Gas Mask, (new) Mark II, mid 30s, example no. 2. Some detail of rubber exhalation (type MII) valve may be discerned, sited between external portion of bifurcated Tissot inlet tube.

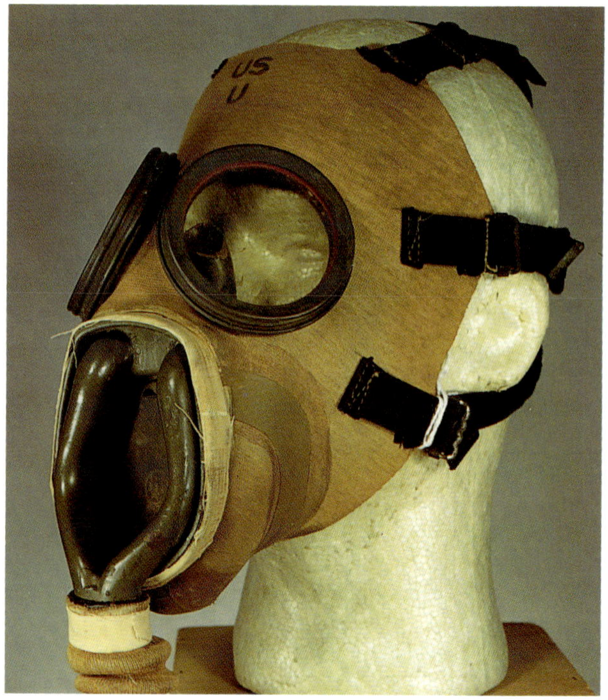

U.S. Navy Diaphragm Gas Mask, (new) Mark II, mid 30s, example no. 2. Detail of chin area and speech diaphragm/inlet block.

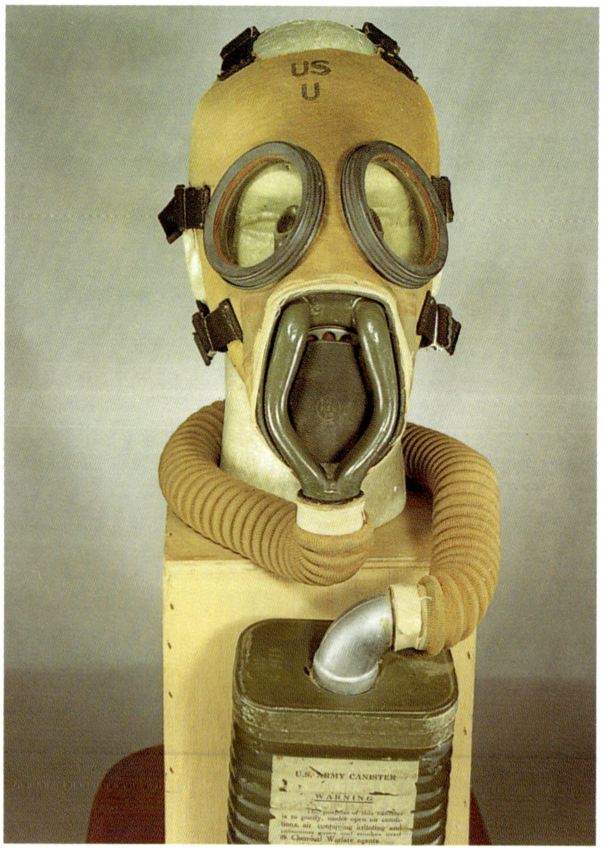

U.S. Navy Diaphragm Gas Mask, (new) Mark II, mid 30s, example no. 2. Good overall view of mask, hose and U.S. Army MVIII filter canister in use with mask. Note the less than perfect placement of the internal Tissot tube channels, which pose a potential visual distraction for the user.

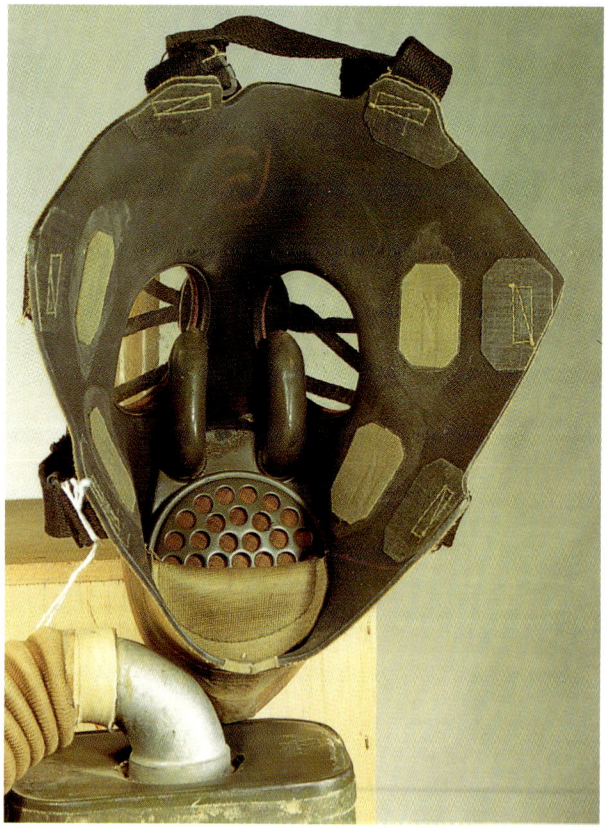

U.S. Navy Diaphragm Gas Mask, (new) Mark II, mid 30s, example no. 2. View of interior of the mask (which also serves to illustrate and exemplify interior of U.S. Army Diaphragm Mask MII), with its bifurcated Tissot inlet tubes and speech diaphragm. Note internal stitching reinforcements on facepiece for (M3 type) head harness attachment and the chin seam area (always considered the weakest part of the MI type masks).

U.S. Army M1A1/M2A1 Training Gas Mask, 1939-40

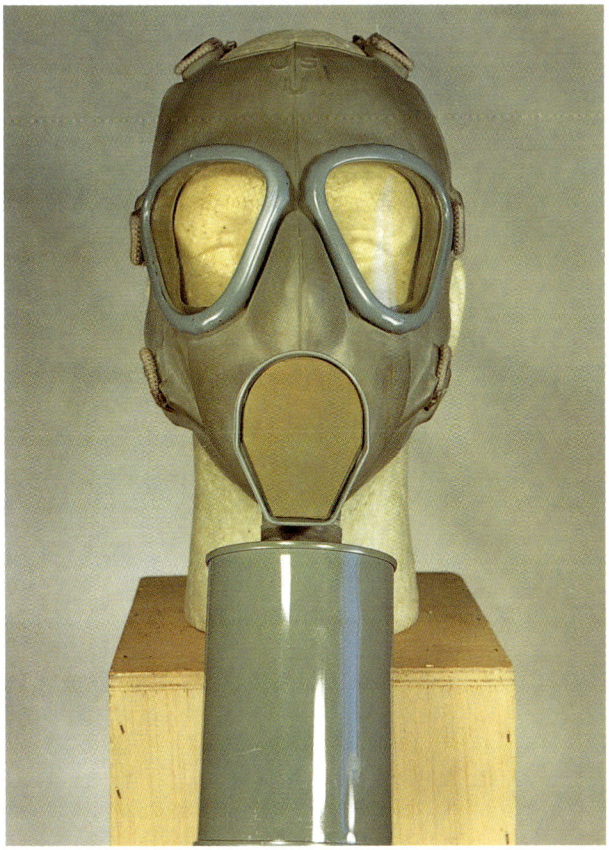

U.S. Army MIA1/M2A1 Training Gas Mask, 1939-40. A well preserved example of the first fully molded rubber facepiece concept for U.S. protective masks. MV exhalation valve and MI Training Filter.

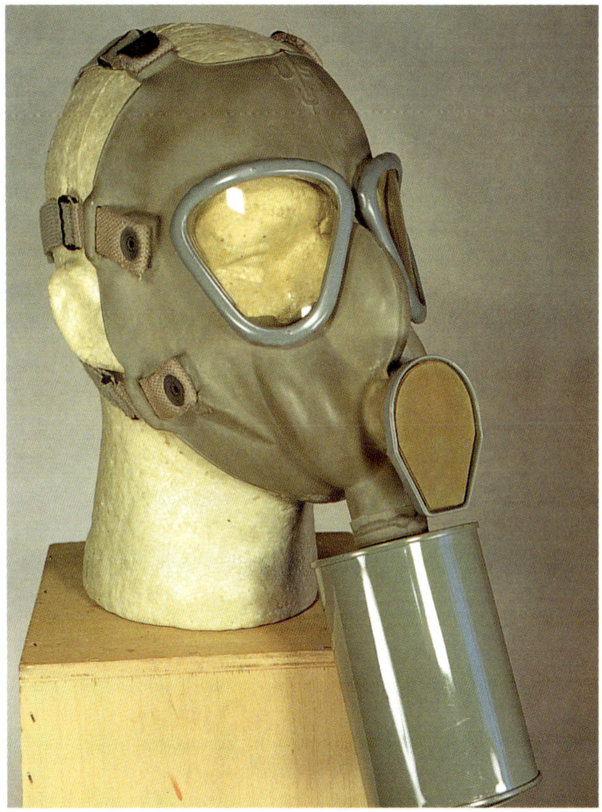

U.S. Army MIA1/M2A1 Training Gas Mask, 1939-40. This specimen in overall 'very good' condition. The vulnerable exposure of the exhalation valve is evident. Note "rifle skid" blocks molded into facepiece in front of lower lateral mask harness attachment points. This was to keep a rifle from catching the harness connection and pulling the mask off, while using a weapon during a CW attack. Eliminated on fully molded rubber facepieces, later in the war.

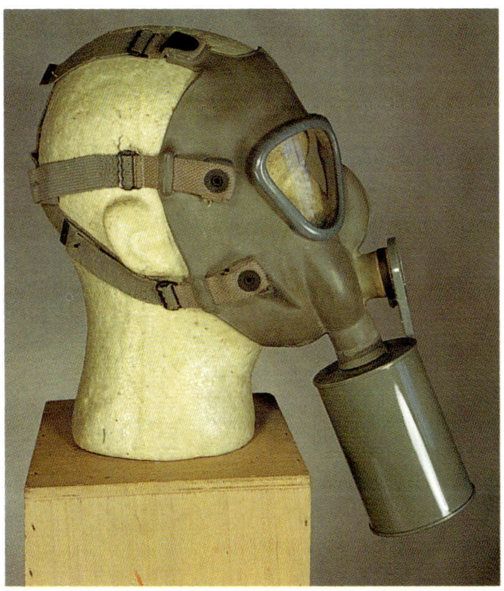

U.S. Army MIA1/M2A1 Training Gas Mask, 1939-40. Note riveted head harness attachment points. These penetrated the rubber facepiece and posed potential failure areas. Straps are all elasticized, except for mask segments, which are non-stretch cotton duck.

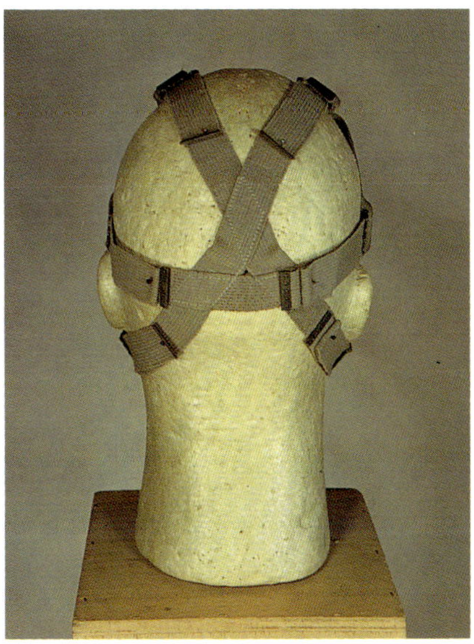

U.S. Army MIA1/M2A1 Training Gas Mask, 1939-40. This style of harness (M4) was first developed and used on early WWI masks (K.T.); it remained in use, with modification, throughout WWII. Straps are pinned for clarity.

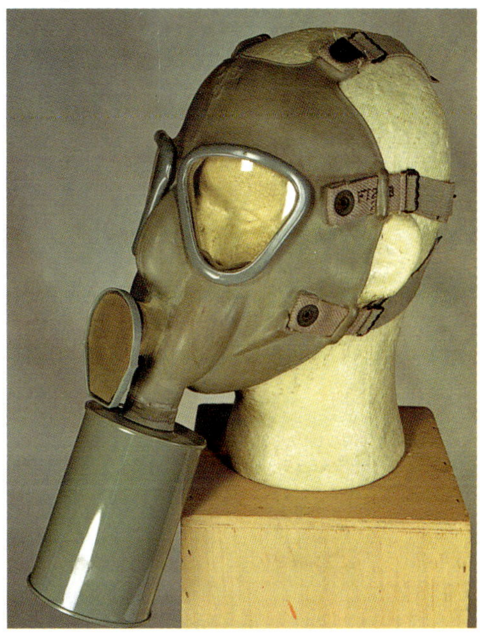

U.S. Army MIA1/M2A1 Training Gas Mask, 1939-40. The relatively bulky cylindrical MI Training Filter was cumbersome. Note clear detail of "rifle skid" moldings.

U.S. Army M2A1 Service Gas Mask (Heavyweight), 1940-41

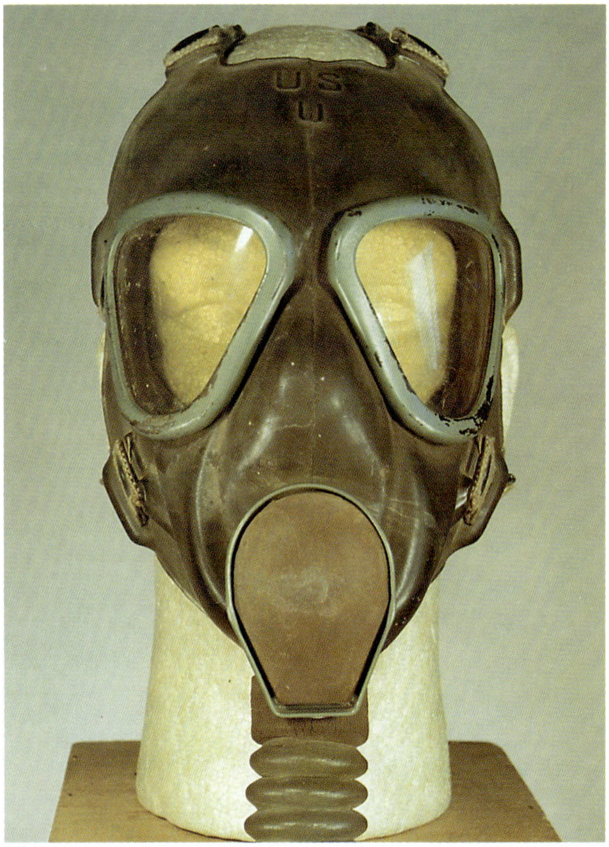

U.S. Army M2A1 Service Gas Mask (Heavyweight), 1940-41. This was the "service" version of the M2 type fully molded facepiece—essentially identical to the MIA1/M2A1 Training Gas Mask facepiece, but with a rectangular filter attached via a corrugated rubber hose. Type MV (Connell) exhalation valve is used (the M2 Service Gas Mask used the MIV (Acushnet) valve, which was button-shaped).

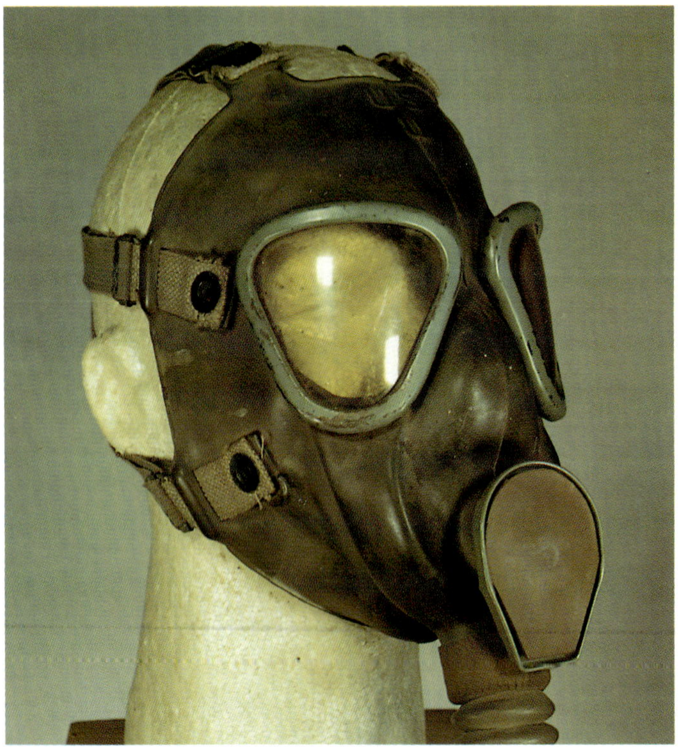

U.S. Army M2A1 Service Gas Mask (Heavyweight), 1940-41. This specimen is in 'good' condition, having all components and parts intact, but exhibits the typical dark discoloration effects of heat and poor storage condition on M2 and later type pure rubber facepieces (original color is lighter green).

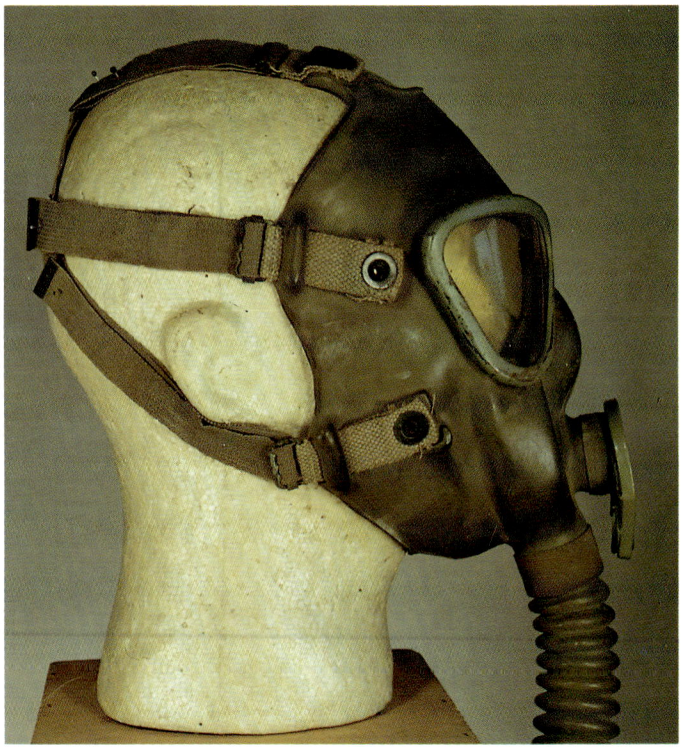

U.S. Army M2A1 Service Gas Mask (Heavyweight), 1940-41. Some deformation of MV exhalation valve mount (made of plastic) is discernible.

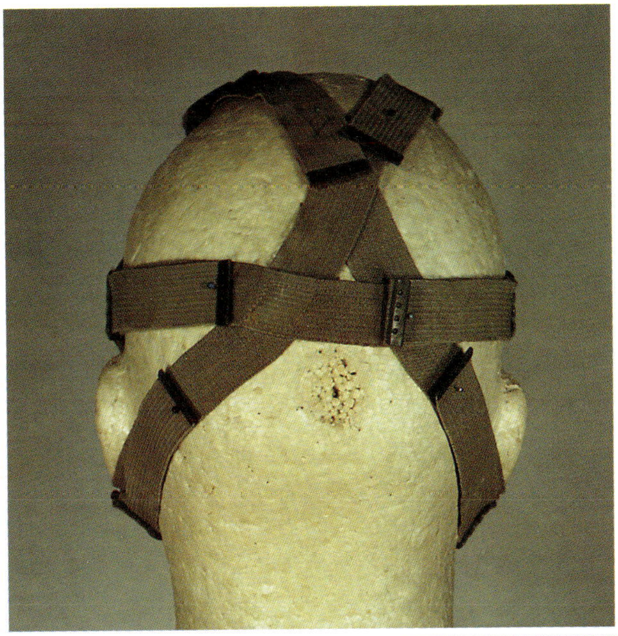

U.S. Army M2A1 Service Gas Mask (Heavyweight), 1940-41. Details of the M4 type elasticized head harness are visible, despite the straps having been pinned for clarity. The M4 harness was also used on the MIA1 Noncombatant Gas Mask, and later on several other masks (M8, etc.).

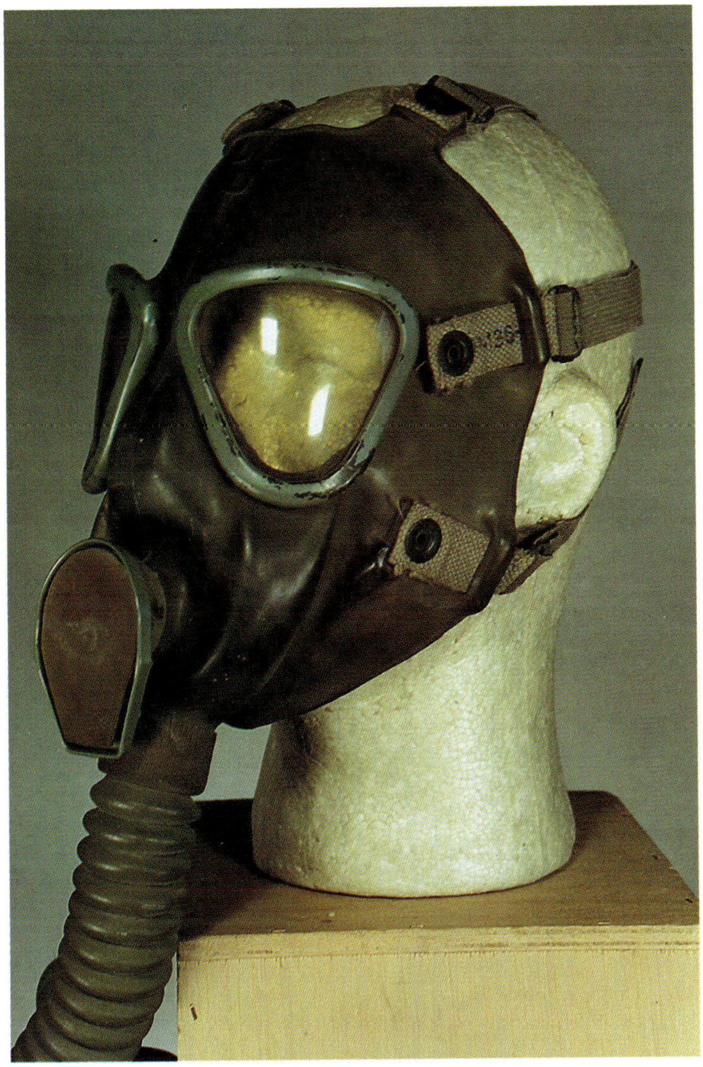

U.S. Army M2A1 Service Gas Mask (Heavyweight), 1940-41. Good view of the type MV exhalation valve, which had a plastic guard backing it.

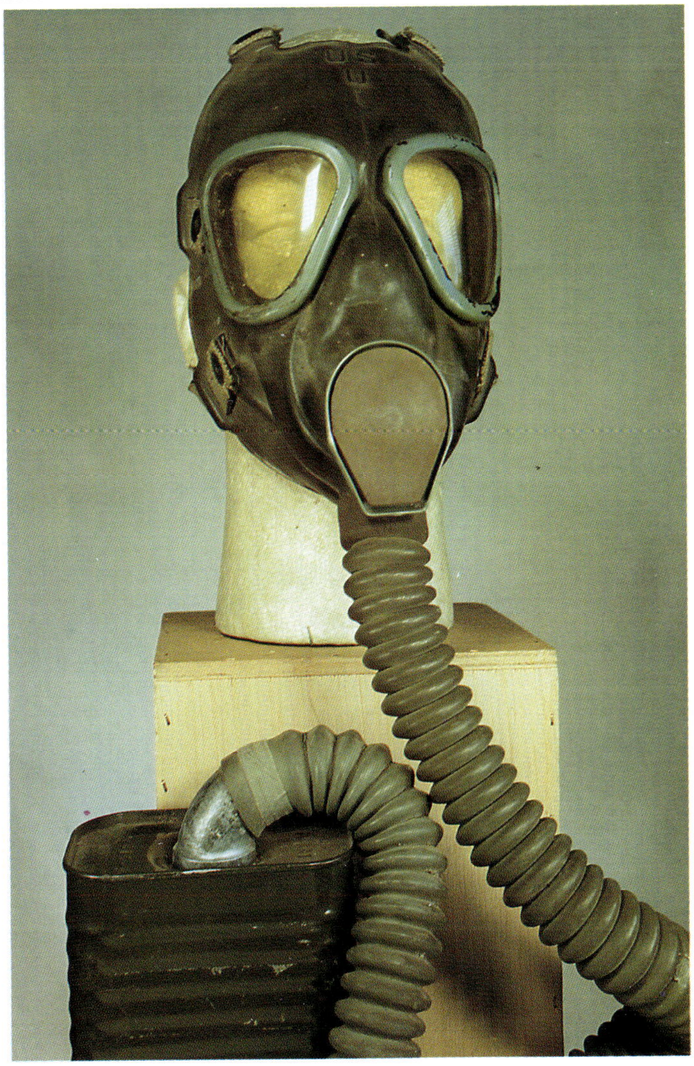

U.S. Army M2A1-IXA1-IVA1 Service Gas Mask (Heavyweight), 1940-41. Original color of facepiece was near that of distal hose end, connected to filter in this image, but became darker with age, exposure to heat, etc.

U.S. Army Diaphragm Gas Mask M3, 1940-41

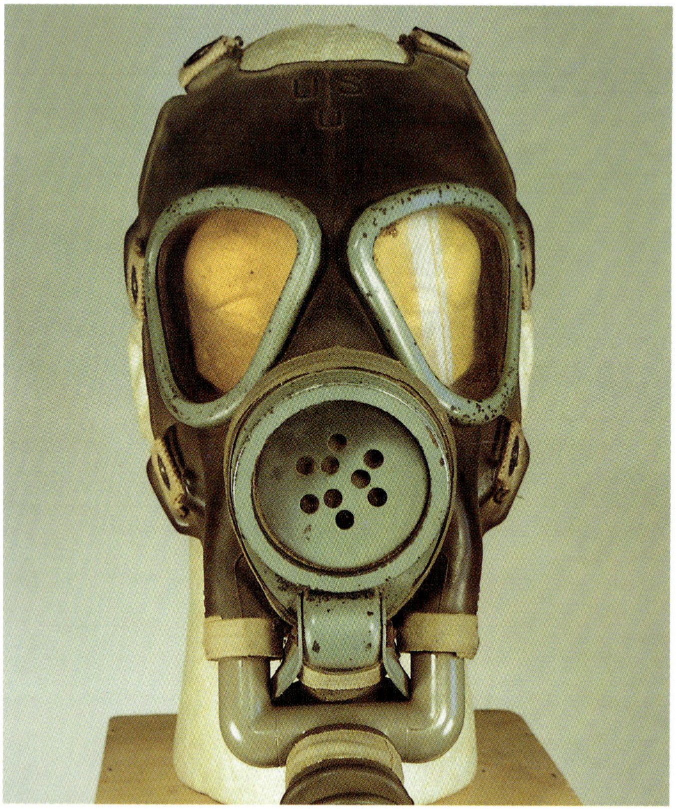

U.S. Army Diaphragm Gas Mask M3, 1940-41, example no. 1. Diaphragm counterpart to the M2A1 Service Gas Mask, the M3 used the type MVI 'spearhead' exhalation valve. This specimen is an early production model in 'good' condition, suffering discoloration effects from age.

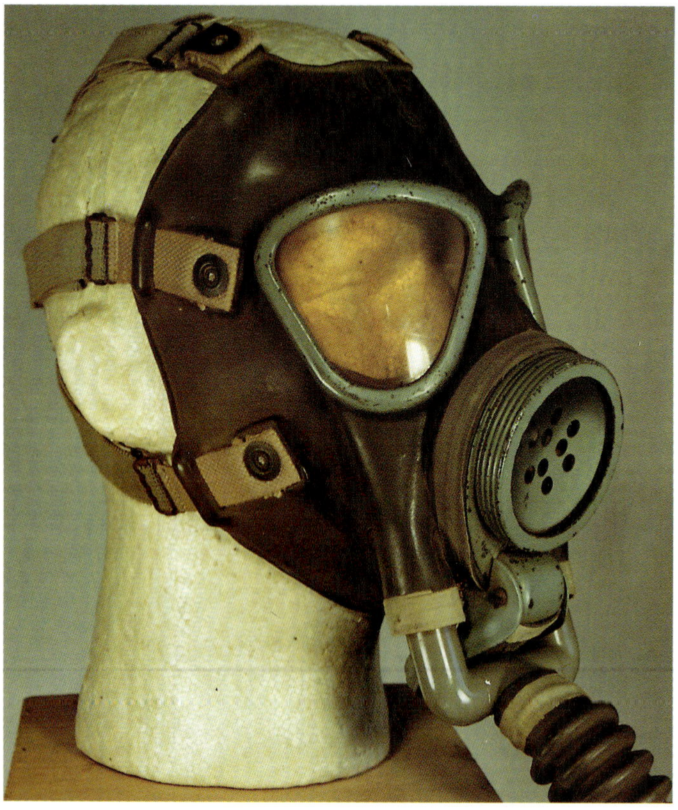

U.S. Army Diaphragm Gas Mask M3, 1940-41, example no. 1. MVI type exhaust valve was aimed rearward and downward, which helped to drain the valve of moisture and to protect it.

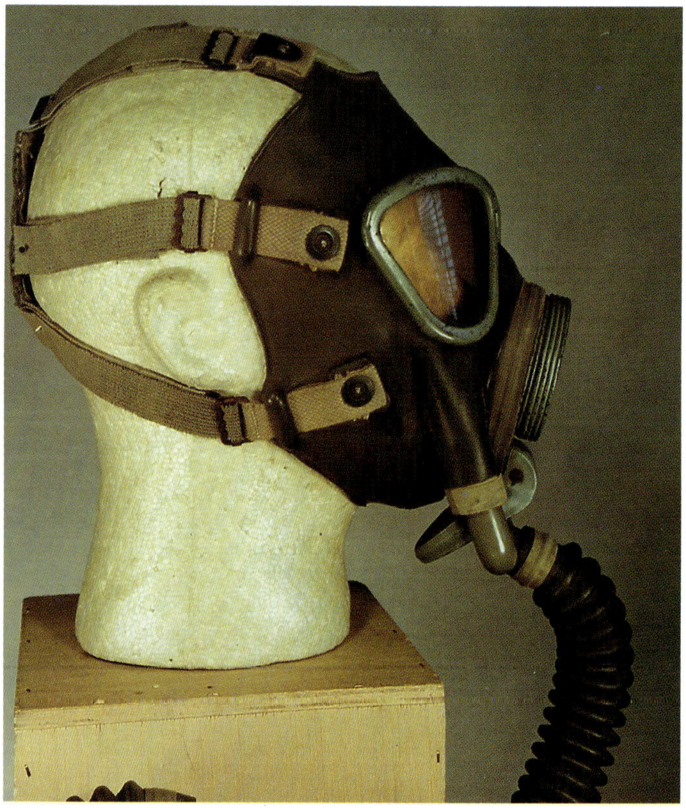

U.S. Army Diaphragm Gas Mask M3, 1940-41, example no. 1. Views of the metal exhalation valve guard and the M2 type head harness buckles (straps pinned for clarity).

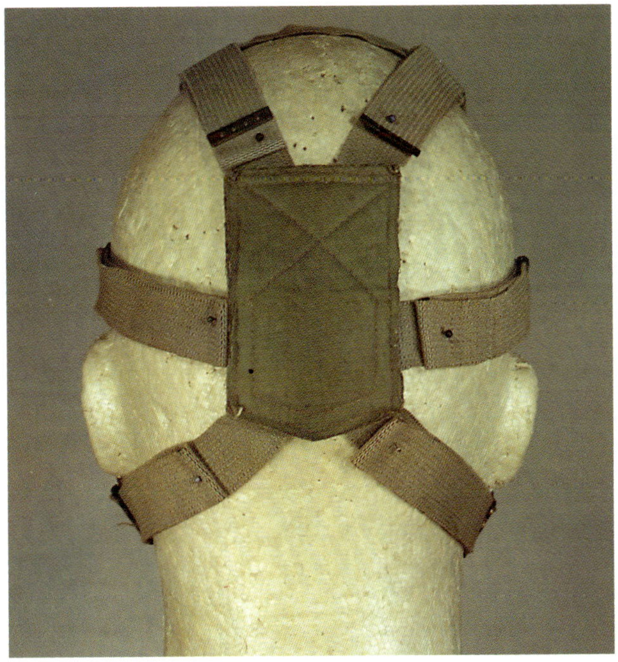

U.S. Army Diaphragm Gas Mask M3, 1940-41, example no 1. The M2 type head harness is clearly viewed.

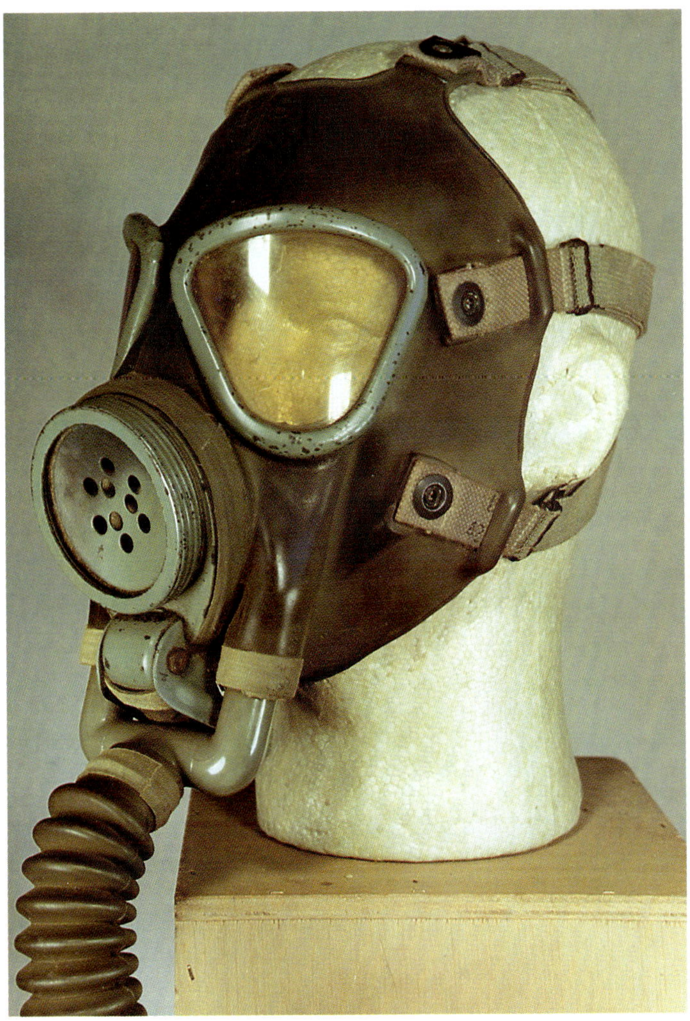

U.S. Army Diaphragm Gas Mask M3, 1940-41, example no. 1. Left profile of M3 mask, showing molded in Tissot tube air channels and bifurcated plastic inlet tube.

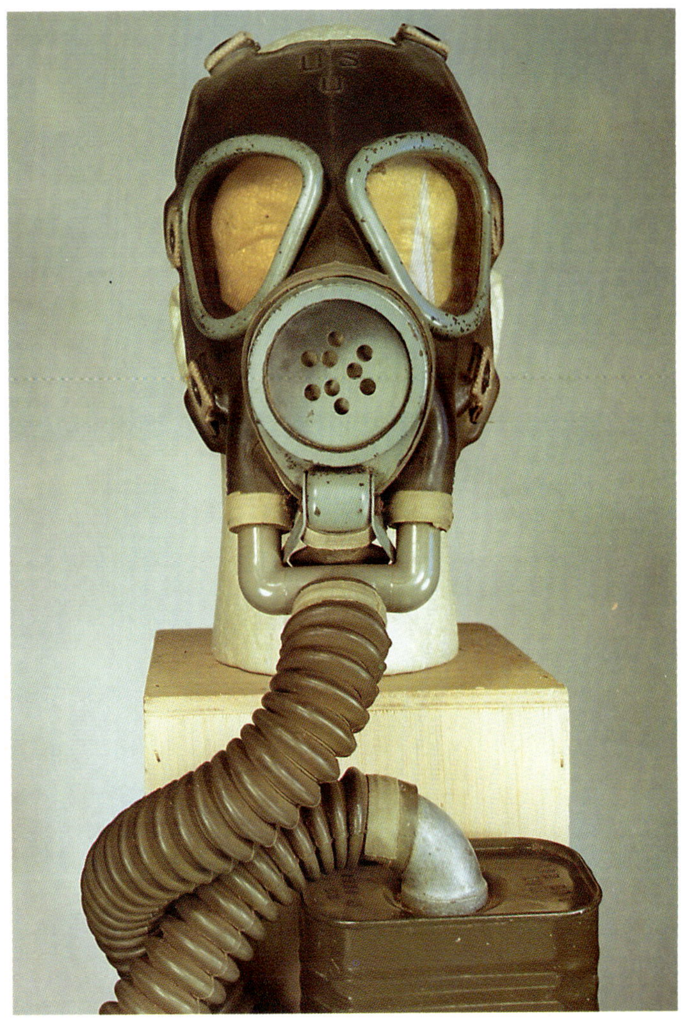

U.S. Army Diaphragm Gas Mask M3, 1940-41, example no. 1. Yellow tint of eye pieces is due to aging effects. Type MIXA1 filter canister is shown clearly.

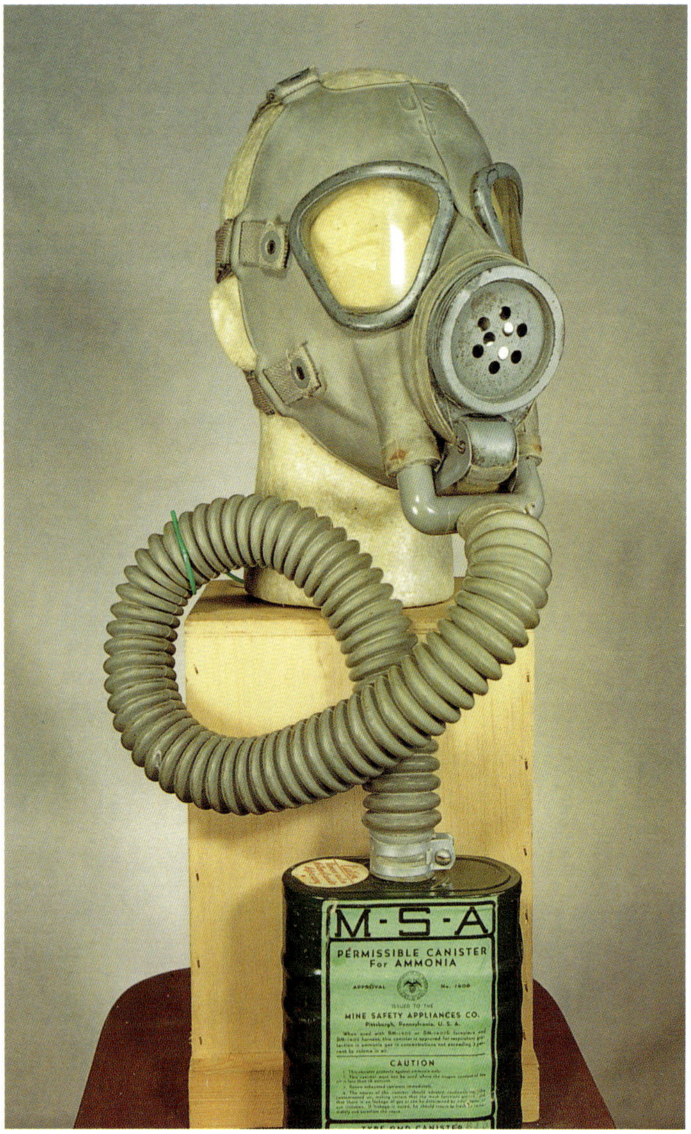

U.S. Army Diaphragm Gas Mask M3, 1940-41, example no. 2. This modification of the M3 used an MSA type GMD (commercial grade) Ammonia filter canister especially for use with that chemical. The type MIVA1 carrying satchel for this mask is marked "Ammonia mask" in stenciled ink, and has a small opening near the filter inlet (made after the carrier was manufactured).

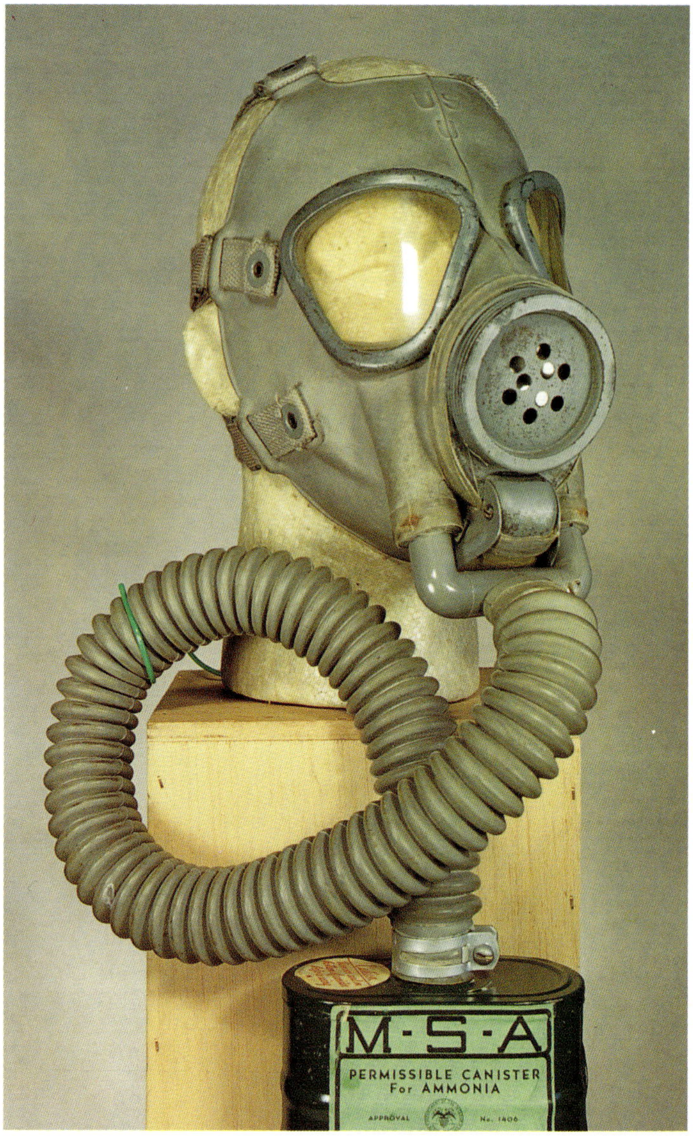

U.S. Army Diaphragm Gas Mask M3, 1941-42, example no. 2. Another image of the 'Ammonia mask.'

U.S. Army Diaphragm Gas Mask M3A1, 1942-43

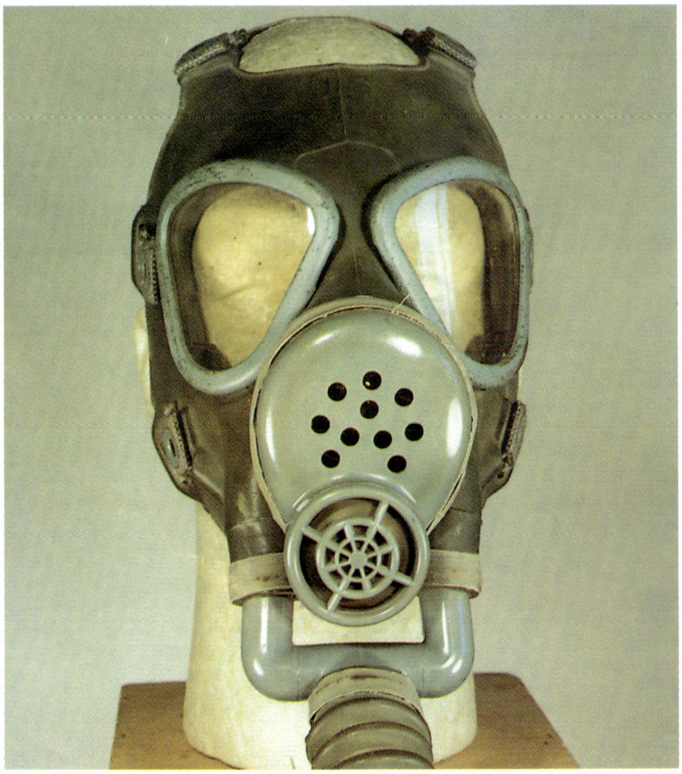

U.S. Army Diaphragm Gas Mask, M3A1, 1942-43. This updated version used the M8 type exhalation valve in a combined plastic diaphragm housing assembly.

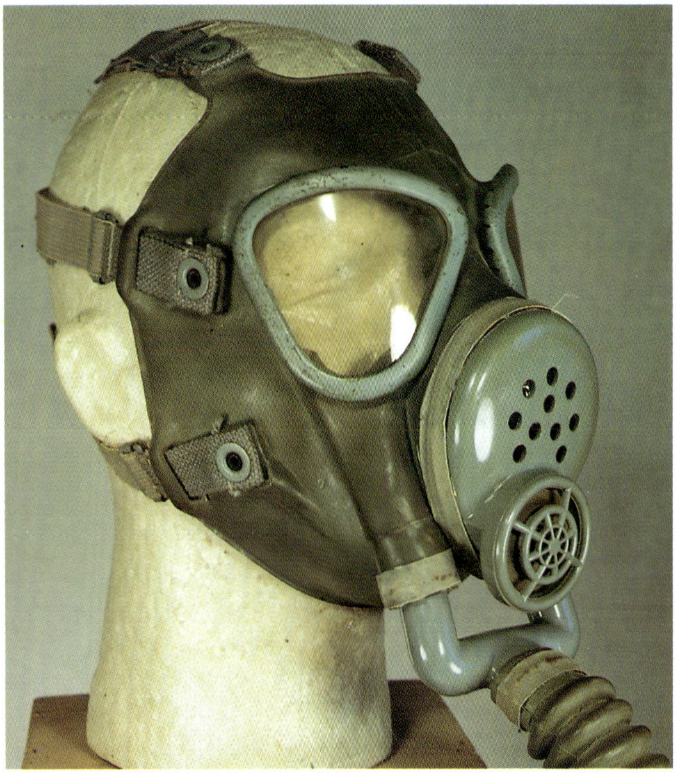

U.S. Army Diaphragm Gas Mask M3A1, 1942-43. Discoloration from age shows in this image but specimen is in 'good' condition overall.

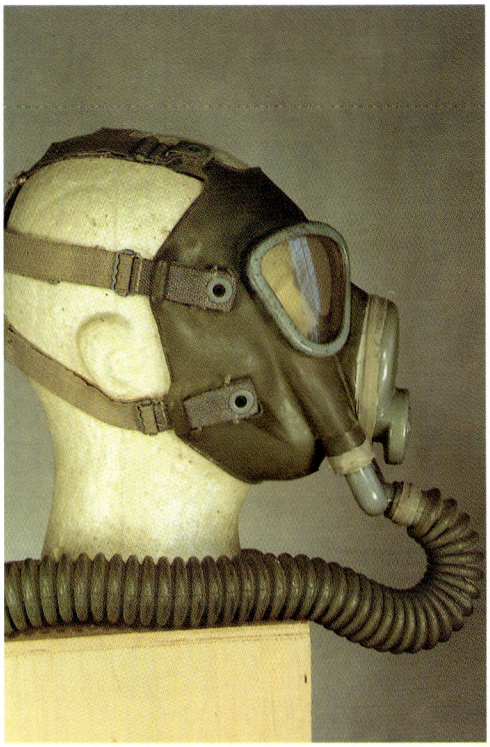

U.S. Army Diaphragm Gas Mask M3A1, 1942-43. Compare this view with the side profile view of the M3 Diaphragm mask. Details of harness are shown.

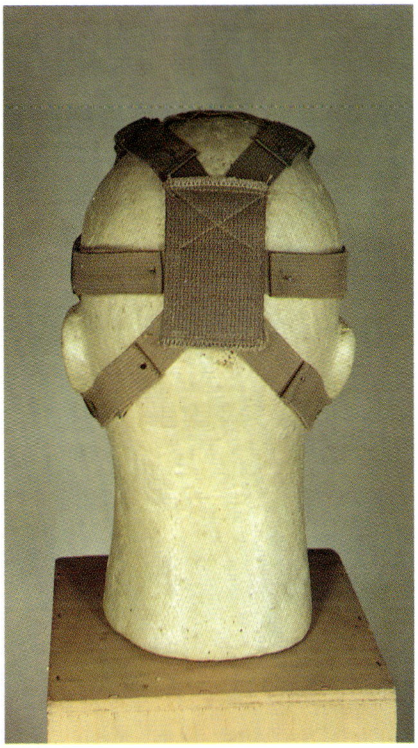

U.S. Army Diaphragm Gas Mask M3A1, 1942-43. Details of M2A1 type head harness are shown (straps pinned for clarity).

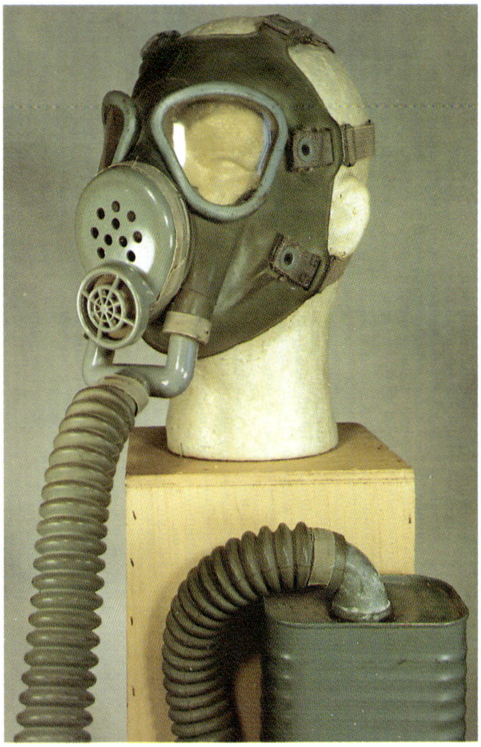

U.S. Army Diaphragm Gas Mask M3A1, 1942-43. Overall view of M3 type facepiece (with M8 valve), 27 inch molded rubber hose, and type MIXA1 filter canister.

U.S. Army Lightweight Gas Mask (neoprene) M3, 1944

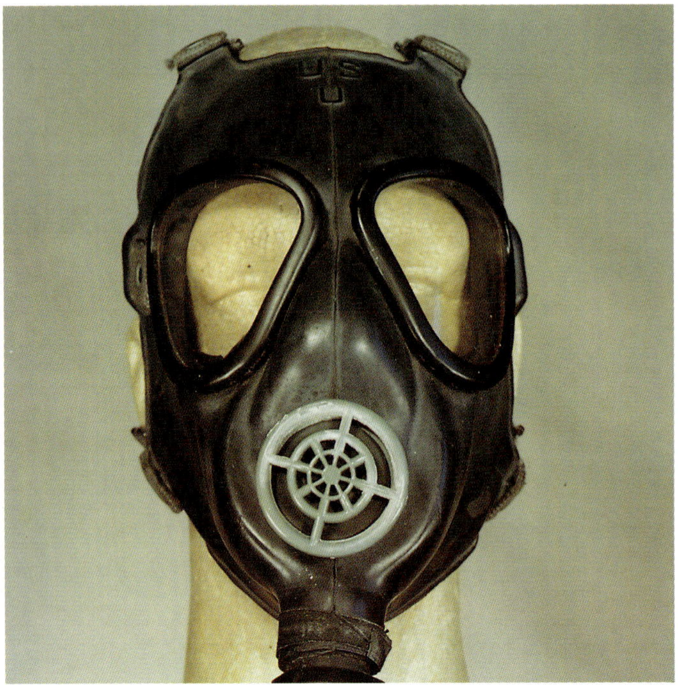

U.S. Army Lightweight Gas Mask (neoprene) M3, 1944, example no. 1. This specimen, with M8 exhalation valve, is one of the early M3 series masks entirely made from neoprene. The M3 was the first mask to feature an oronasal internal cup to enhance demisting control.

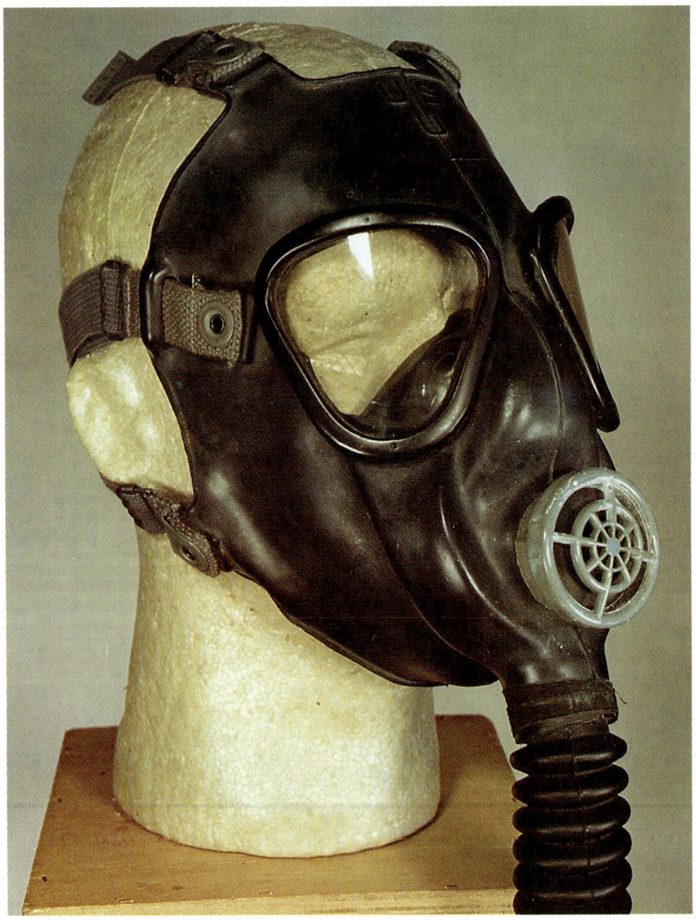

U.S. Army Lightweight Gas Mask (neoprene) M3, 1944, example no. 1. Internal oronasal cup may be seen through right lens. This specimen is in 'excellent' condition throughout, which considering the problems with neoprene's "cold set" tendencies, is remarkable.

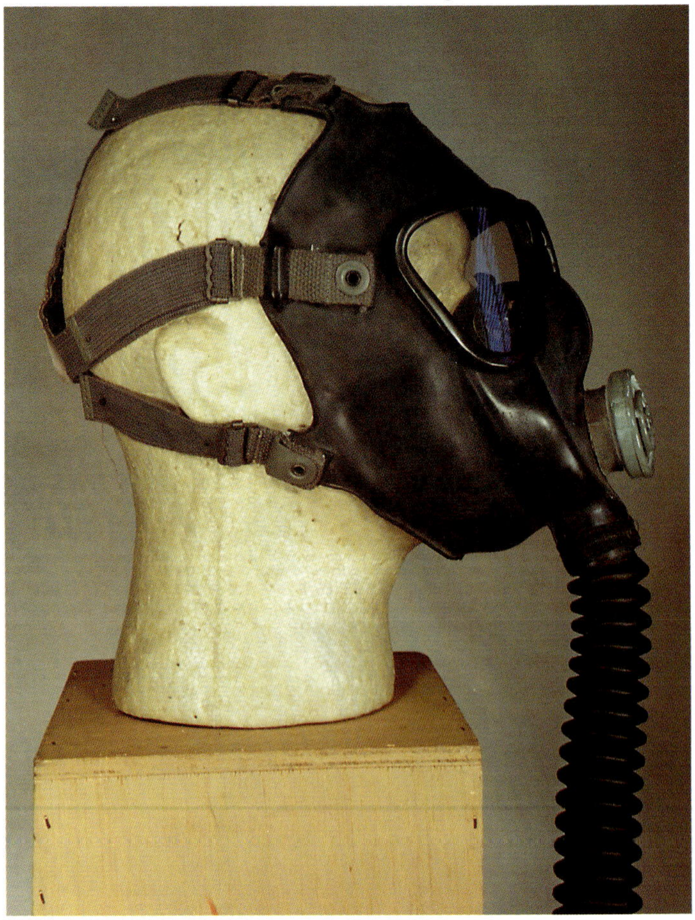

U.S. Army Lightweight Gas Mask (neoprene) M3, 1944, example no. 1. Side view of M3 service mask shows M7 type head harness detail.

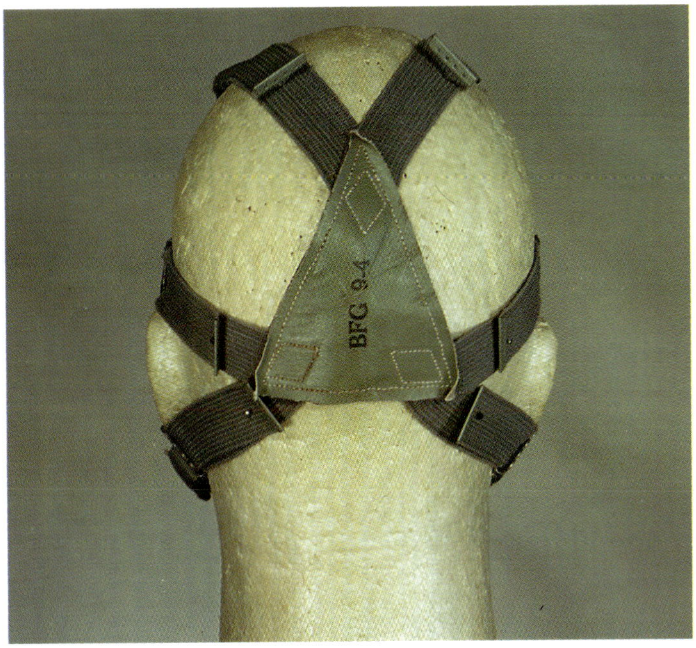

U.S. Army Lightweight Gas Mask (neoprene) M3, 1944, example no. 1. Rear view of type M7 head harness with mfg. ID and date shown(B.F.Goodrich, 9/44).

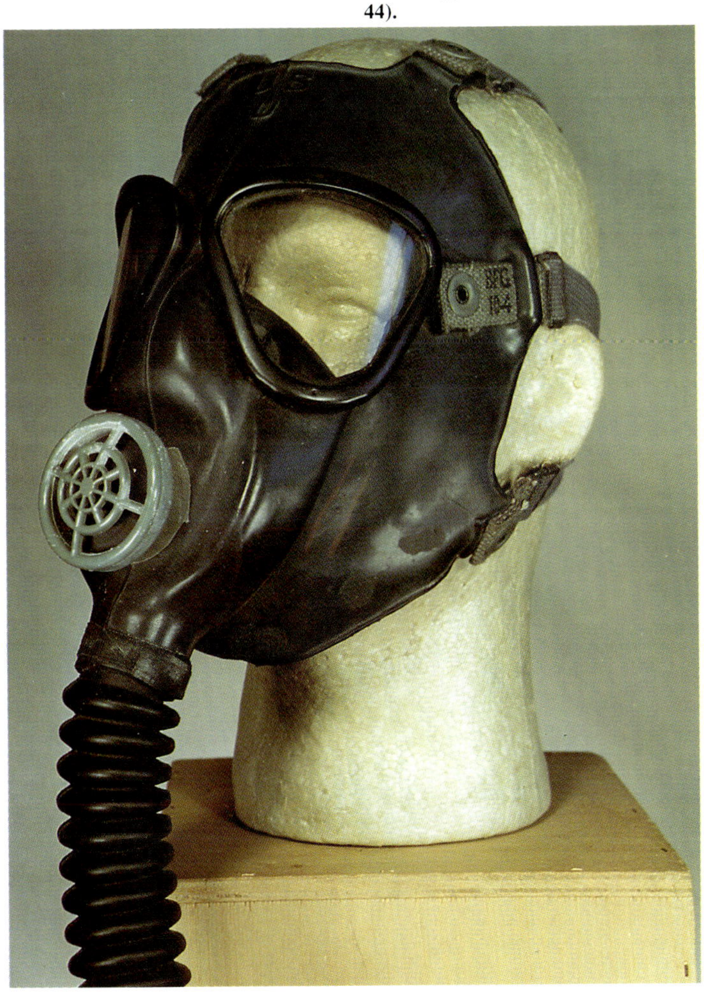

U.S. Army Lightweight Gas Mask (neoprene) M3, 1944, example no. 1. A left oblique view. Note mfg. ID and date on left lateral strap attachment (BFG, 10/44).

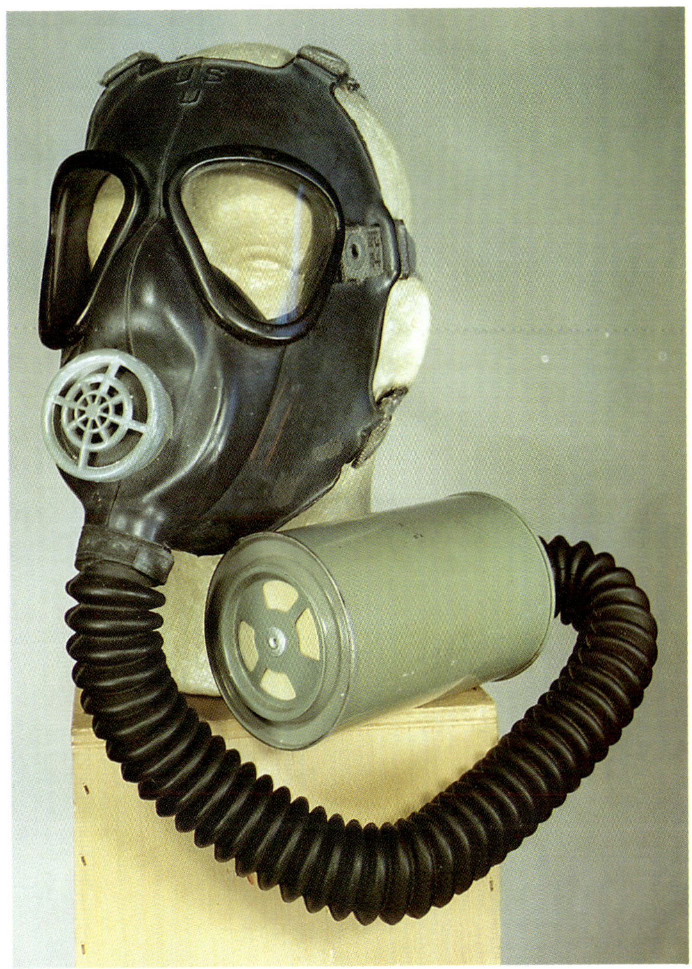

U.S. Army Lightweight Gas Mask (neoprene) M3, 1944, example no. 1. Shown is the complete assembly of neoprene facepiece, hose and type M10A1 filter canister. Excellently preserved and never issued or used.

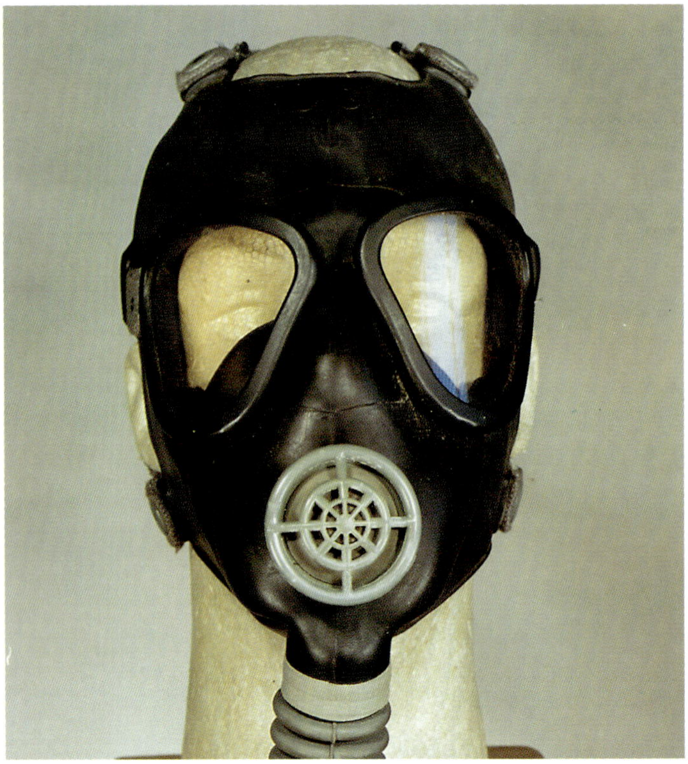

U.S. Army Lightweight Gas Mask (neoprene/natural rubber) M3, 1944, example no. 2. Specimen shown has natural rubber hose and neoprene facepiece, a not atypical configuration given the unpredictable rubber supply problems of the war. Also in 'excellent' (unissued) condition.

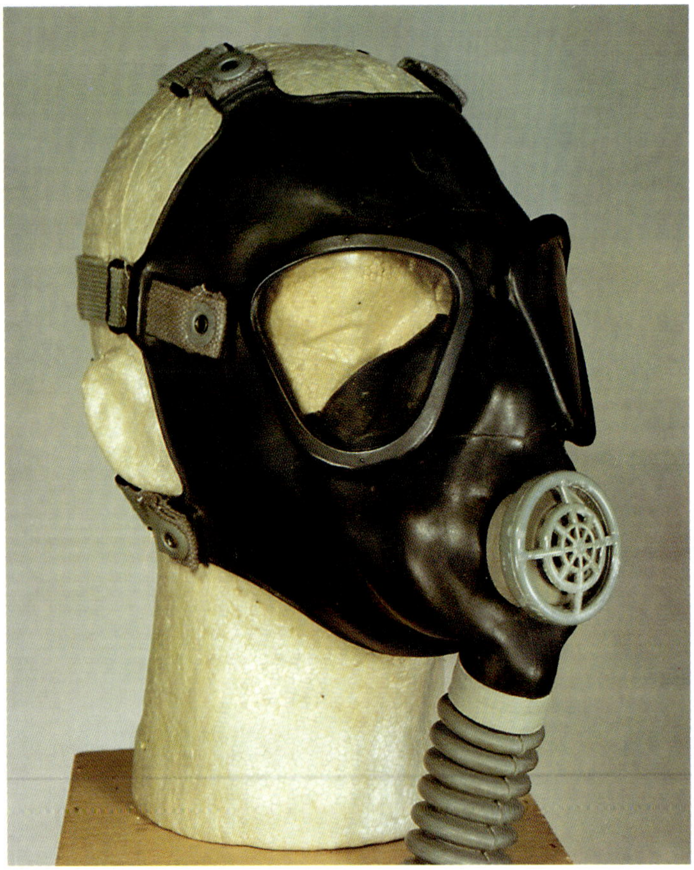

U.S. Army Lightweight Gas Mask (neoprene/natural rubber) M3, 1944, example no. 2. 'Cold-set' problems experienced during winter of 1944-45 made this type of neoprene constructed mask unusable.

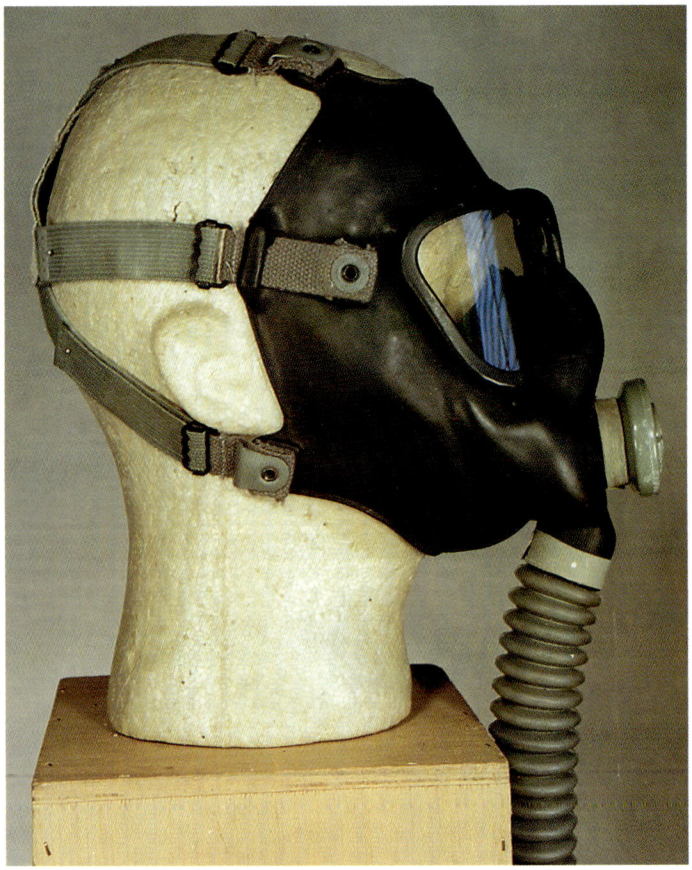

U.S. Army Lightweight Gas Mask (neoprene/natural rubber) M3, 1944, example no. 2. Side view shows M7 harness details, which was a modified and sturdier expression of the earlier M4 design used on the M2 training mask. Rearward angulation of mask inlet at chin is due to cold-set 'memory' (compare with previous specimen, same profile view).

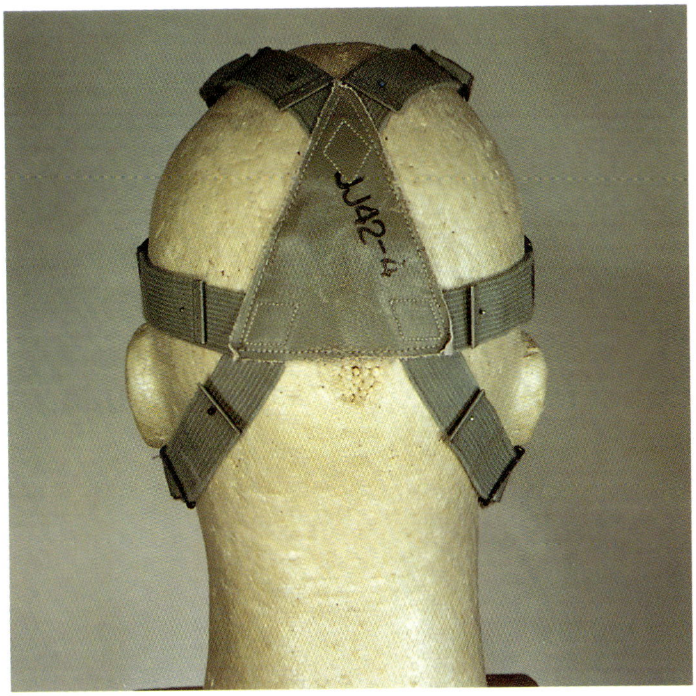

U.S. Army Lightweight Gas Mask (neoprene/natural rubber) M3, 1944, example no. 2. Detail of typical M7 head harness with mfg. ID and date.

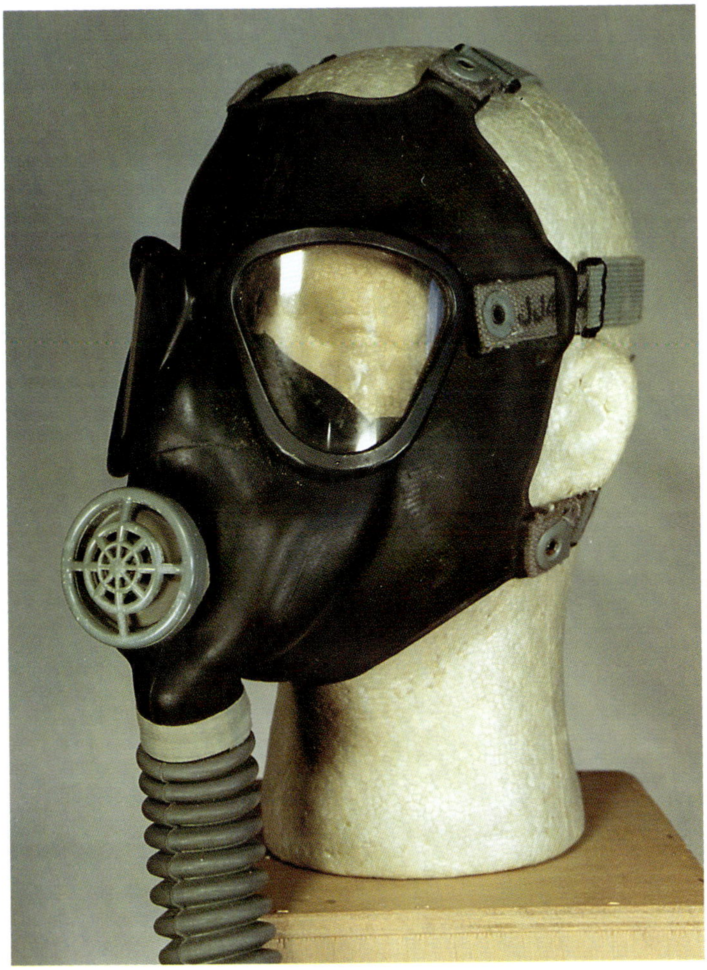

U.S. Army Lightweight Gas Mask (neoprene/natural rubber) M3, 1944, example no. 2. Whitish, powder-like substance on M8 exhalation valve is waxy solution used as a preservative.

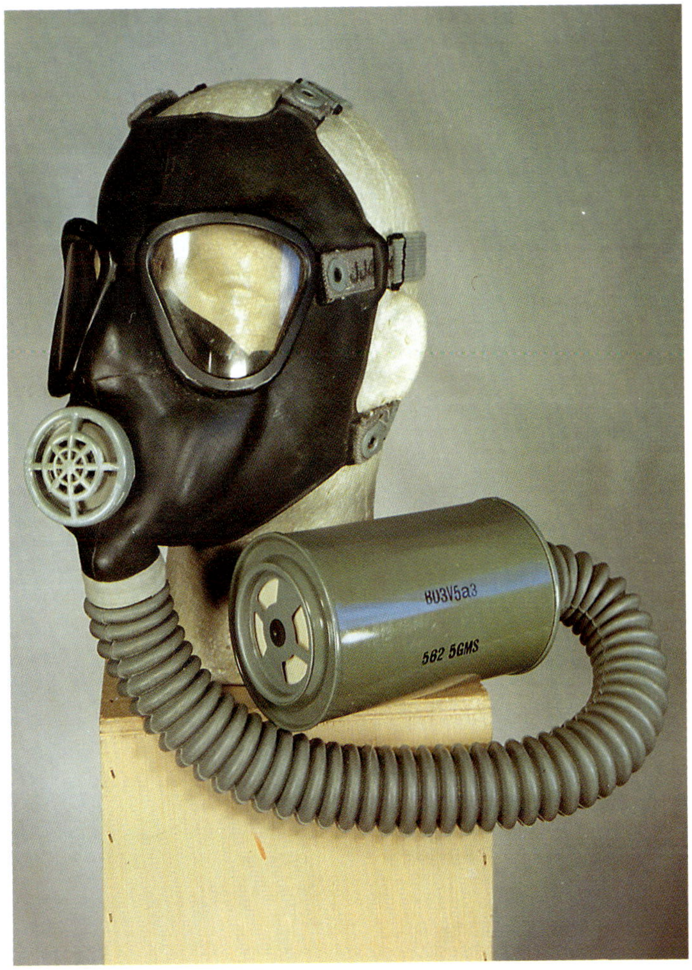

U.S. Army Lightweight Gas Mask (neoprene/natural rubber) M3, 1944, example no. 2. Left profile view reveals overall 'excellent' (unissued) condition of this specimen, with natural rubber hose and M10A1 filter canister. Note perfect condition of thin rubber filter inlet valve.

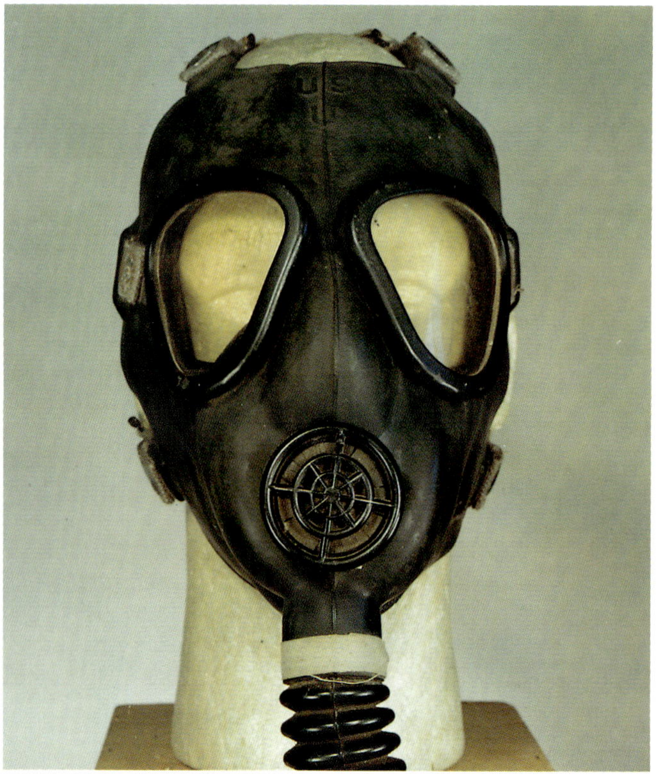

U.S. Army Lightweight Gas Mask (neoprene) M3, 1944, example no. 3. Specimen is in overall 'very good' condition, although some desiccation of (M8) valve rubber is noted, harness is in 'average/ fair' condition, and mask is somewhat dusty.

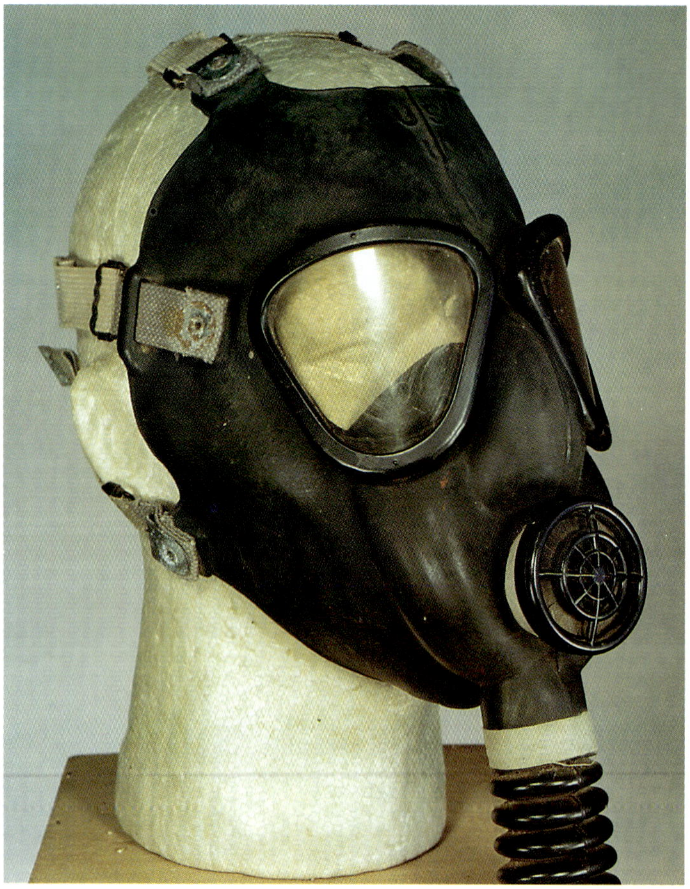

U.S. Army Lightweight Gas Mask (neoprene) M3, 1944, example no. 3. Despite the fact that the M3 design had been developed in 1942, and started production in 1943, only about 15,000 were made prior to 1944 due to problems with the M3 eye-rings, M6 type carrier and M10 type filter canister.

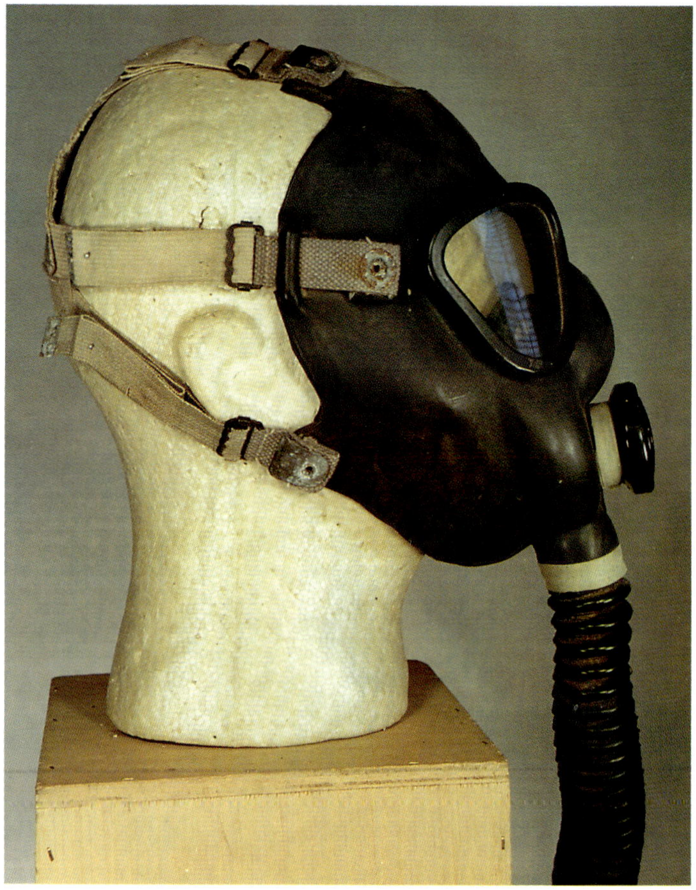

U.S. Army Lightweight Gas Mask (neoprene) M3, 1944, example no. 3. The somewhat deteriorated harness straps may be discerned, as well as some corrosion of the mask strap fittings. The facepiece itself and hose are in excellent condition.

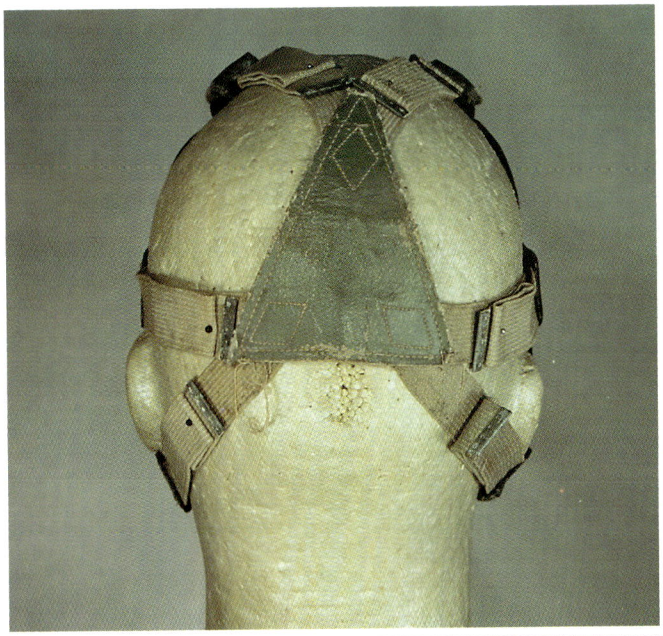

U.S. Army Lightweight Gas Mask (neoprene) M3, 1944, example no. 3. The major distinction between the M3 and the succeeding M3A1 was substitution on the latter mask of the newer C15 exhalation valve assembly. Head harness may be seen here in 'average/fair' condition.

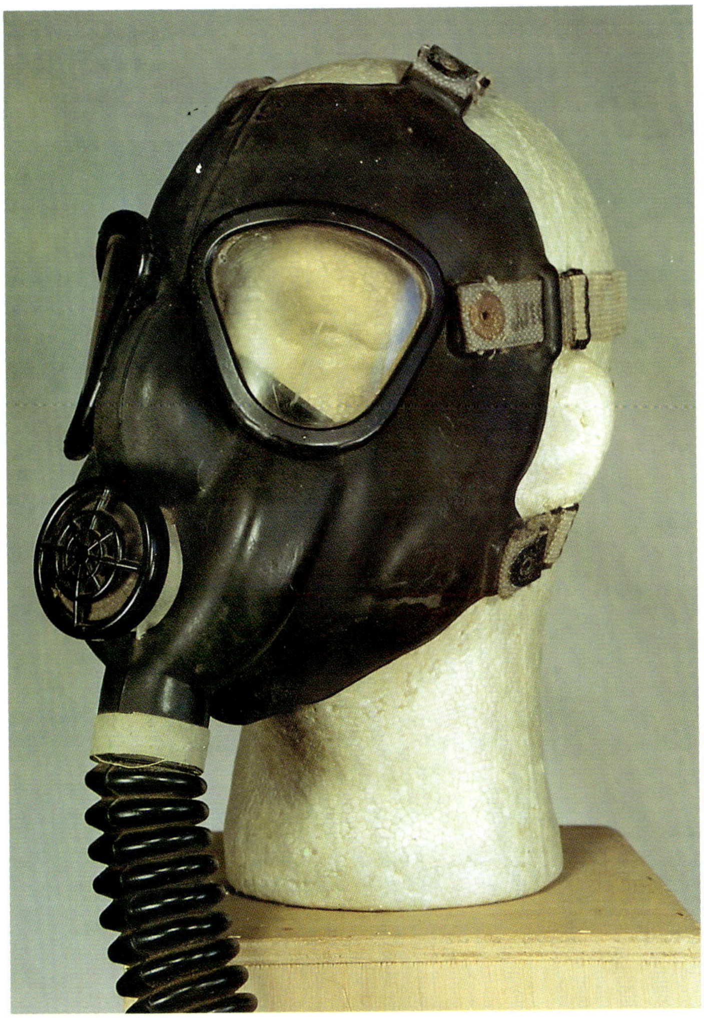

U.S. Army Lightweight Gas Mask (neoprene) M3, 1944, example no. 3. Another view of the left oblique aspect of this specimen. Note mfg. ID and date mark on temple strap attachment piece. The plastic used in this specimen's M8 type exhalation valve is black, instead of green.

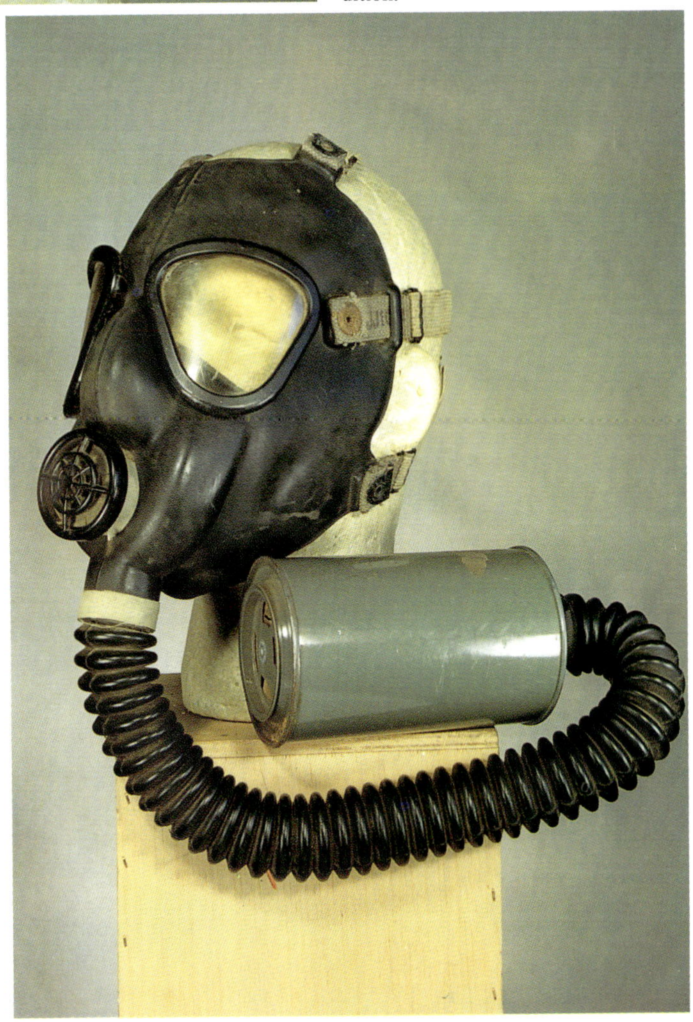

U.S. Army Lightweight Gas Mask (neoprene) M3, 1944, example no. 3. Overall view shows some corrosion on M10A1 filter canister, deteriorated filter inlet valve, and facepiece harness strap attachment hardware corrosion. The standard "Lightweight" mask hose length was 18 inches (compared to 27 for the "Heavyweight" masks).

U.S. Army Lightweight Gas Mask (neoprene, natural rubber) M3A1, 1944

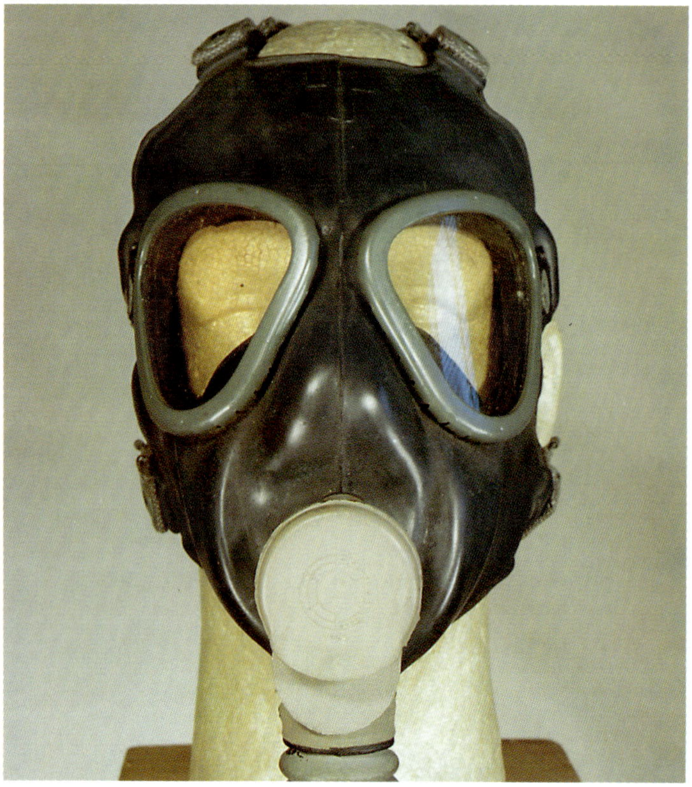

U.S. Army Lightweight Gas Mask (neoprene/natural rubber) M3A1, 1944. Addition of C15 exhalation valve assembly resulted in M3A1 designation; otherwise identical to M3. Note natural rubber hose.

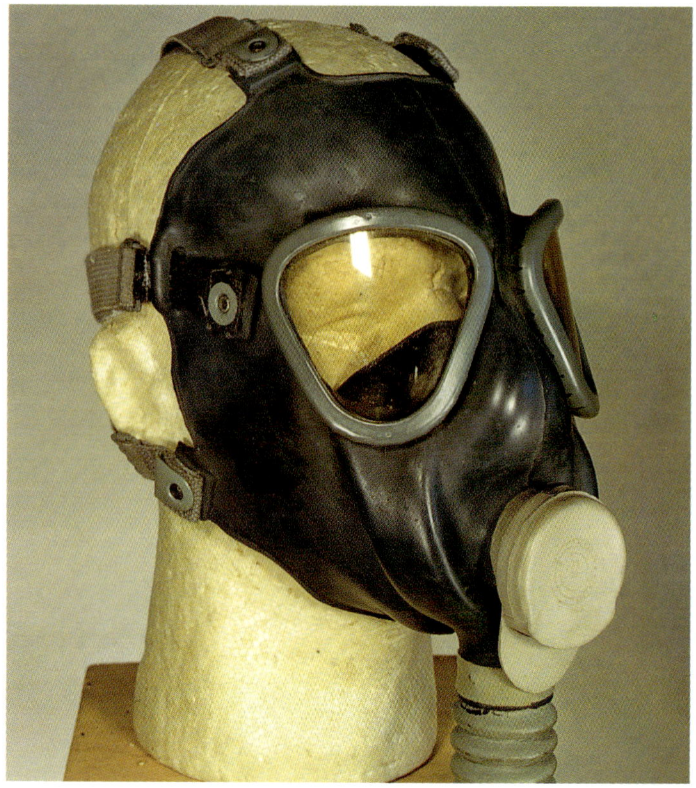

U.S. Army Lightweight Gas Mask (neoprene/natural rubber) M3A1, 1944. Note use of black woven cotton duck on facepiece portion of temple strap (instead of gray/green). This specimen is in overall 'very good' condition.

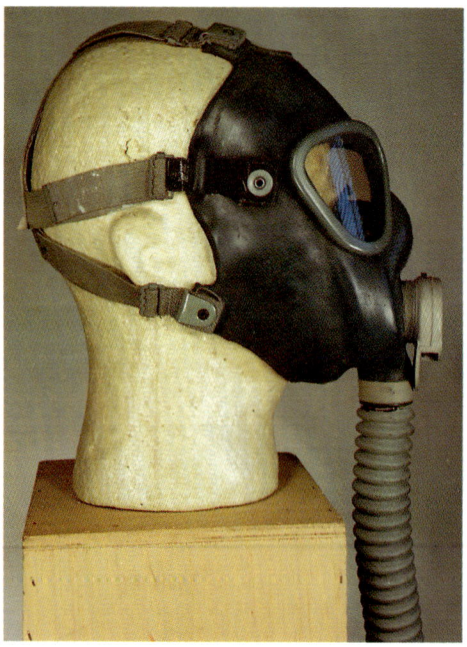

U.S. Army Lightweight Gas Mask (neoprene/natural rubber) M3A1, 1944. Hose vertical exit attitude from facepiece is normal (no cold-set 'memory' from storage in M6 carrier).

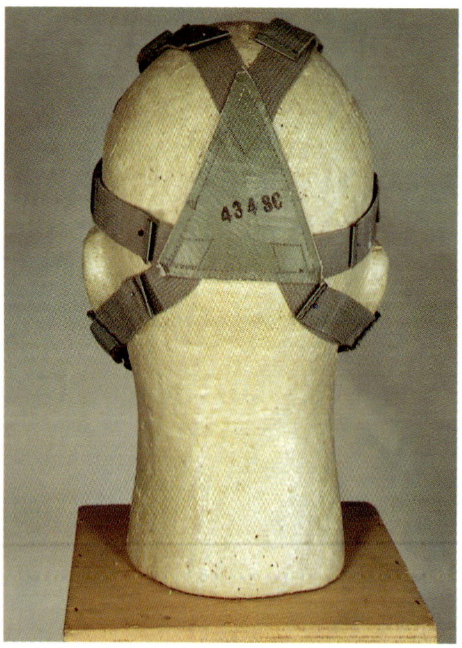

U.S. Army Lightweight Gas Mask (neoprene/natural rubber) M3A1, 1944. Details of M7 type head harness may be observed. Straps are pinned to head form for clarity. Mfg. ID & date on triangular pad of harness.

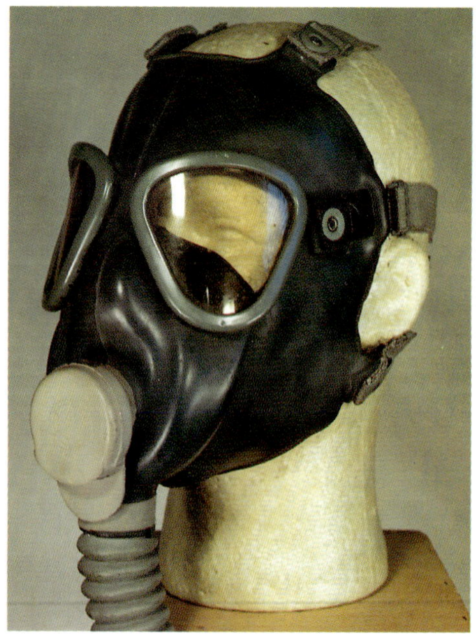

U.S. Army Lightweight Gas Mask (neoprene/natural rubber) M3A1, 1944. A good left oblique view of this specimen and C15 style exhalation valve. 18 inch hoses for the M3 and M4 were not infrequently made by cutting down older M2 style service mask 27 inch hoses, and give the misleading appearance of having been "field-rigged." In actuality, they were thus configured during initial fabrication.

U.S. Army Lightweight Gas Mask, M4, 1944

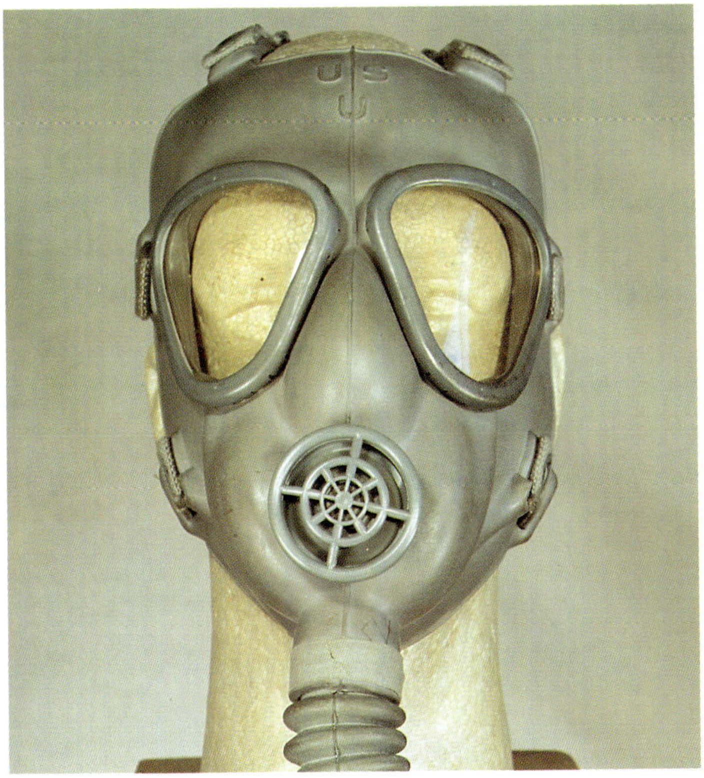

U.S. Army Lightweight Gas Mask M4, 1944. This specimen is made from an M2A2 rubber facepiece and hose and utilizes the M8 exhalation valve. Overall condition is 'excellent' and it appears as if this specimen was issued but never used. Color of rubber is very close to original (no aging effects).

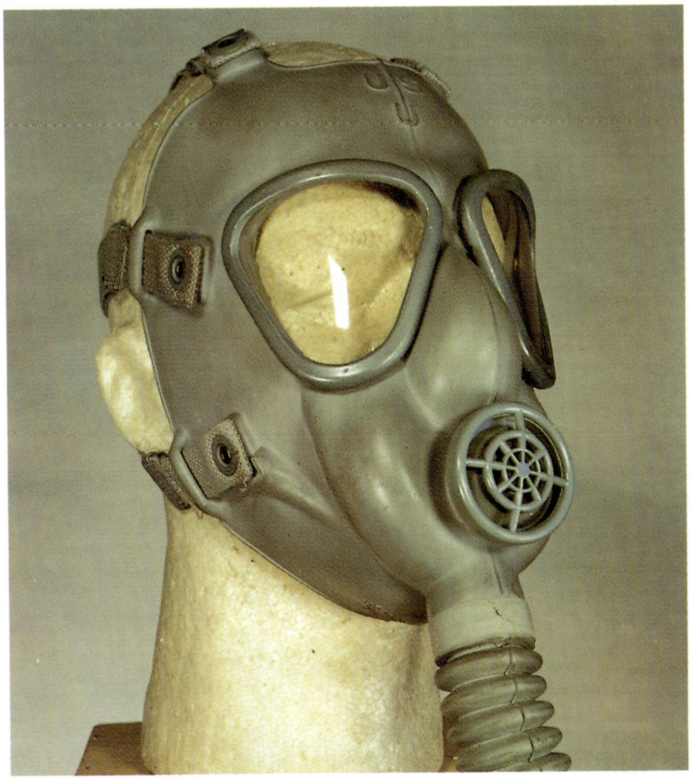

U.S. Army Lightweight Gas Mask M4, 1944. Eye frames are characteristic of earlier facepieces. Note clear detail of 'rifle skids' on facepiece's lower lateral harness attachment points. M4A1 used C15 exhalation valve instead of M8.

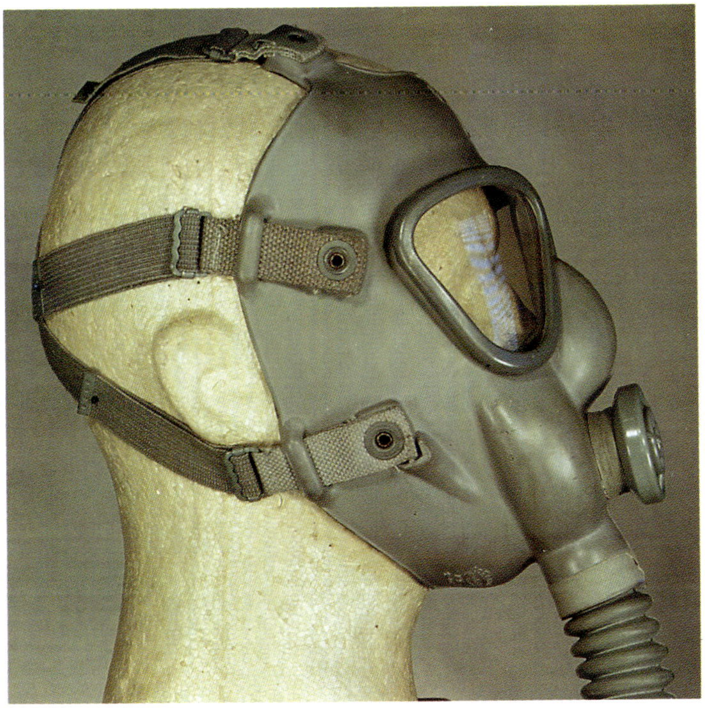

U.S. Army Lightweight Gas Mask M4, 1944. Note that this specimen has not been modified with the addition of an internal oronasal cup, which was later bonded into M4 masks. Lower strap attachments are characteristic of older M2 style facepieces.

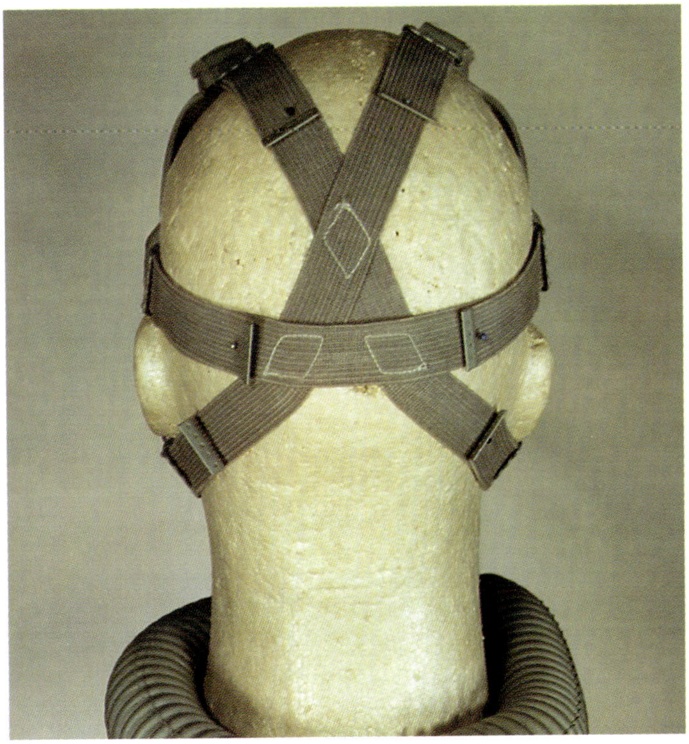

U.S. Army Lightweight Gas Mask M4, 1944. Good view of older M2 facepiece style head harness (M4 type), which is further evidence of M4 mask identification. The M7 head harness was retrofitted, when circumstances required replacement.

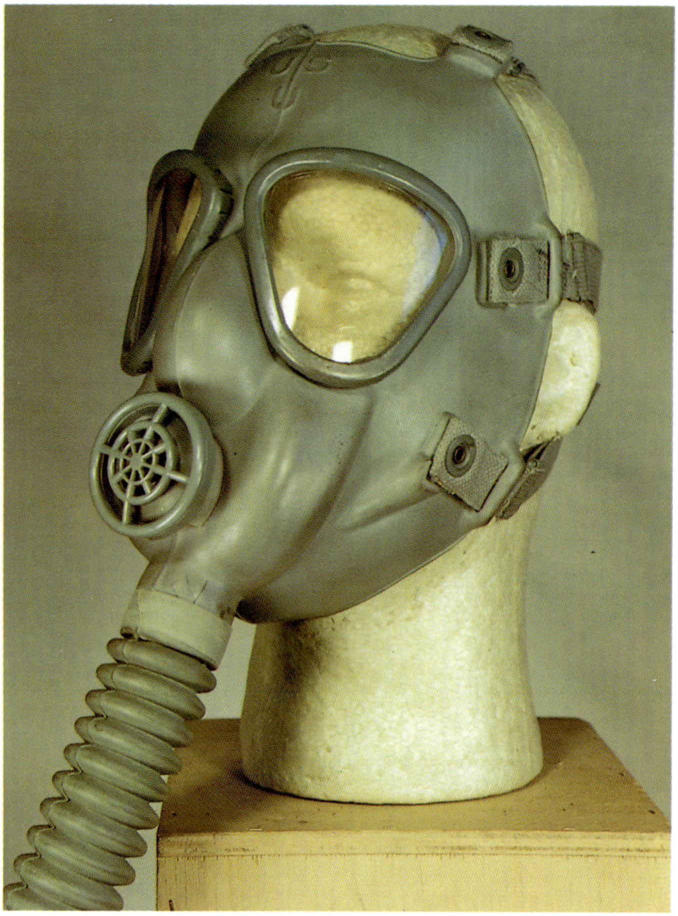

U.S. Army Lightweight Gas Mask M4, 1944. Good left oblique view of M4 mask facepiece (M2A1 type, retrieved and reclaimed).

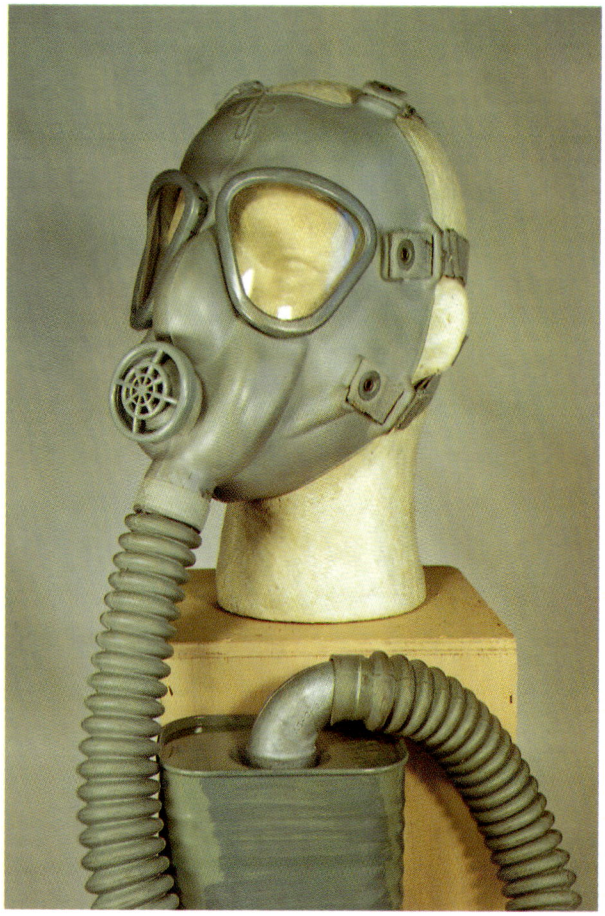

U.S. Army Lightweight Gas Mask M4, 1944. Overall view, showing facepiece, hose and type MIXA1 filter canister (gray paint has been inexplicably brushed on side of filter).

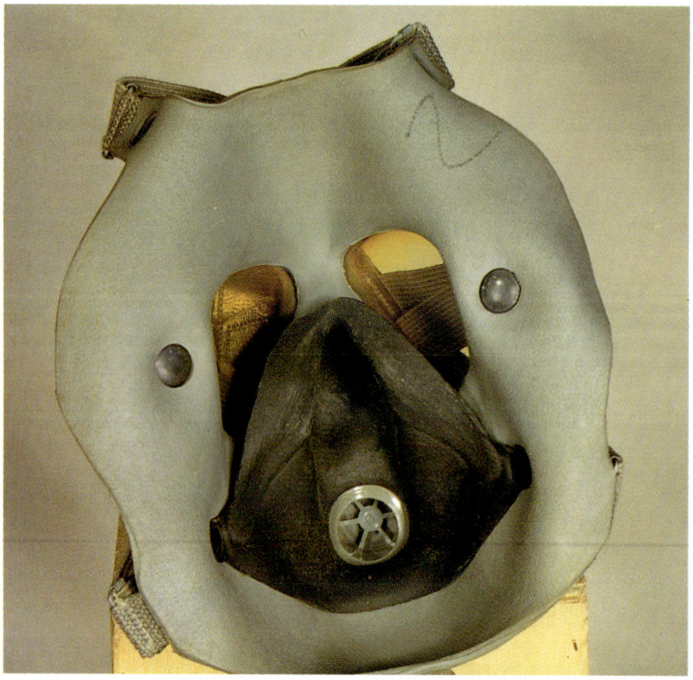

U.S. Army Lightweight Gas Mask M4A1. View of interior of an M4A1 mask which has had the internal oronasal cup fitted to it during (re)manufacturing process. Compare to next photo.

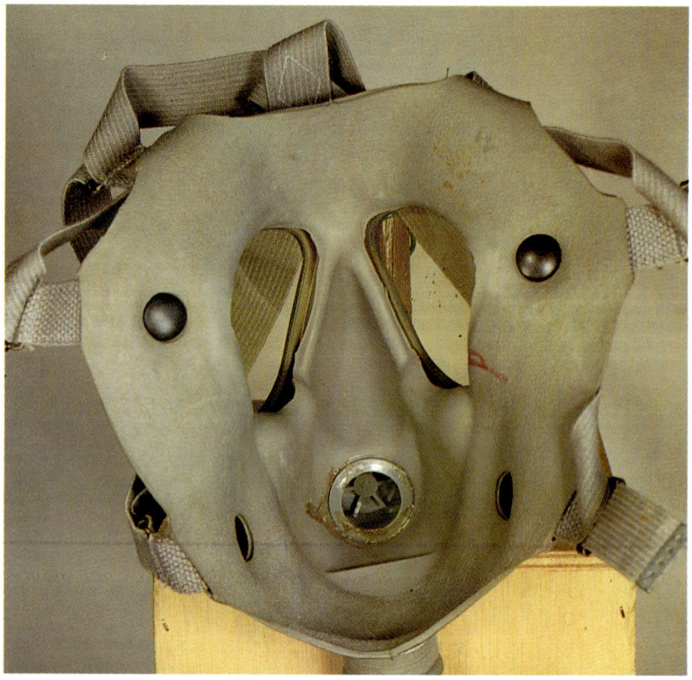

U.S. Army Lightweight Gas Mask M4. View of interior of mask which has not been fitted with the internal oronasal cup. The M3 series masks were fabricated with the cup at onset of assembly, as were later M4A1 series masks.

U.S. Army Assault Gas Mask (Combat Service Gas Mask) M5-11-7, 1944

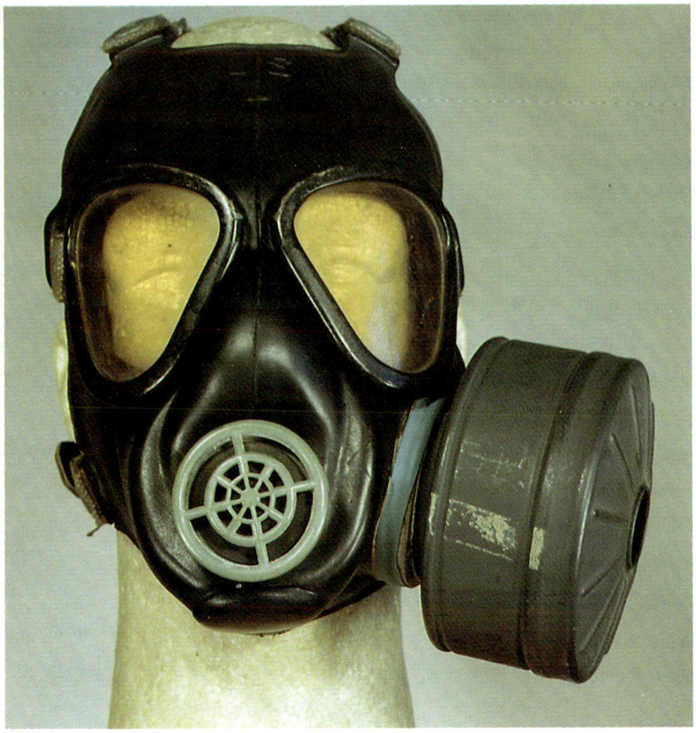

U.S. Army Assault Gas Mask (Combat Service Gas Mask) M5-11-7, 1944. Possibly one of the most interesting, and certainly one of the rarer, respirators ever produced by the United States, this specimen features a neoprene facepiece and an M8 exhalation valve, despite Army TM-3-205 / C5 references to its being properly fitted with a C15 exhalation valve.

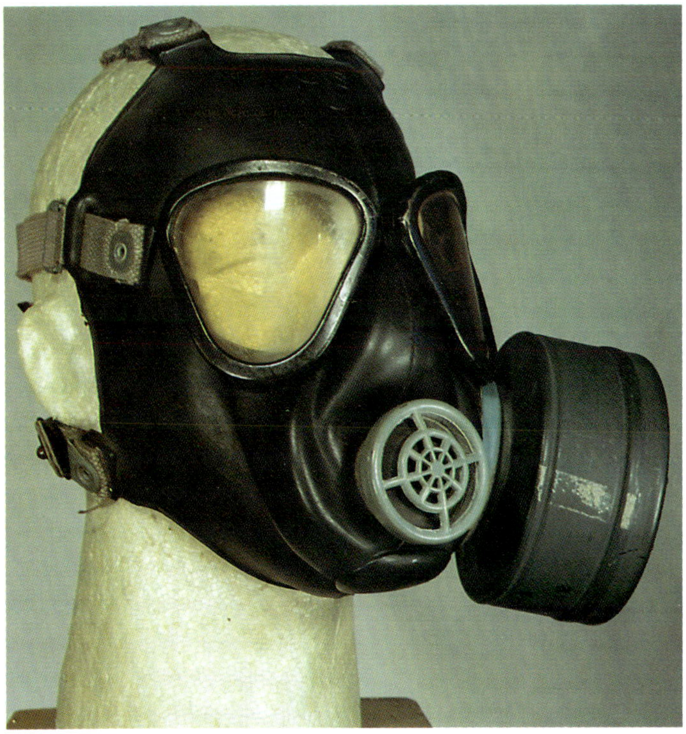

U.S. Army Assault Gas Mask (Combat Service Gas Mask) M5-11-7, 1944. This specimen is in overall 'excellent' condition, considering its relative rarity, and was used with the early M11 drum filter (which was modeled after the German FE-42 filter).

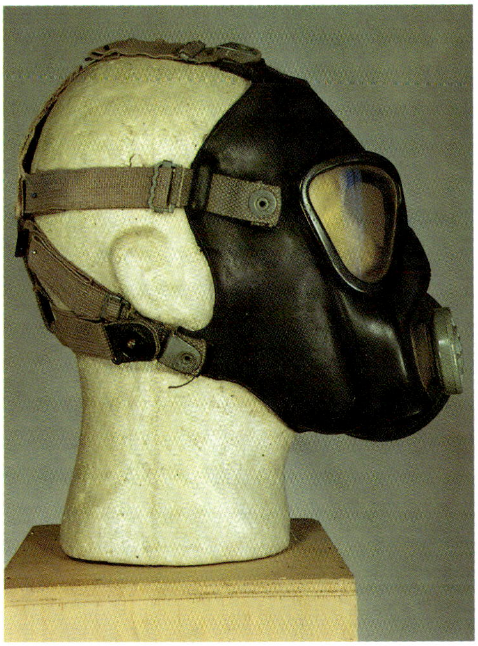

U.S. Army Assault Gas Mask (Combat Service Gas Mask) M5-11-7, 1944. It is evident from this view that there is no internal oronasal cup fitted, as in the M3 series. The M5 production program was plagued with difficulties from the onset and as a result only a limited number of the masks were ever completed before the contract was terminated at the end of 1944.

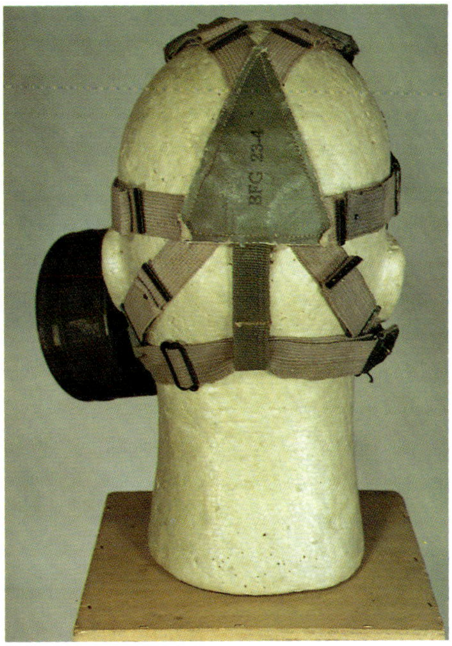

U.S. Army Assault Gas Mask (Combat Service Gas Mask) M5-11-7, 1944. A good view of the C4 type head-harness fitted to the M5 masks shows the nape strap which was added to the M7 type design. Mfg. ID (BFG) and date of fabrication mark on center pad.

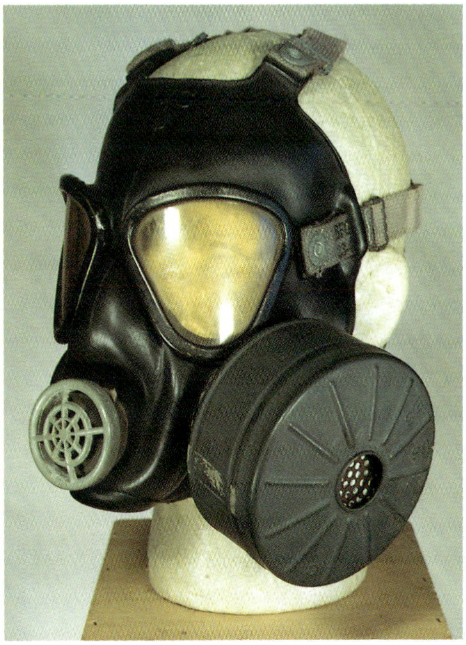

U.S. Army Assault Gas Mask (Combat Service Gas Mask) M5-11-7, 1944. A good view of the M11 canister as fitted to the left side of the neoprene facepiece. Date and mfg. ID on left temple strap fitting. The early M11 canisters incorporated asbestos as part of the particulate filtering component!

U.S. Army Snout-type Gas Mask M8-11-10, 1945

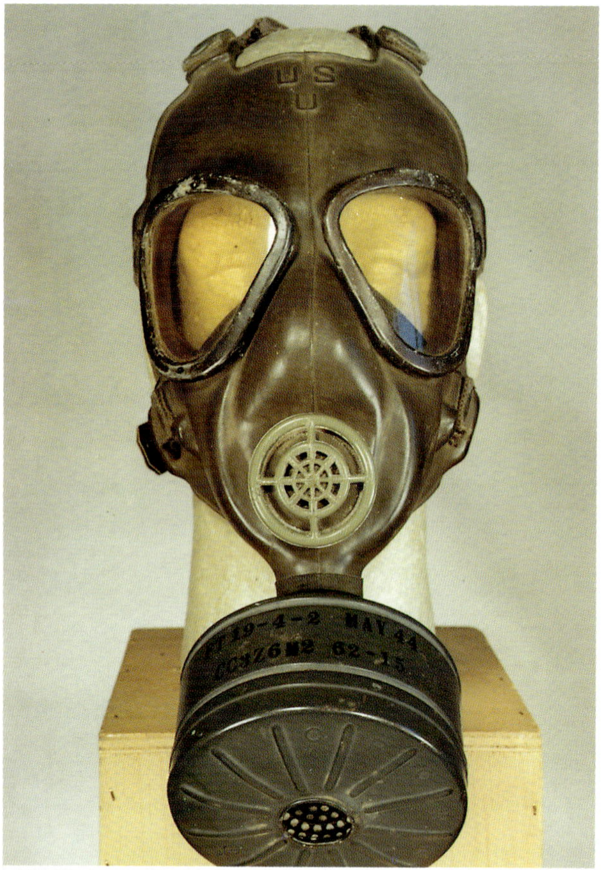

U.S. Army Snout-type Gas Mask M8-11-10, 1945. The other rare U.S. Army mask of this era, two variants of the M8 were common. One used earlier style rubber facepieces and the second used later style rubber (not neoprene) facepieces. Date on the M11 filter is clear (May 44).

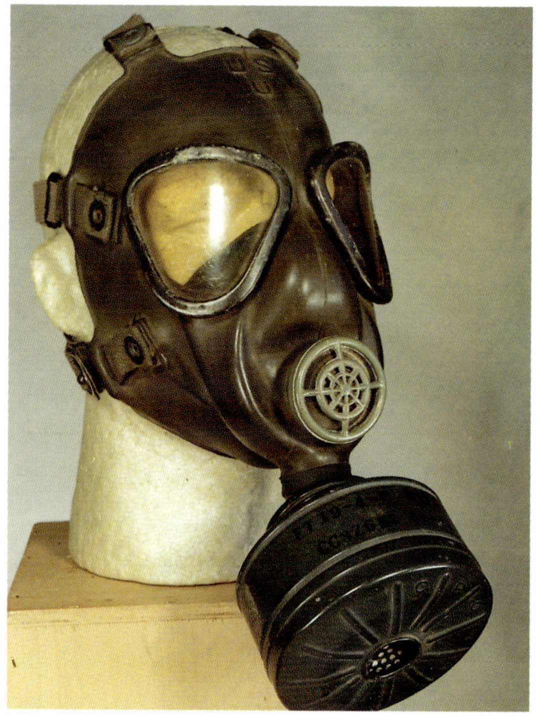

U.S. Army Snout-type Gas Mask M8-11-10, 1945. The 'rifle skid' moldings are just discernible in this photo. U.S. Army TM 3-205 (3/51) indicates the C15 exhalation valve was standard on this mask; the specimen here has the M8 valve fitted, and therefore was made using an older facepiece. Overall condition of this example is 'very good', despite some discoloration from effects of heat and age. The internal oronasal cup is evident, as well.

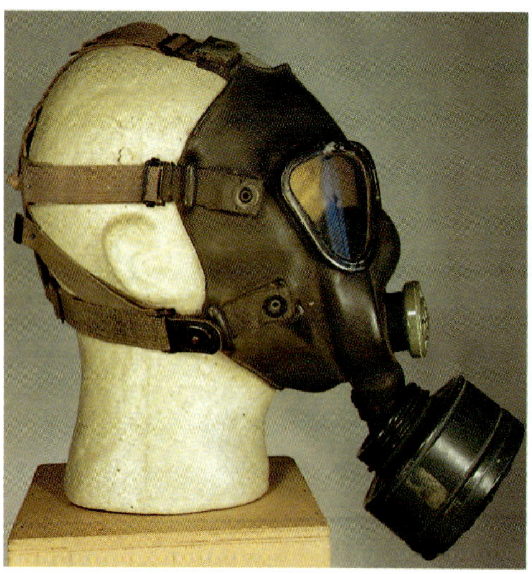

U.S. Army Snout-type Gas Mask M8-11-10, 1945. Produced too late in the war to be distributed to any extent, the M8 mask was intended to be a 'stop-gap' item, following failure of the M5 series. Of interest here is the angulation of the chin-mounted M11 filter. The filter adapter is a simple metal assembly, which was easy to retrofit to older faceblanks.

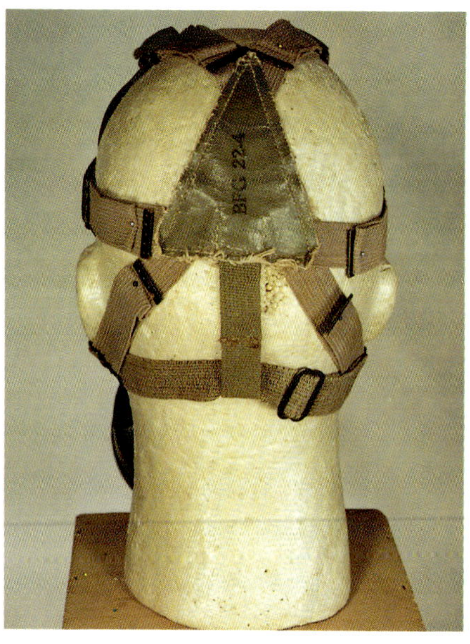

U.S. Army Snout-type Gas Mask M8-11-10, 1945. Good view of the C4 type head harness (also used on the M5 mask). Straps are pinned for clarity.

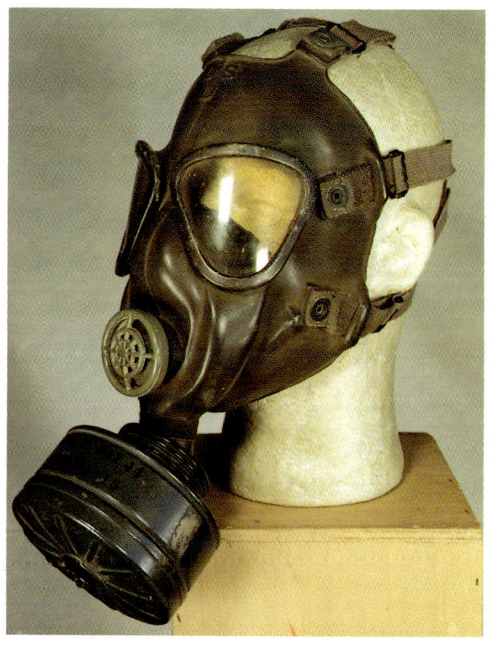

U.S. Army Snout-type Gas Mask M8-11-10, 1945. Definitely one of the scarcer type U.S. Army respirators to be found today, existing examples are usually in poor condition. The M10 carrier bore a vague resemblance to the early WWII MI/M2 Training Gas Mask carrier.

U.S. Navy NDO Mark I Optical Gas Mask, 1941

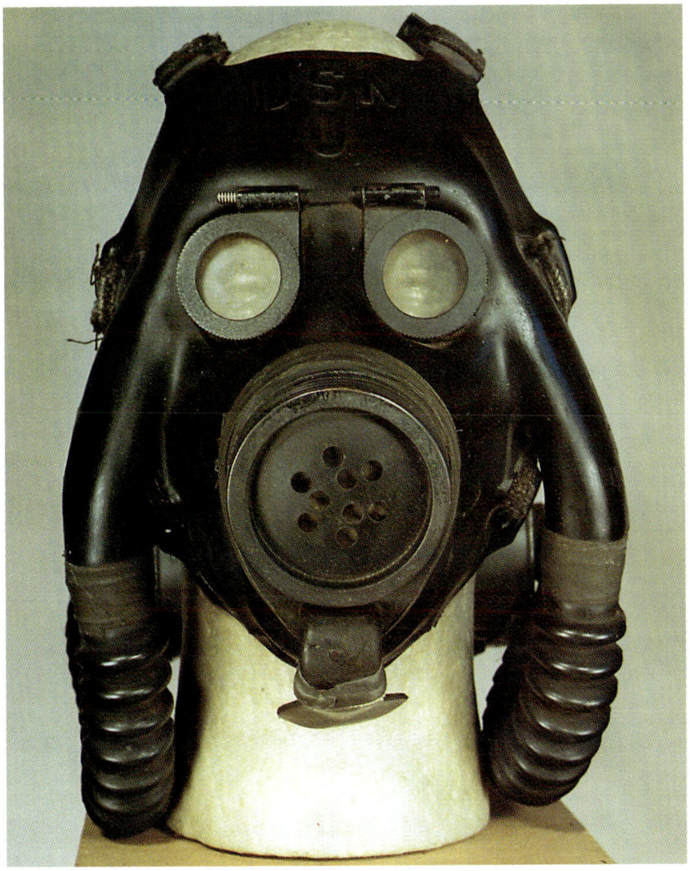

U.S. Navy NDO Mark I Optical Gas Mask, 1941. Essentially a Navy version of the U.S. Army Optical Gas Mask MI, the small lenses were adjustable for use with weapons sighting systems.

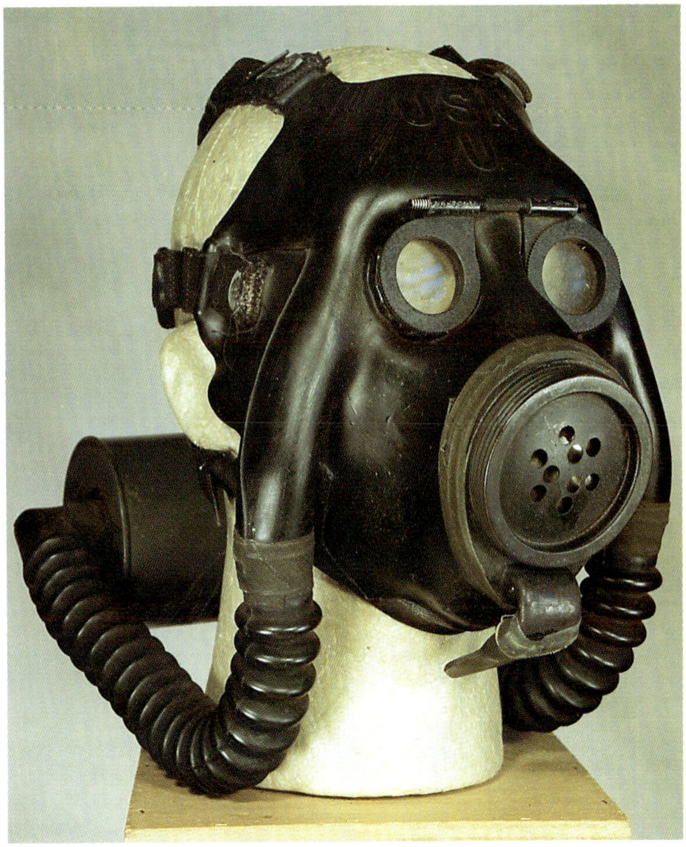

U.S. Navy NDO Mark I Optical Gas Mask, 1941. The type MVI 'spearhead' exhalation valve was precariously exposed, not well protected, and consequently the rubber part of the valve is often missing.

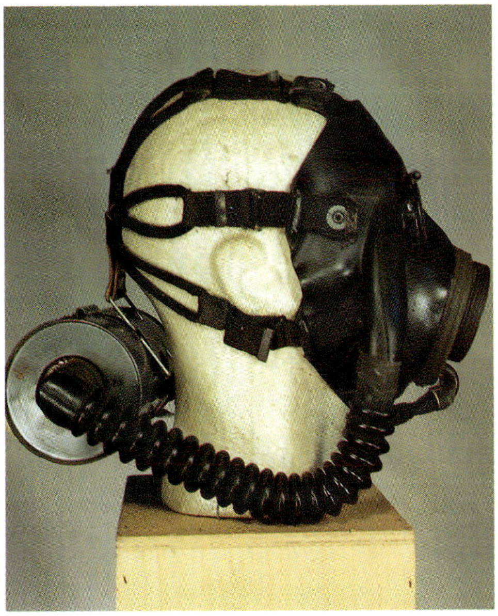

U.S. Navy NDO Mark I Optical Gas Mask, 1941. A good view of many components of the mask assembly, the filter canister was quite heavy and this explains the need for the reinforced coil-spring head harness (M3) from which the filter was suspended at the rear of the head.

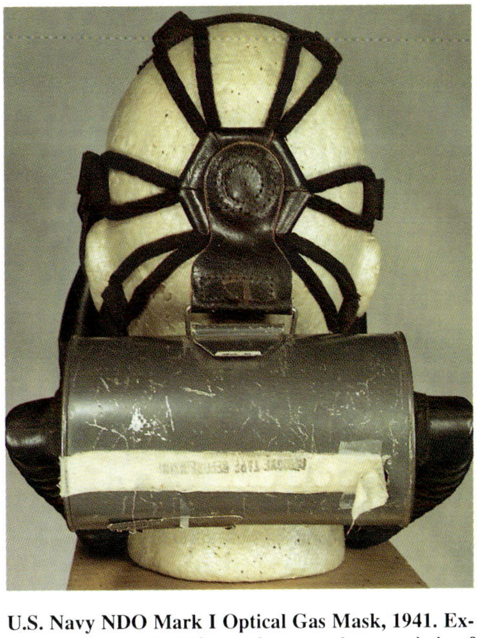

U.S. Navy NDO Mark I Optical Gas Mask, 1941. Excellent view of the M3 type harness characteristic of both Army and Navy optical masks. The white tape covers the inlet holes on the filter (legend on it say: "Remove Tape Before Using"). The Army version of this mask was molded of gray-green rubber, similar to service style masks.

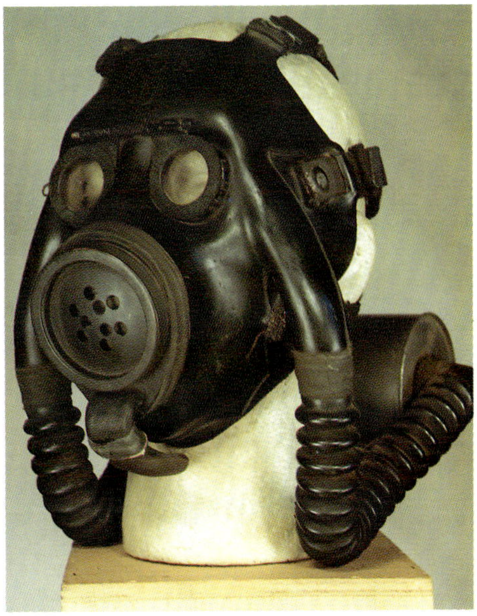

U.S. Navy NDO Mark I Optical Gas Mask, 1941. This specimen is in overall 'very good' condition, having all components, but needing a clean-up to remove dust.

U.S. Navy ND Mark III Diaphragm Gas Mask, 1942-43

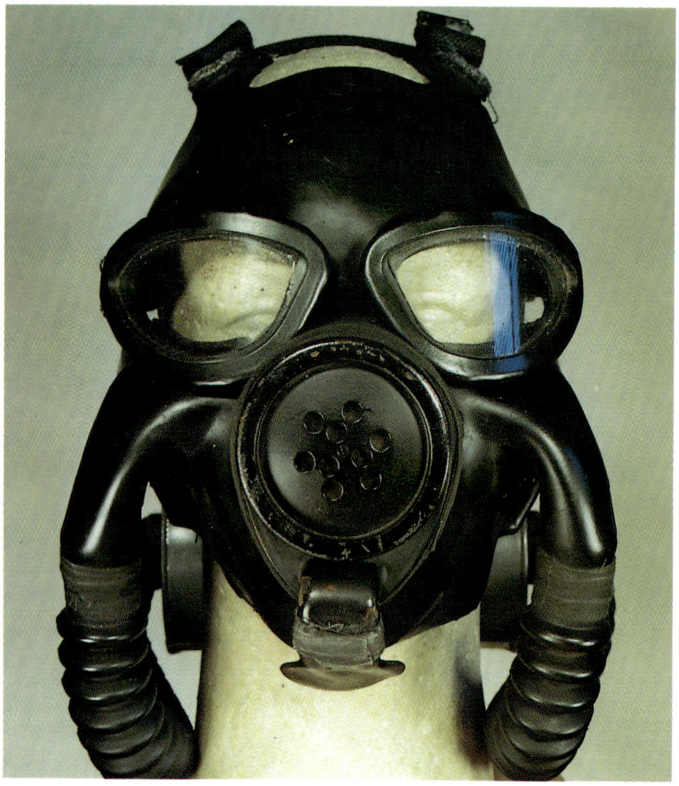

U.S. Navy ND Mark III Diaphragm Gas Mask, 1942-43. A modification and improvement of the original optical mask design, the Mark III featured larger lenses that bring to mind the latest U.S. Army M43A1 helicopter mask. This example is in overall 'very good' condition.

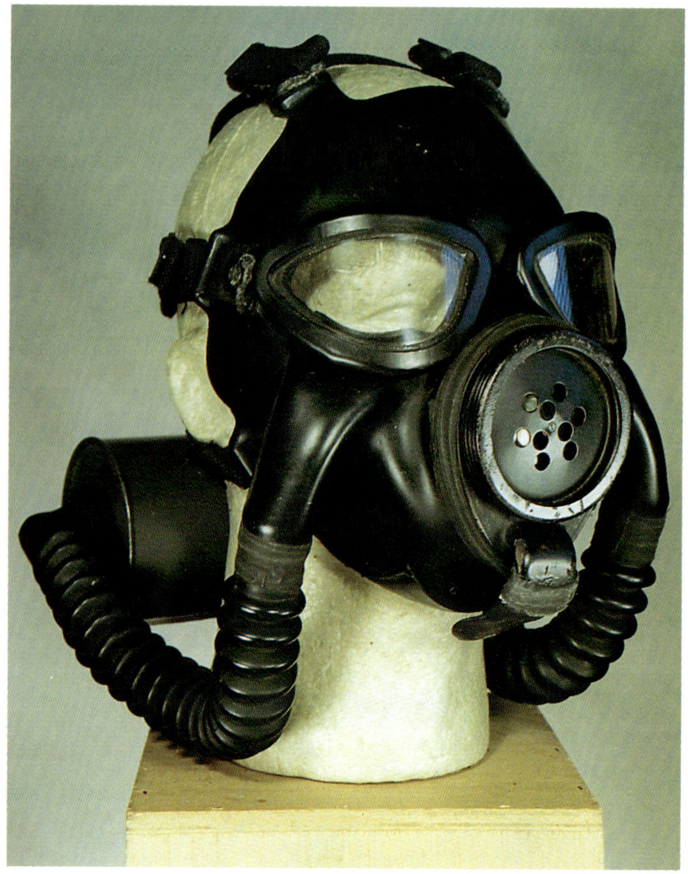

U.S. Navy ND Mark III Diaphragm Gas Mask, 1942-43. A good view of the diaphragm type 'voicemitter,' which functioned identically to those used on Army diaphragm gas masks. There was no oronasal cup internally to control misting but rather a 'speech cone' that merely served to focus speech into the voicemitter element.

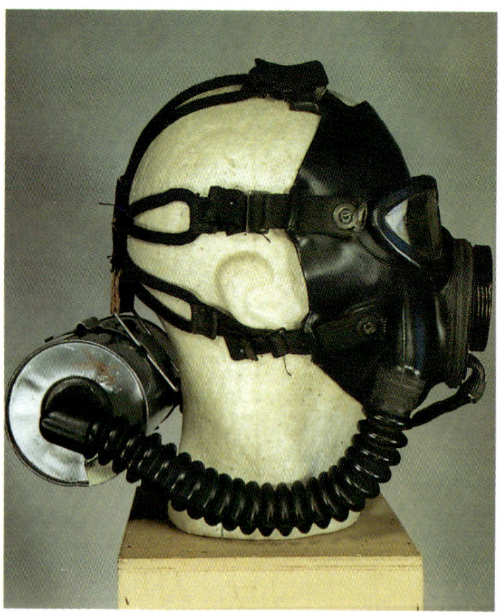

U.S. Navy ND Mark III Diaphragm Gas Mask, 1942-43. Compare the profile of this mask to the NDO Mark I (Optical Gas Mask). The obviously exposed position of the type MVI spearhead exhalation valve is easily seen. This valve was frequently subject to damage when being reinstalled into the carrier, after use. Filter inlet holes were relocated on this mask to the bottom of the canister, where they were less likely to entrain water, while in use on ships.

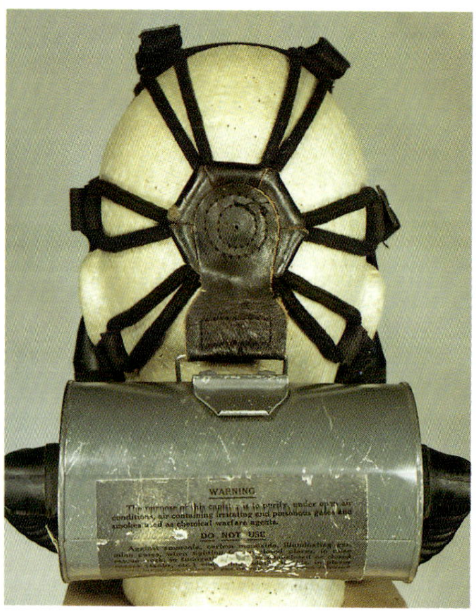

U.S. Navy ND Mark III Diaphragm Gas Mask, 1942-43. Good view of improved M3 type harness. Inlet holes are positioned at bottom of filter, with tape covering them prior to use.

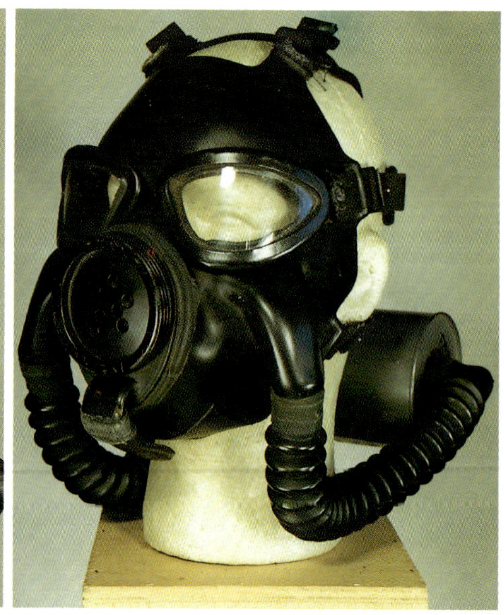

U.S. Navy ND Mark III Diaphragm Gas Mask, 1942-43. The Mark IV mask was identical, except for its larger eye lenses.

U.S. Navy ND Mark IV Diaphragm Gas Mask, 1943-44

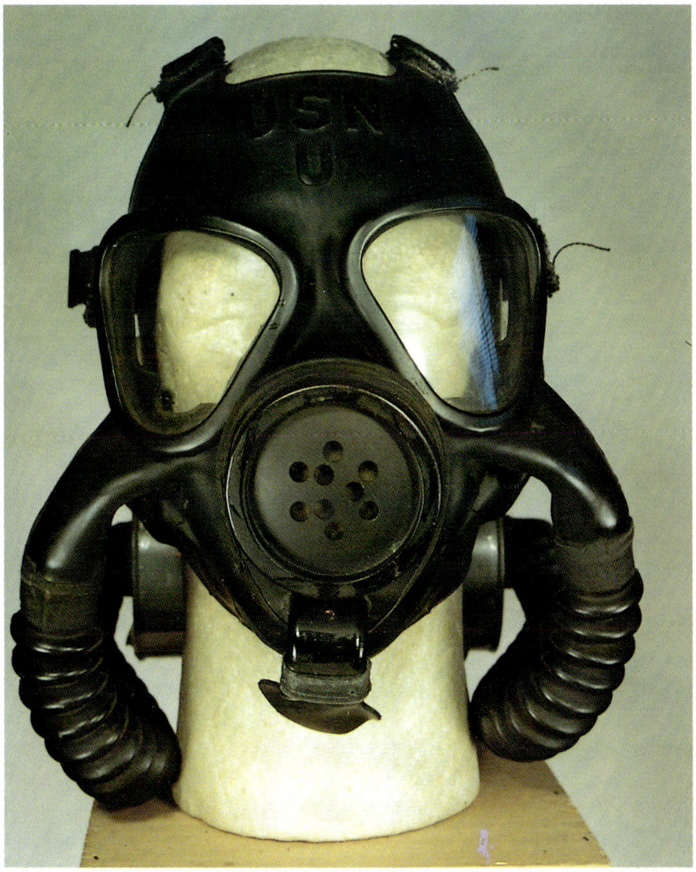

U.S. Navy ND Mark IV Diaphragm Gas Mask, 1943-44. The Mark IV mask featured improved fields of vision through use of larger lenses (similar to U.S. Army service mask lenses), but was otherwise identical to the Mark III in every aspect.

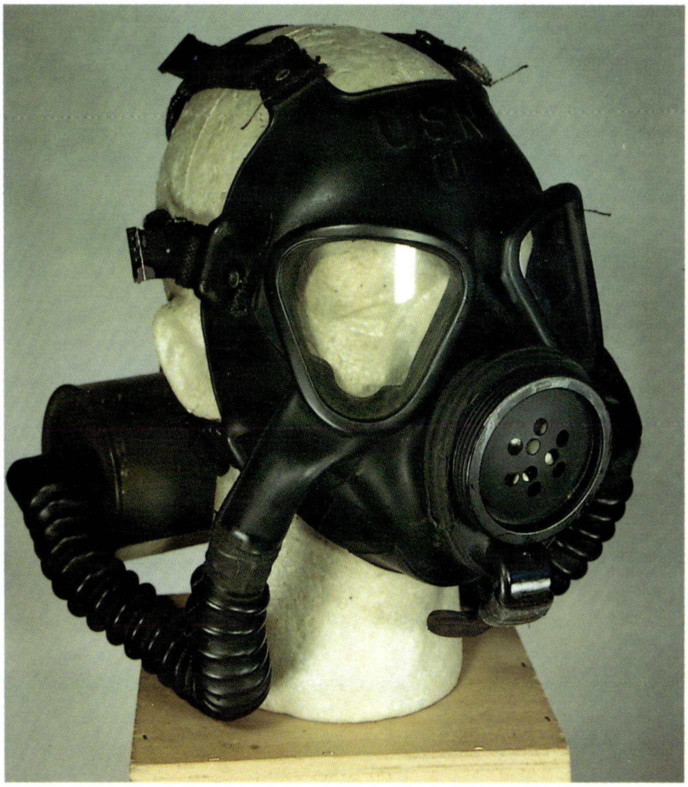

U.S. Navy ND Mark IV Diaphragm Gas Mask, 1943-44. The good oblique view which shows off the exposed and fragile MVI 'spearhead' exhalation valve. This specimen is in overall 'very good' condition,' with all components intact. The common ancestry with the original U.S. Navy WWI "Head Mask and Canister" design is obvious.

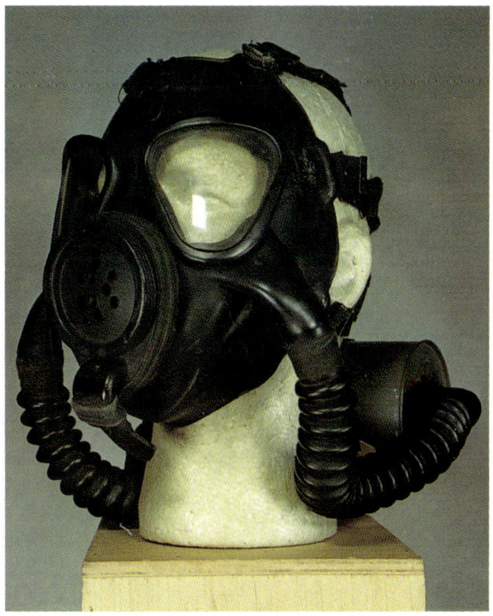

U.S. Navy ND Mark IV Diaphragm Gas Mask, 1943-44. The Navy masks were all issued with either a metal or a fiberboard face-form which provided good protection against deforming of facepiece during stowage. Unlike the Army fiberboard service mask face formers, which tended to be thrown away after some use, the Navy stringently required that the ND/NDO mask face forms be refitted before they were stowed in their carriers.

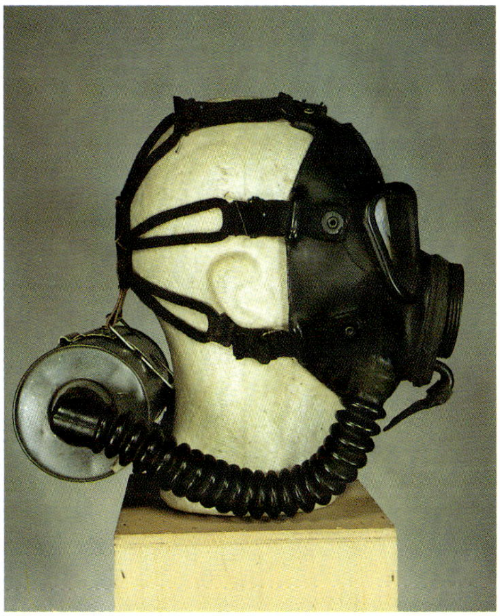

U.S. Navy ND Mark IV Diaphragm Gas Mask, 1943-44. This profile view invites comparisons with both earlier ND Mark III mask and the NDO Mark I (Optical Mask).

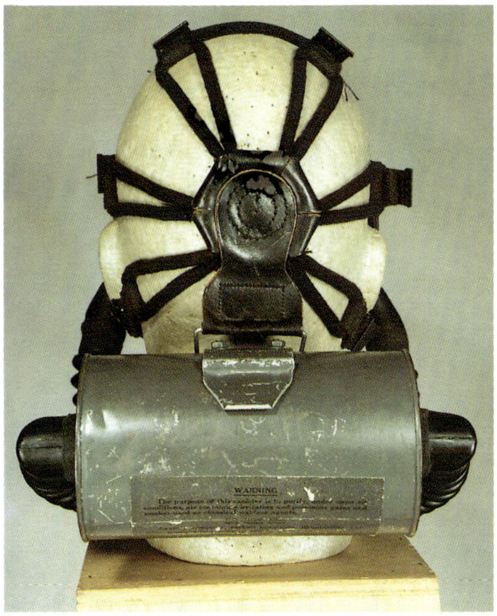

U.S. Navy ND Mark IV Diaphragm Gas Mask, 1943-44. Two position catch-clip on filter allowed some adjustment of canister position behind neck.

U.S. Navy Mask, Chemical and Biological, ND Mark V, 1957

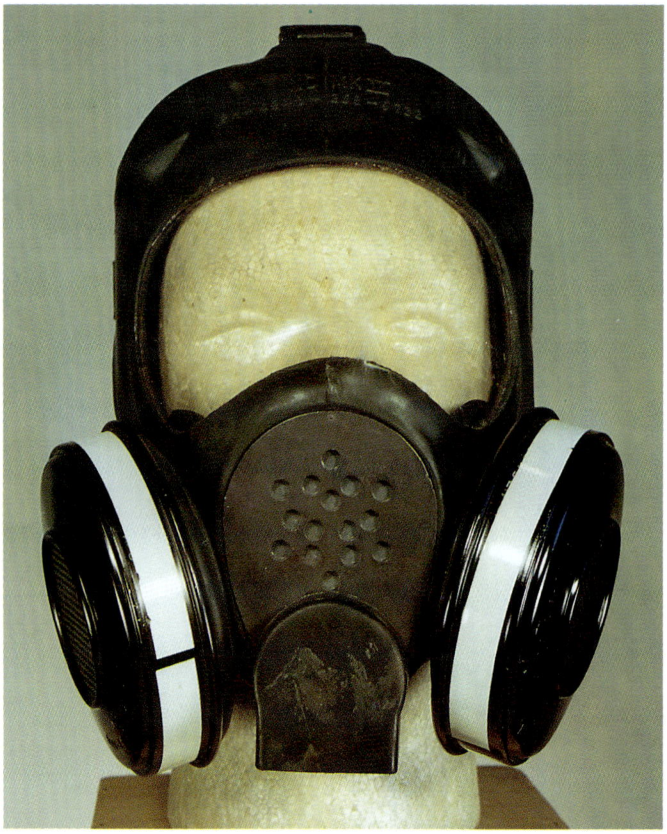

U.S. Navy Mask, Chemical and Biological, ND Mark V, 1957. An interesting design, this mask used two C1 bilateral filters, held in place on mounting discs attached to the mask by rubber collars. The field of vision was excellent, although no internal oronasal cup was used.

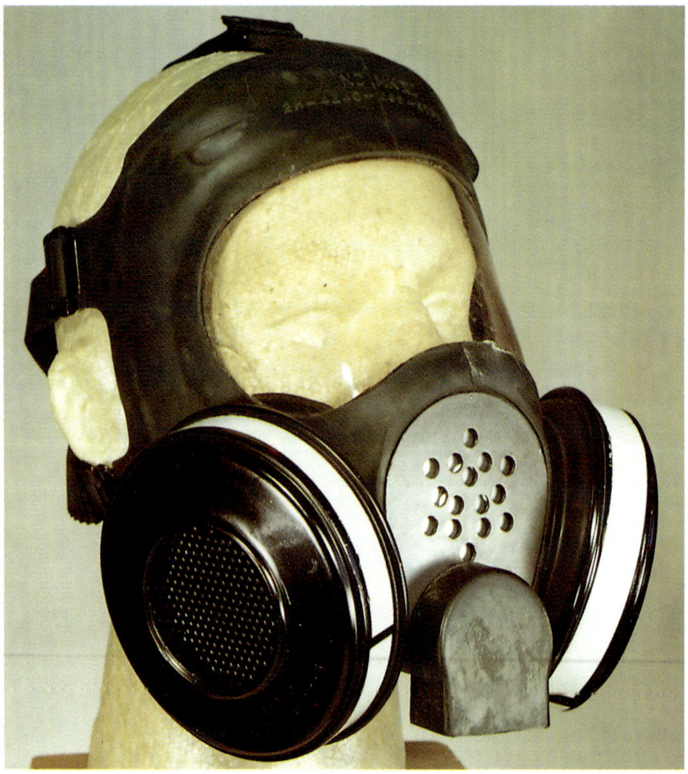

U.S. Navy Mask, Chemical and Biological, ND Mark V, 1957. White stripes on filters were for enhanced visibility. Internal facial contact area of mask featured an inflated bladder for enhanced sealing, a design aspect shared with the British S-6 mask.

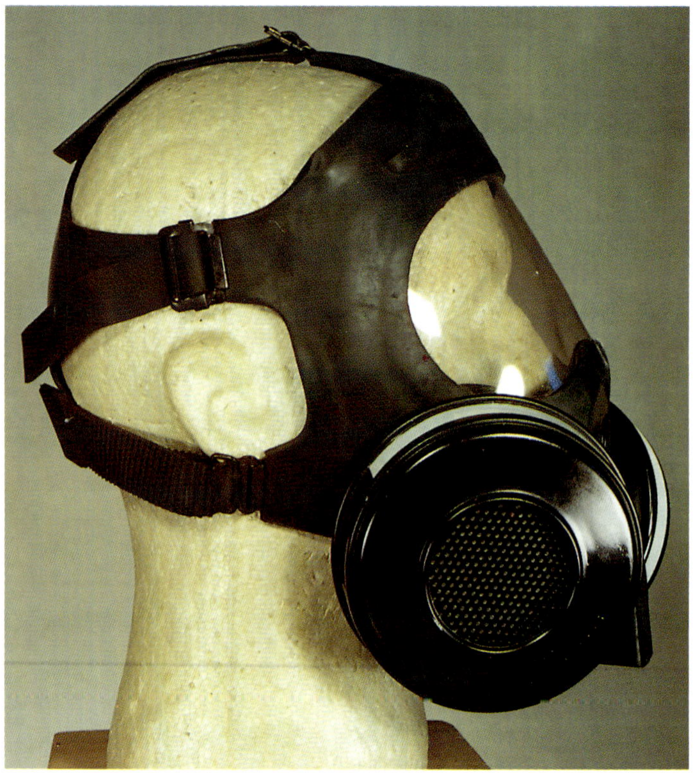

U.S. Navy Mask, Chemical and Biological, ND Mark V, 1957. Protected exhalation valve position between the filter is seen. The head retention component consisted of a 5 strap rubber harness assembly, with easily adjustable quick release buckles below ears on both sides.

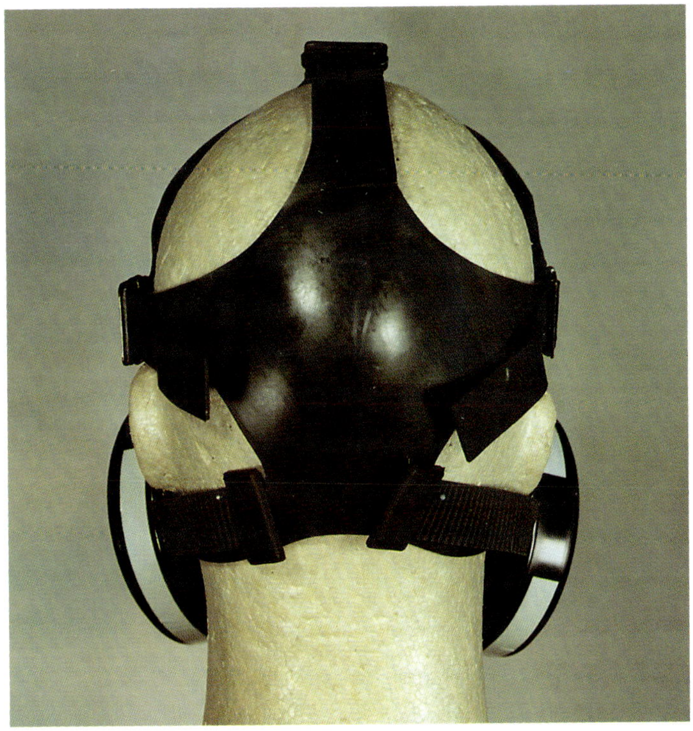

U.S. Navy Mask, Chemical and Biological, ND Mark V, 1957. Good view of molded rubber head harness, which was comfortable and held mask in position quite well.

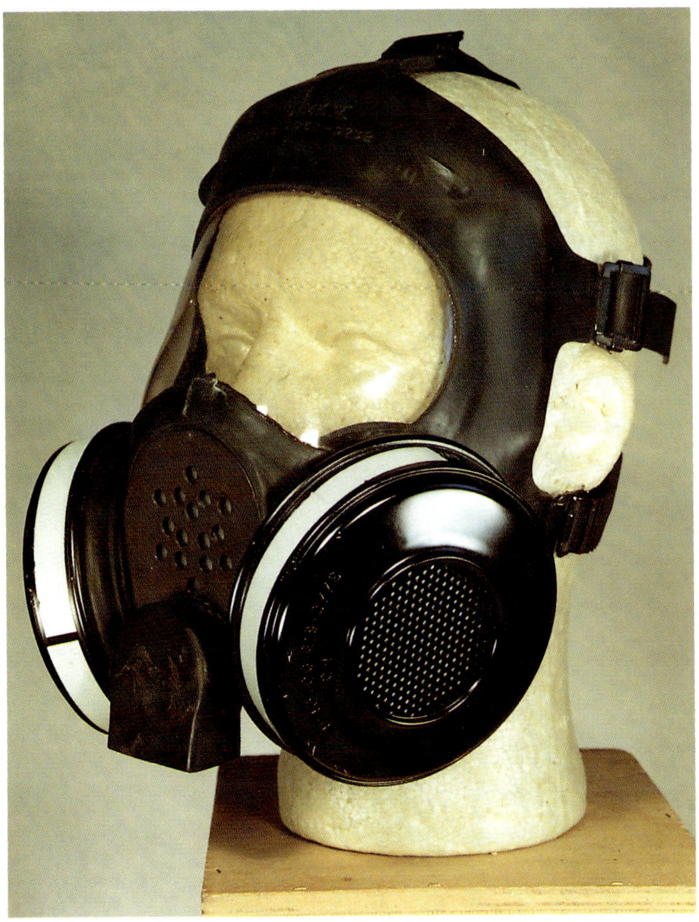

U.S. Navy Mask, Chemical and Biological, ND Mark V, 1957. This specimen is in 'excellent' condition, with all components, face seal bladder intact, no corrosion of fittings, and clear, unyellowed, flexible plastic face lens.

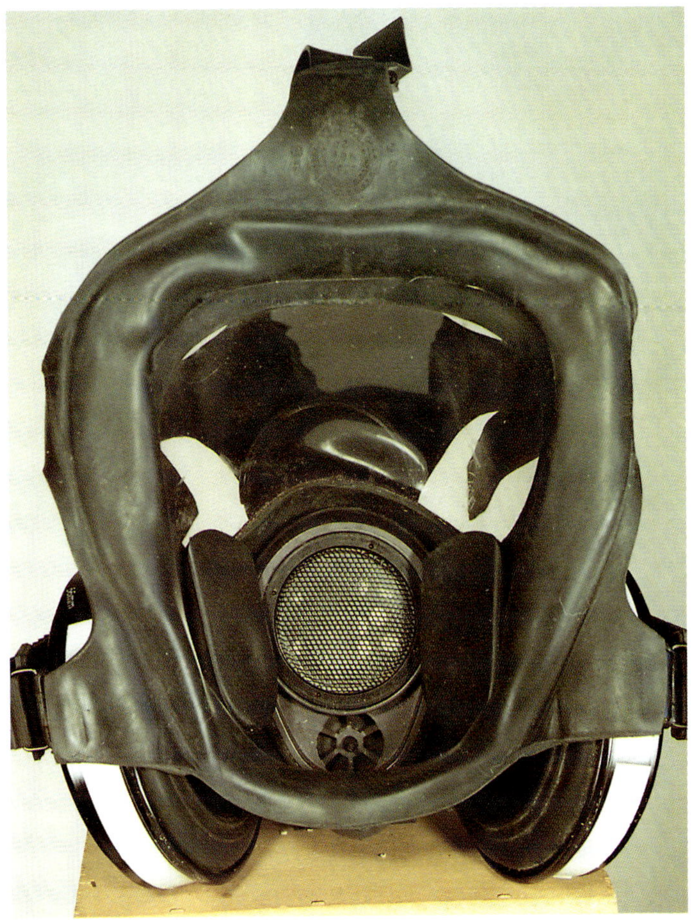

U.S. Navy Mask, Chemical and Biological, ND Mark V, 1957. View of interior of mask, showing inflated face-contact bladder for enhanced sealing, voicemitter diaphragm, air deflectors, and exhalation valve outlet.

U.S. Navy Civilian Gas Mask NC-1, 1941

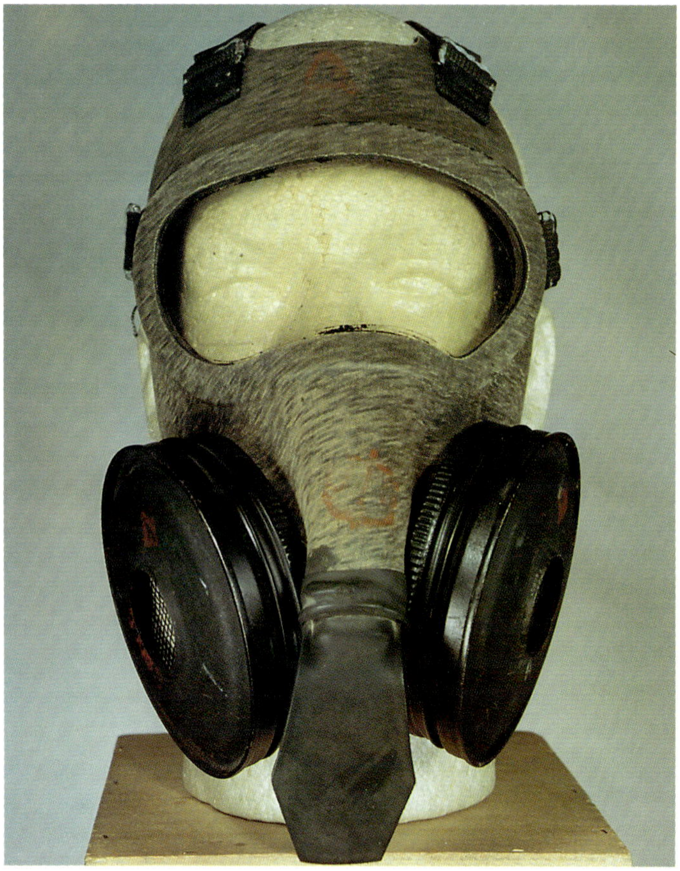

U.S. Navy Civilian Gas Mask NC-1, 1941. Surprisingly similar in concept to the later generation Navy NBC mask Mark V, the NC-1 mask was intended for civilian workers employed by the Navy.

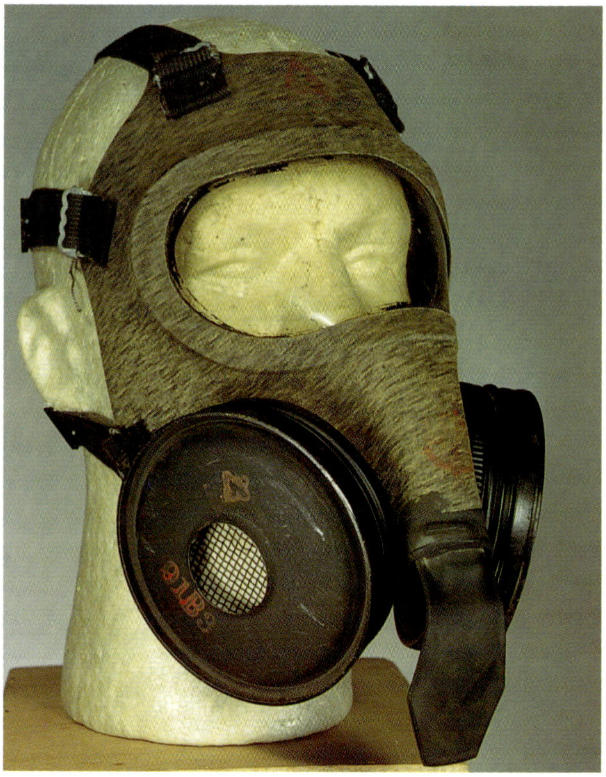

U.S. Navy Civilian Gas Mask NC-1, 1941. The facepiece was made of rubber sheet, covered by stockinet fabric and a flapper type (similar to U.S. Army MI) exhalation valve was used. A flexible plastic visor provided an excellent field of vision.

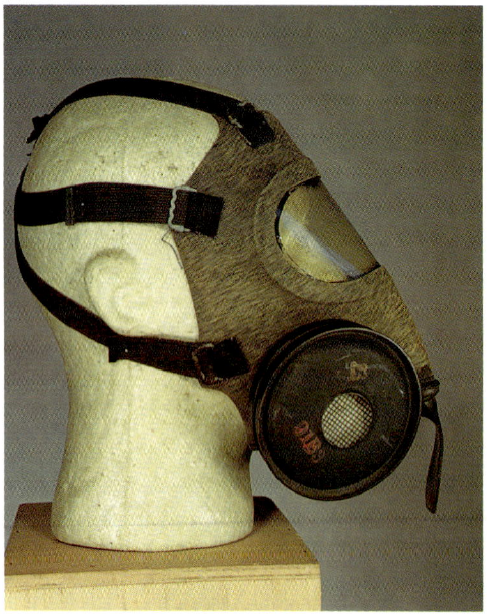

U.S. Navy Civilian Gas Mask NC-1, 1941. Surprisingly simple in construction, with a single chin seam, the NC-1 provided a good face fit for most faces. Red numeral and markings on filters and mask are identifying designations.

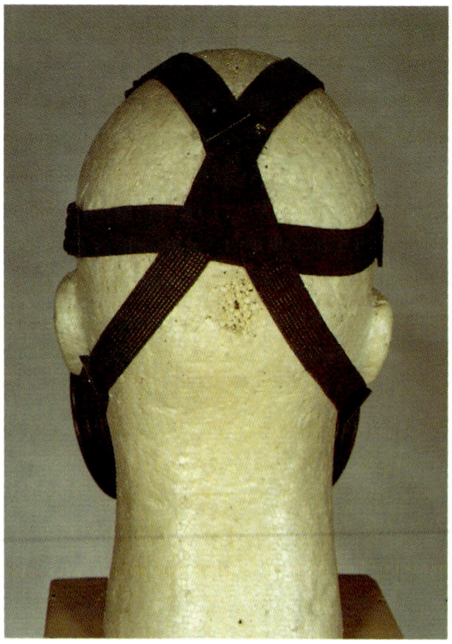

U.S. Navy Civilian Gas Mask NC-1, 1941. The all elasticized head harness was similar to the U.S. Army M4 head harness.

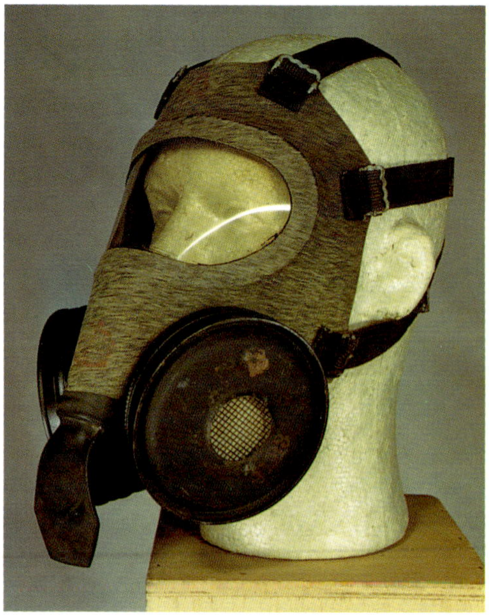

U.S. Navy Civilian Gas Mask NC-1, 1941. circular filter pods unscrewed to allow replacement of filters, in a manner similar to some MSA commercial respirators of the period. The exhalation flapper valve looks precariously positioned, but most examples today have survived with the rubber intact. This specimen is in 'very good' to 'excellent' condition.

U.S. Noncombatant Gas Mask MIA2, 1943

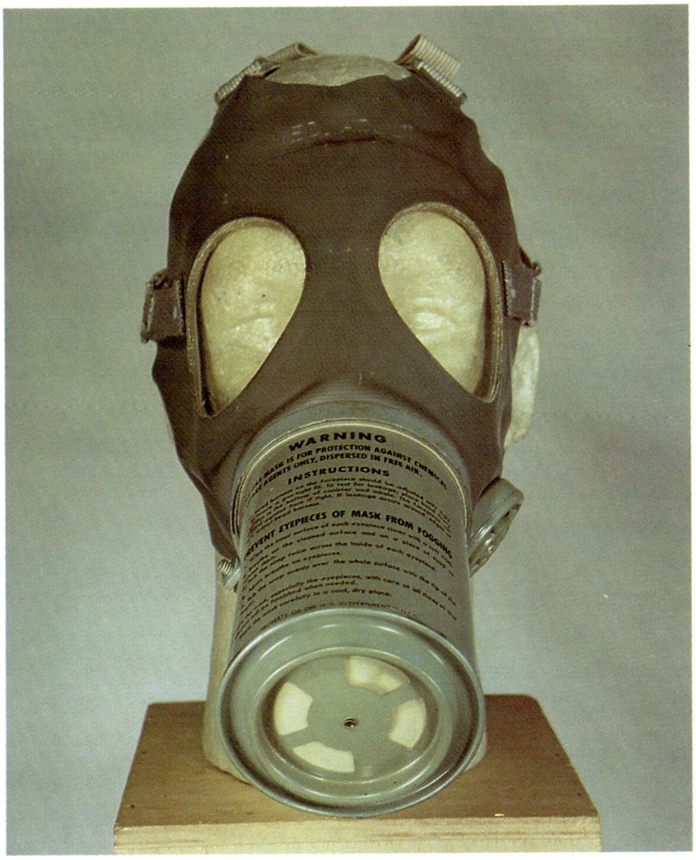

U.S. Noncombatant Gas Mask MIA2, 1943. Somewhat more complicated in fabrication than it appears, the MIA2 mask was produced in substantial numbers, many of which were sent overseas to Australia. They are very common today, many still in their original sealed boxes; this specimen is in 'excellent,' unissued condition.

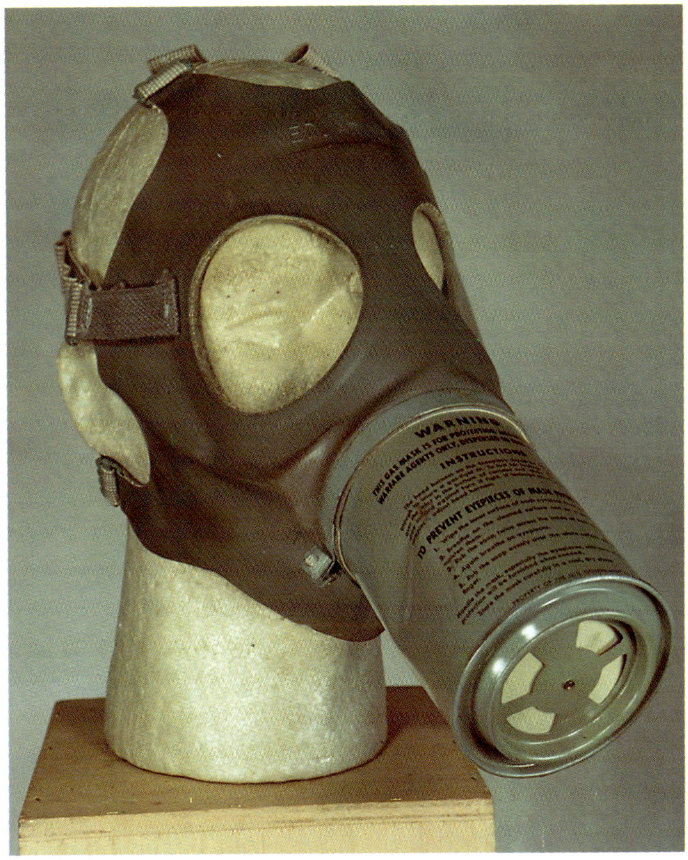

U.S. Noncombatant Gas Mask MIA2, 1943. Using the same MI type filter found on the MI/M2 Training Mask, the MIA2 was preceded was two earlier versions (MI and MIA1). It featured two large circular flexible plastic lenses and a flexible plastic coated facepiece, with an M8 exhalation valve.

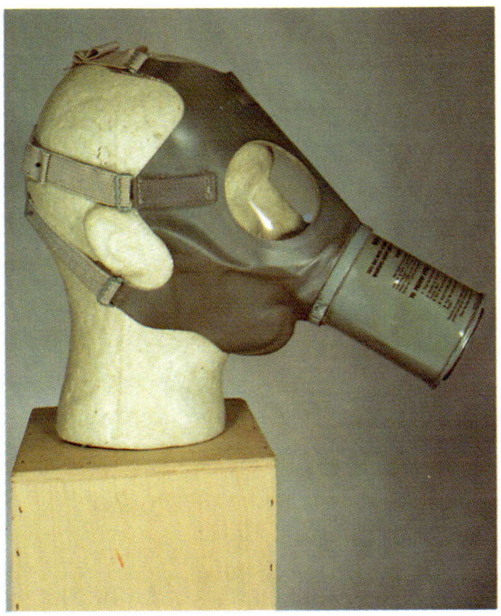

U.S. Noncombatant Gas Mask MIA2, 1943. Filter was permanently attached to the facepiece, although it could be removed and replaced with special tools. The face-fit was not as good as might be desired although the mask was made in several adult and child sizes.

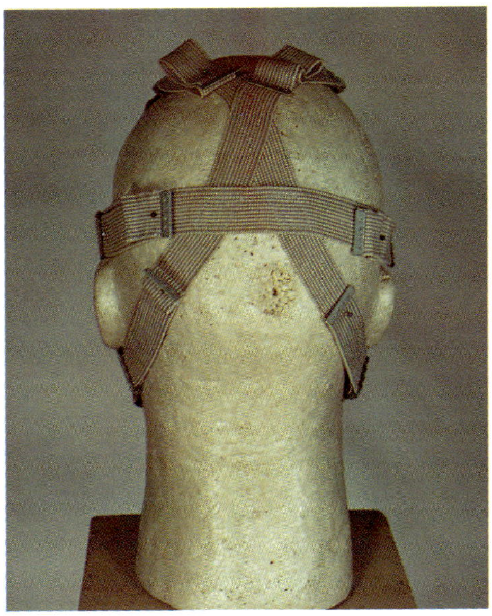

U.S. Noncombatant Gas Mask MIA2, 1943. The details of the all elastic M4 type head harness are viewable. Early version of this civilian mask (the MI Noncombatant mask) featured the MVII exhalation valve on left side. Straps of harness are pinned for clarity.

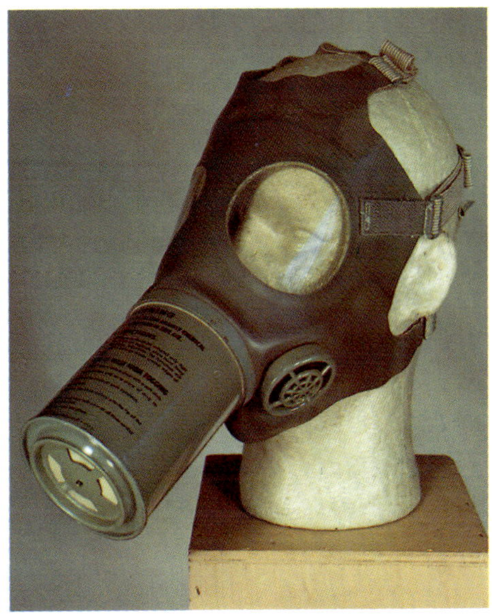

U.S. Noncombatant Gas Mask MIA2, 1943. Good oblique view of the left side of the facepiece with M8 valve and MI training type filter attached.

U.S. Noncombatant Gas Mask, MIA2, Child, 1943

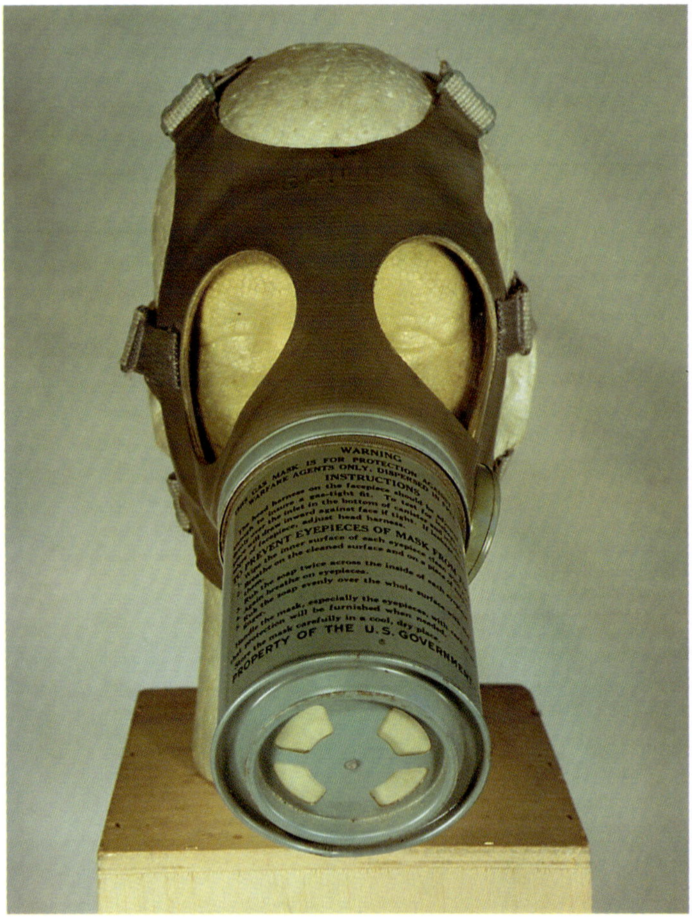

U.S. Noncombatant Gas Mask, MIA2, Child, 1943. Essentially identical in all respects to MIA2 adult noncombatant gas mask but sized to child's face.

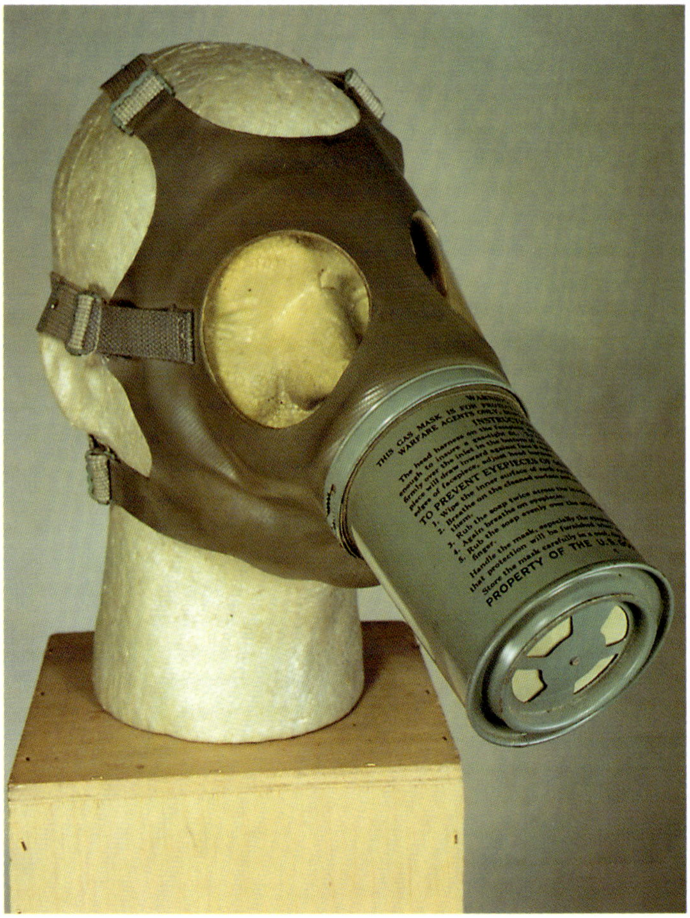

U.S. Noncombatant Gas Mask, MIA2, Child, 1943. The head form in use is an adult size, showing the relatively smaller sizing of the mask for children.

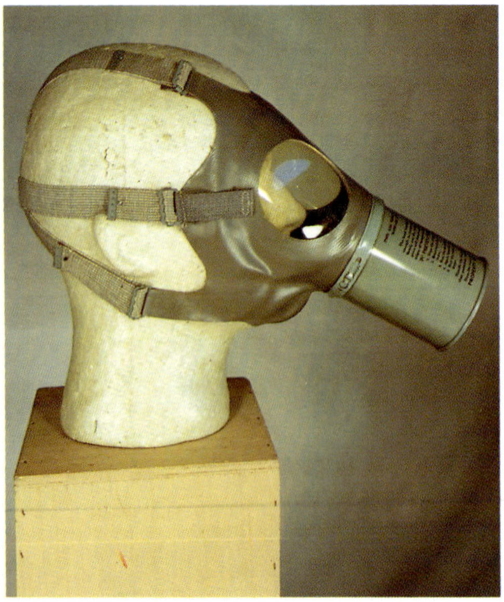

U.S. Noncombatant Gas Mask, MIA2, child, 1943. Again, profile shows the child's mask fitted to an adult sized head form, for comparative visualization. Good visual fields in children's masks help alleviate possible claustrophobic anxieties in children.

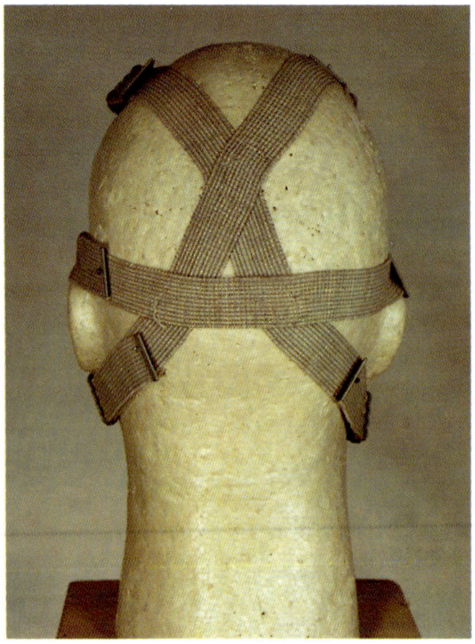

U.S. Non Combatant Gas Mask, MIA2, Child, 1943. View of the M4 type all-elasticized head harness. This specimen of the child's mask is in 'excellent,' unissued condition.

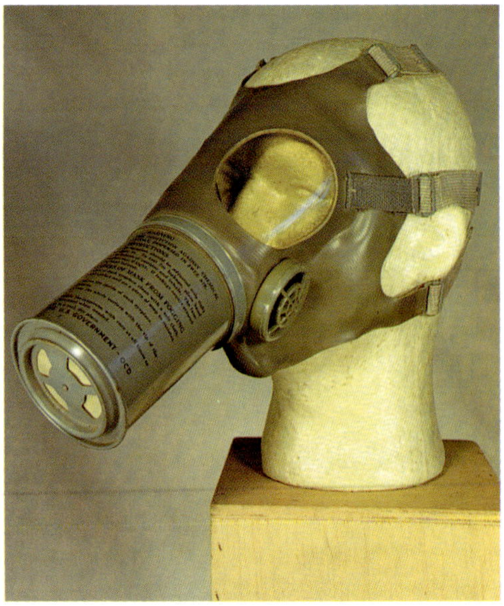

U.S. Noncombatant Gas Mask, MIA2, Child, 1943. View of the left oblique aspect, with M8 exhalation valve and MI training type filter (permanently) fitted.

U.S. Noncombatant Gas Mask, M2-2-1, Small Child, 1943

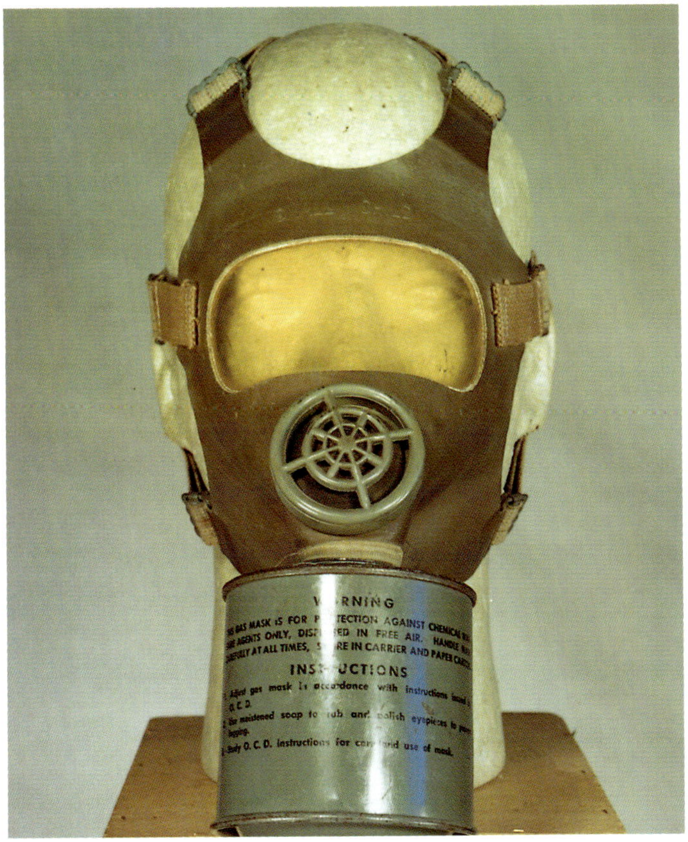

U.S. Noncombatant Gas Mask, M2-2-1, Small Child, 1943. An adaptation of the MIA2 type civilian mask for small children, the M2 Child's Gas Mask featured a single flexible plastic lens to reduce anxieties. The M8 type exhalation valve was mounted at the front of the facepiece, above the M2 type filter.

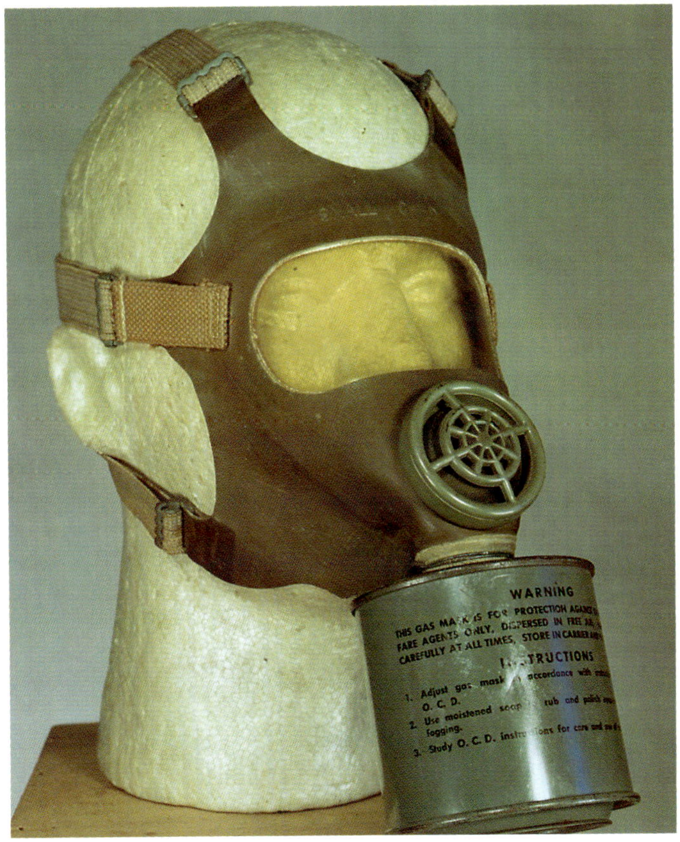

U.S. Noncombatant Gas Mask, M2-2-1, Small Child, 1943. A Walt Disney collaboration with the U.S. Army produced a proposal for what is known as the "Mickey Mouse Mask." Illustrations of the Mickey Mouse Mask show it as being similar in intended functional structure to the M2 Small Child Mask, but having a faceblank molded with a rubber Mickey Mouse face—certainly a mask unique among CBW protective equipment designs!

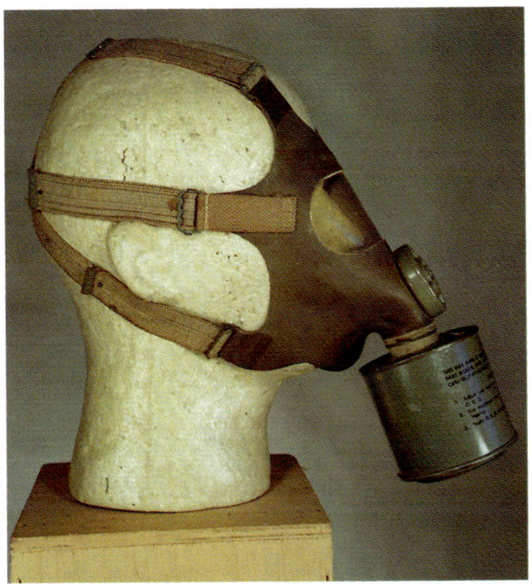

U.S. Noncombatant Gas Mask, M2-2-1, Small Child, 1943. The specimen shown here is in 'good' condition, with some obvious deterioration from storage and aging effects.

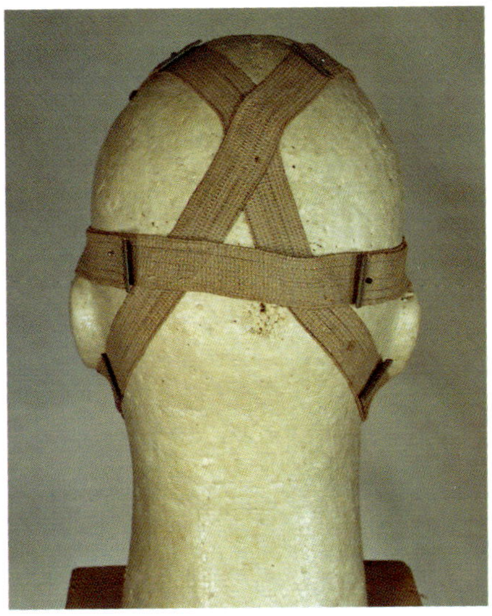

U.S. Noncombatant Gas Mask, M2-2-1, Small Child, 1943. Typical civilian mask M4 style all elasticized harness.

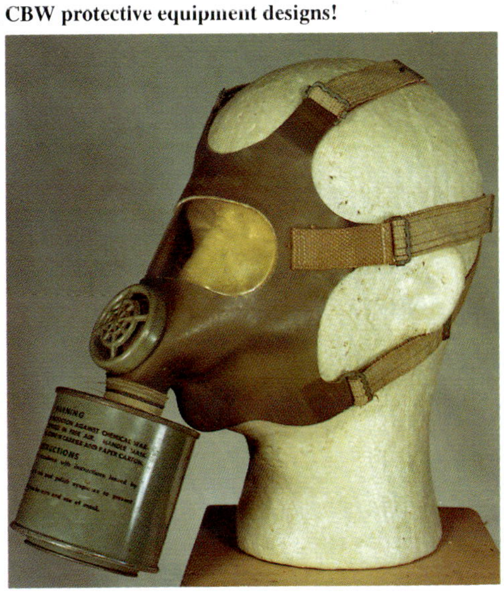

U.S. Noncombatant Gas Mask, M2-2-1, Small Child, 1943. Good left oblique view of this mask intended for smaller children. Infants and babes-in-arms were provided for with the MI Infant Protector, which was a large sack like enclosure of proofed material that used a hand-operated bellows fitted to a filter to provide fresh air.

U.S. M16 Civilian Defense Mask (CD V-800), 1957

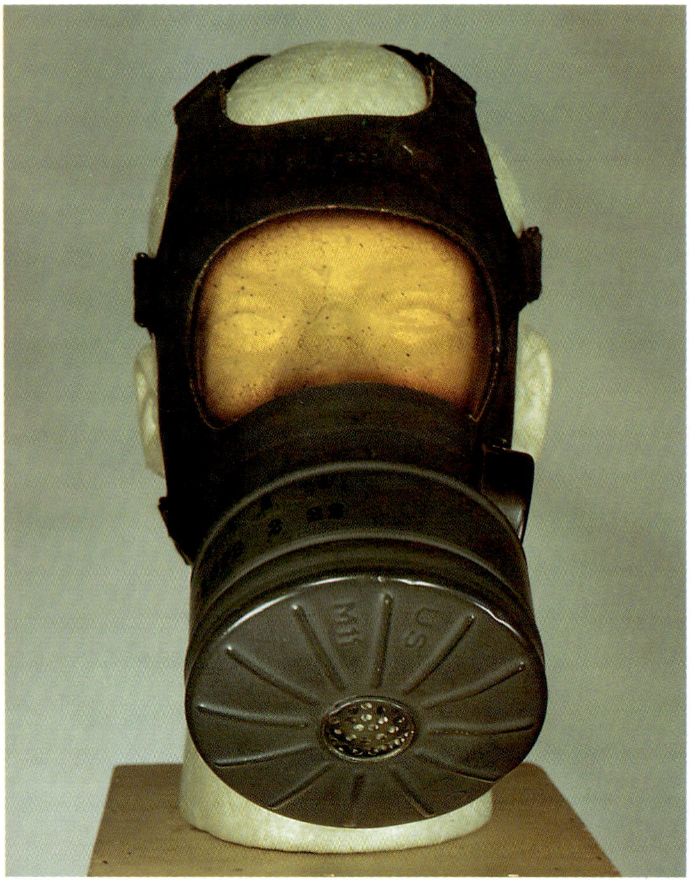

U.S. M16 Civilian Defense Mask (CD V-800), 1957. Very similar in concept to earlier noncombatant designs, this mask had a proofed flexible fabric faceblank with a C15 type exhalation valve fitted to left side and an M11 filter canister screw mount on its chin section. The mask was produced in substantial numbers for civilian defense use.

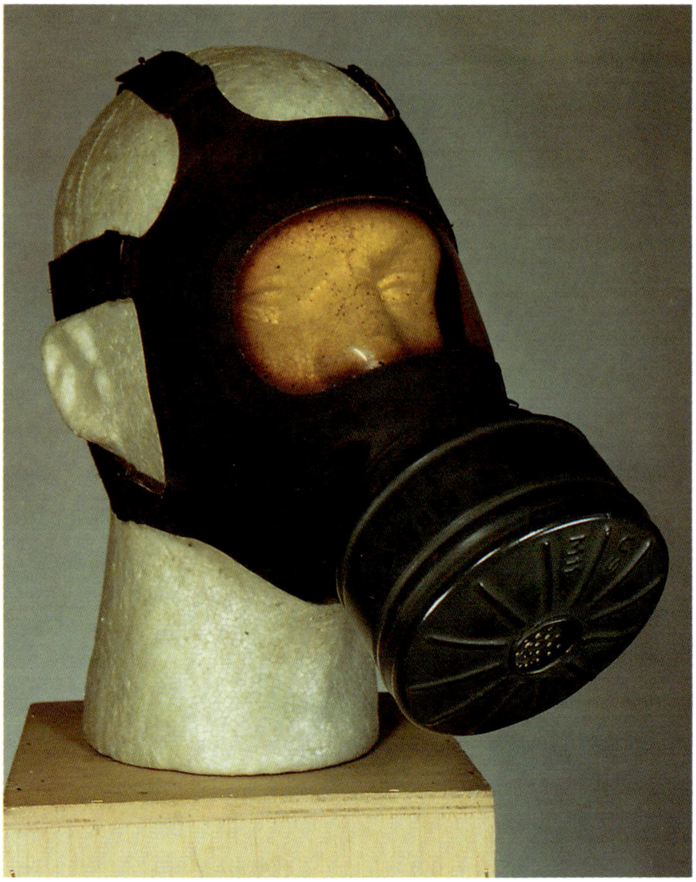

U.S. M16 Civilian Defense Mask (CD V-800), 1957. The flexible transparent plastic used for a visor on this mask very easily becomes yellowed with time, and excellent specimens are hard to find, although none of the surviving examples (of which there are many) were ever actually used.

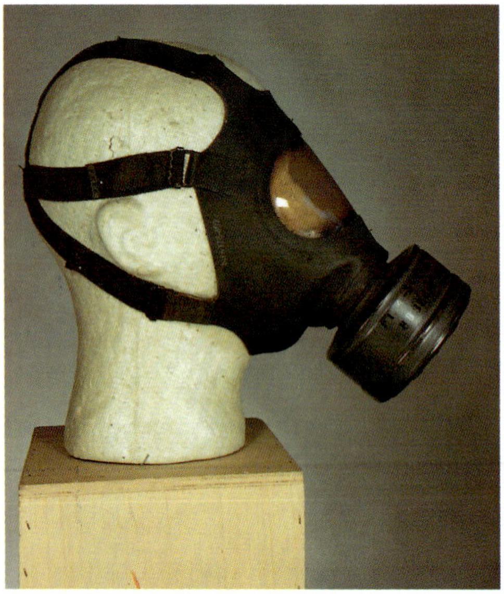

U.S. M16 Civilian Defense Mask (CD V-800), 1957. The CD V-800 used the same standard M11 axial flow filter as the military M9 and M9A1 masks then in use.

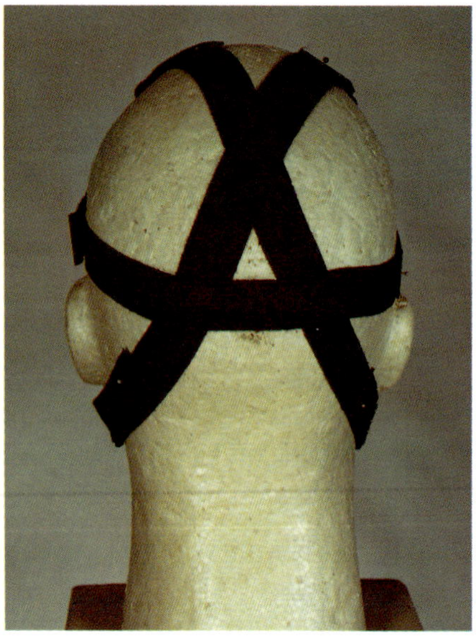

U.S. M16 Civilian Defense Mask (CD V-800), 1957. The all elastic head harness, of black material, is essentially identical to the earlier M4 type military harness. Straps are pinned for clarity.

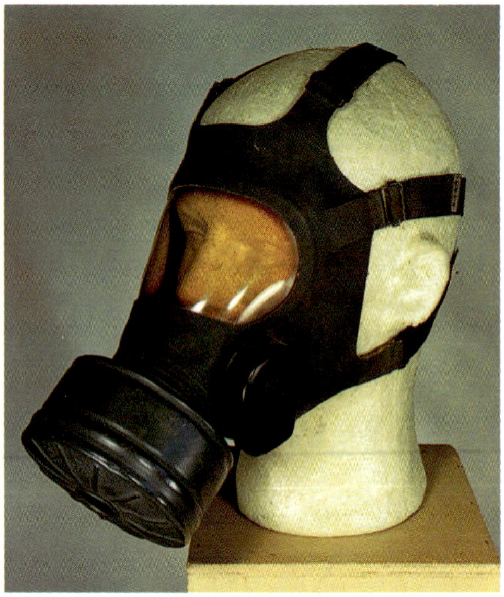

U.S. M16 Civilian Defense Mask (CD V-800), 1957. Left oblique view of the mask that would have been used to protect American civilians from nuclear and CBW attacks, had they occurred during the Cold War years.

U.S. M22 Civilian Defense Mask (CD V-805), 1975

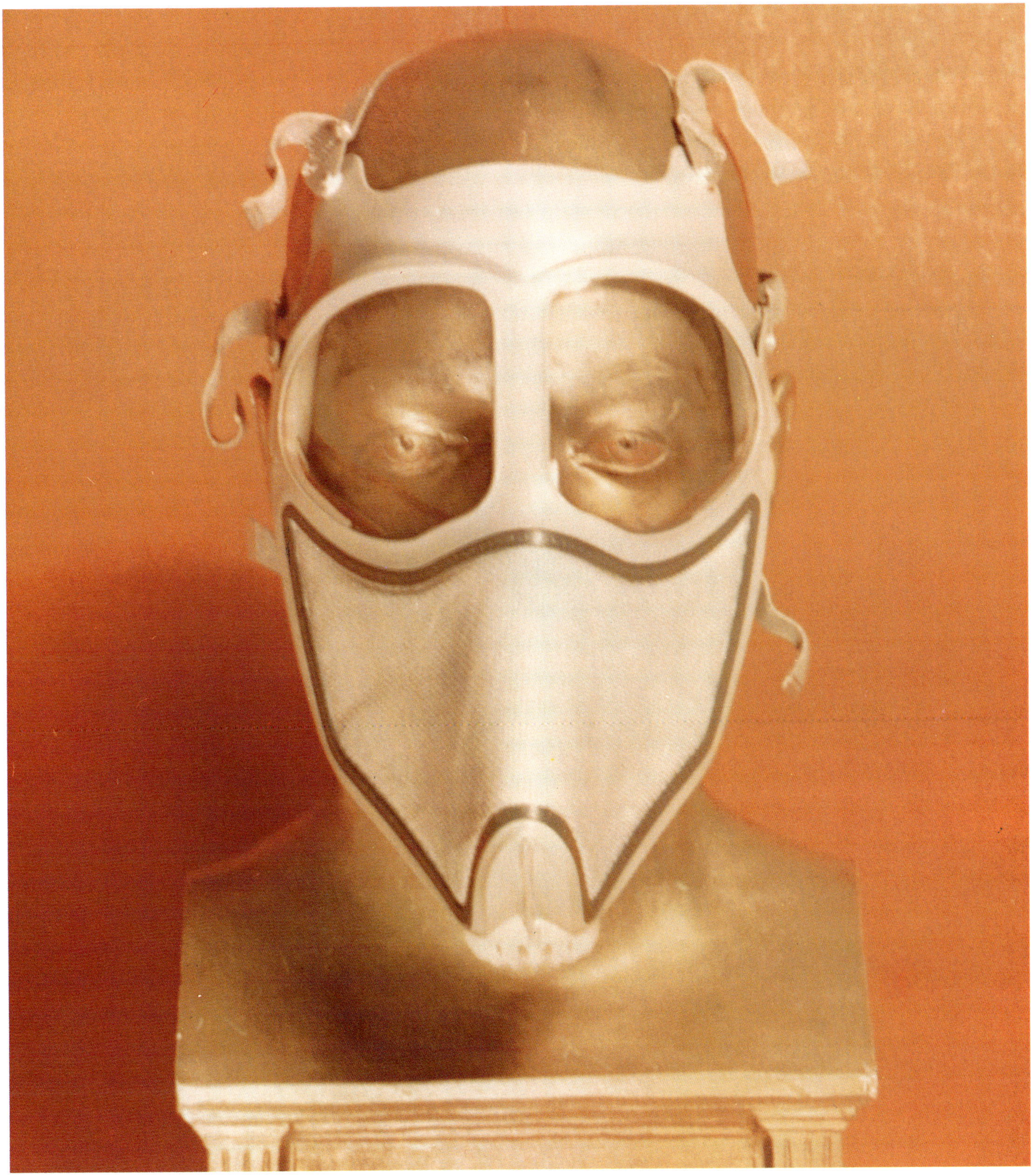

U.S. M22 Civilian Defense Mask (CD V-805), 1975. A much later civilian NBC defense mask, produced along similar lines as the military M28 "grasshopper" mask (silicone facepiece). Very hard to find respirator today, the development and production of this mask was fraught with controversy and production difficulties. Originally known as the experimental E52R27 type mask, during development, the filter pads were permanently molded into the facepiece. Exhaust valve is located in front, below.

U.S. Army Optical Gas Mask M2-10A1-6, 1952

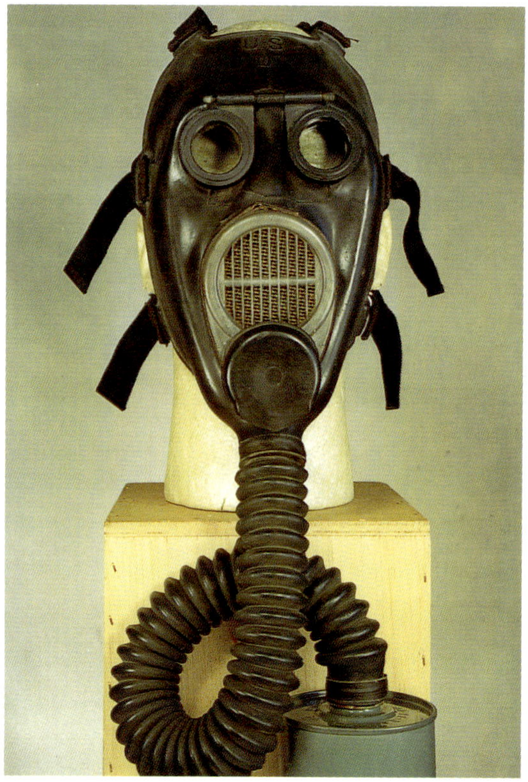

U.S. Army Optical Gas Mask M2-10A1-6, 1952. When this mask was first introduced (1944) it was listed (in TM 3-205/C1, 1944) as having an M8 type exhalation valve, but the correct designation for the combination diaphragm/exhalation valve assembly is given as C11 in later TM releases.

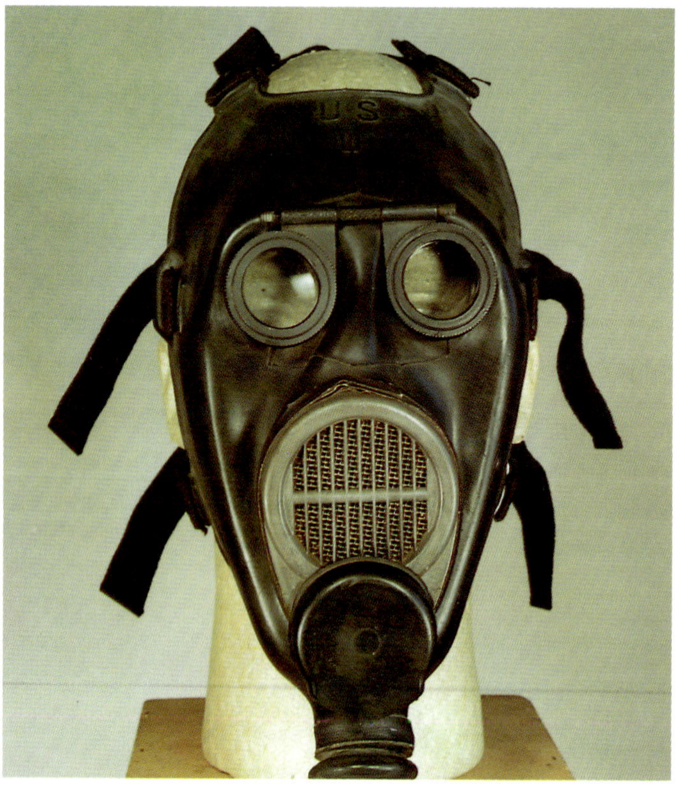

U.S. Army Optical Gas Mask M2-10A1-6, 1952. A closer view of the M2 optical mask; some detail of the adjustable intraocular distance mechanism is viewable. First produced in 1944, the M2 mask was manufactured and remained in use over a period of many years (from the mid 40s into the 60s).

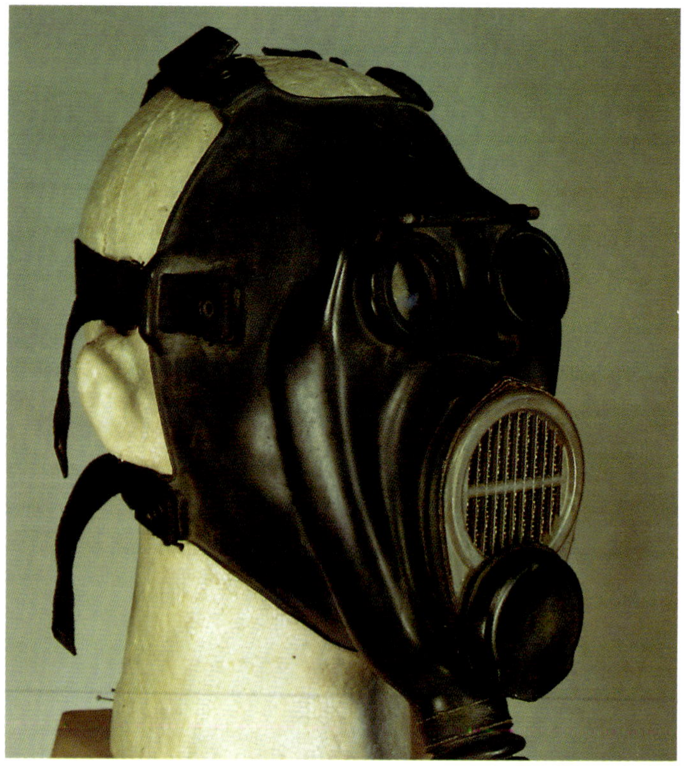

U.S. Army Optical Gas Mask M2-10A1-6, 1952. The M2 mask's eye lenses are very small, typical of specialized weapons sighting systems respirators. Some Russian (ex-Soviet Bloc) masks have the same feature and are used in the same manner. The field of view is (necessarily) very small and induces a claustrophobic feeling in some, when worn for any other than optical sighting applications.

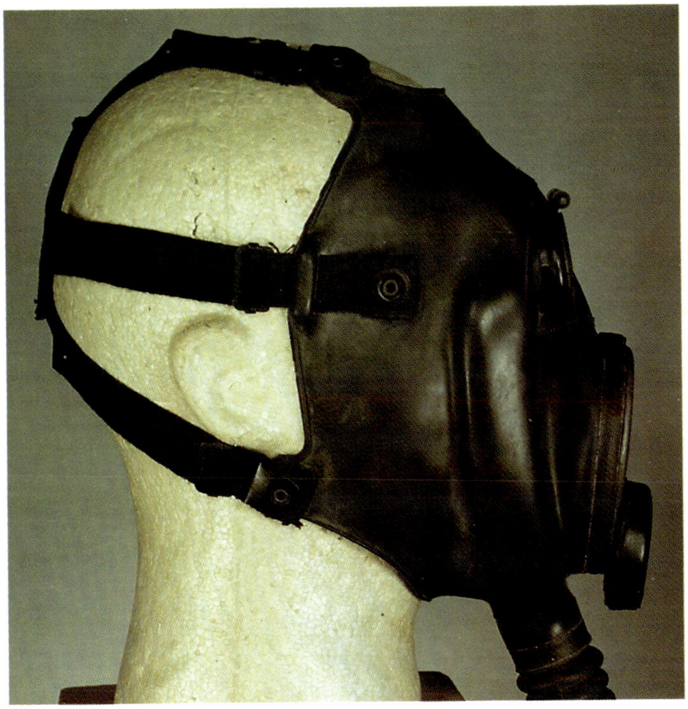

U.S. Army Optical Gas Mask M2-10A1-6, 1952. M7 type head harness is used. Detail of the molded in Tissot air distribution tubes is visible in this profile view.

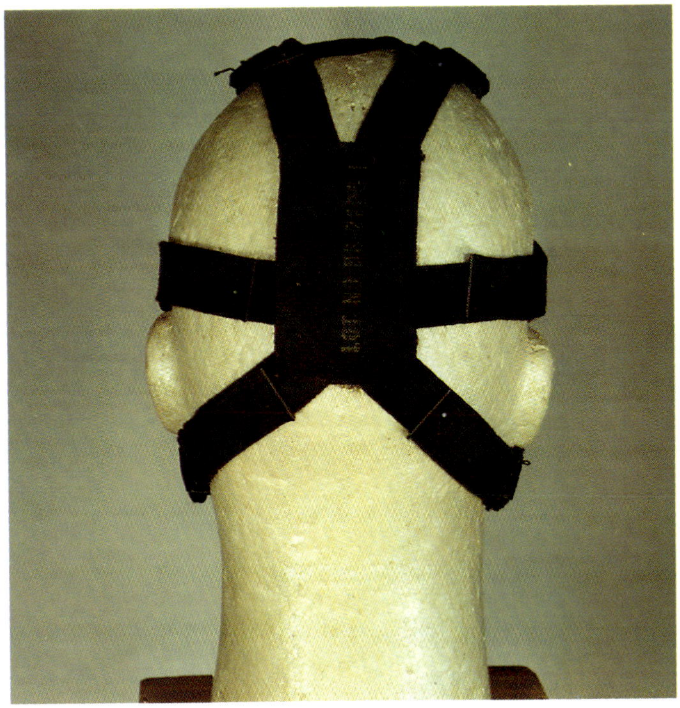

U.S. Army Optical Gas Mask M2-10A1-6, 1952. Rear view of M7 elasticized head harness.

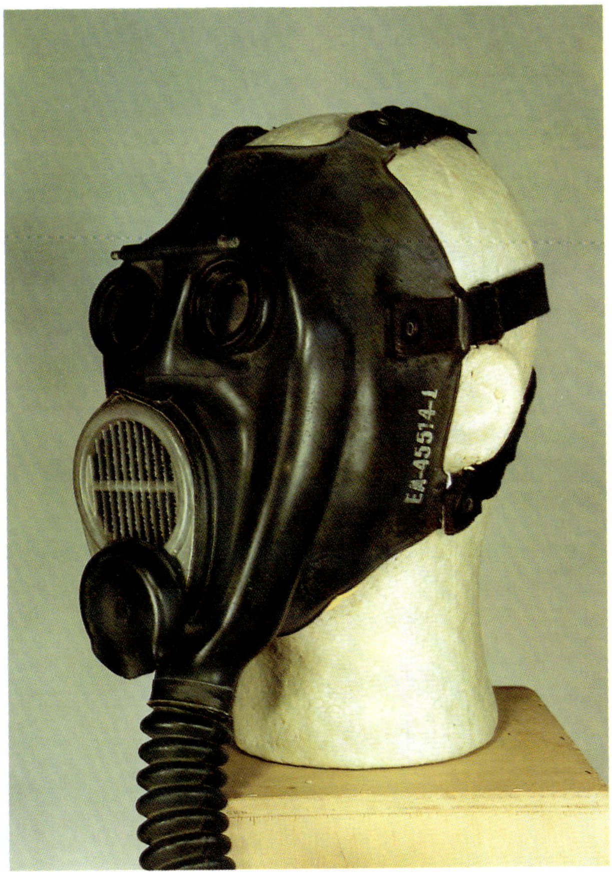

U.S. Army Optical Gas Mask M2-10A1-6, 1952. Left oblique view shows lot number on edge of faceblank. The exhalation valve cover had small bead-like rubber protrusions on the inner surface to aid in deicing the valve, if necessary.

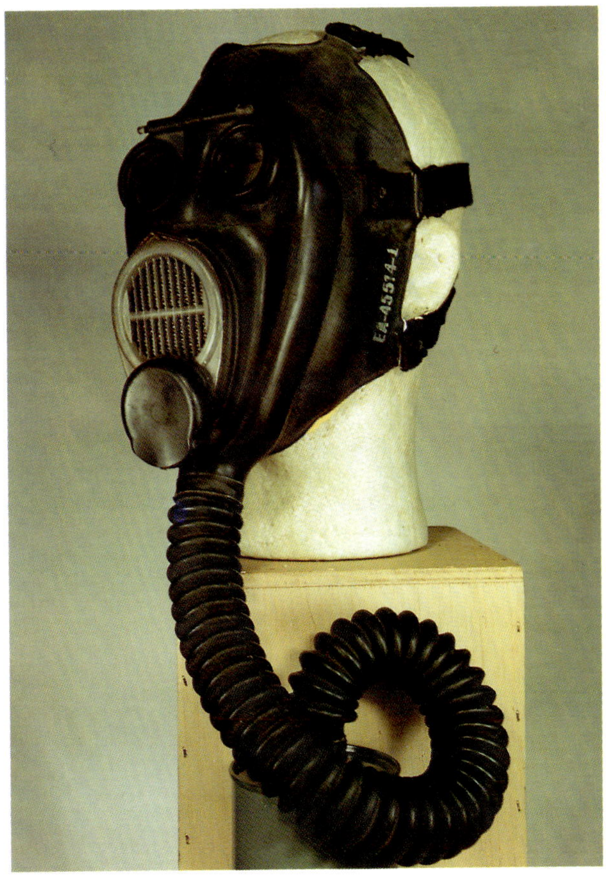

U.S. Army Optical Gas Mask M2-10A1-6, 1952. This specimen, seen here with M3 hose and M10A1 filter, is in overall 'excellent' condition, although examples may be found, without too much difficulty, still sealed in their original metal (tin) packing cans.

U.S. Army Field Protective Mask M9, 1952

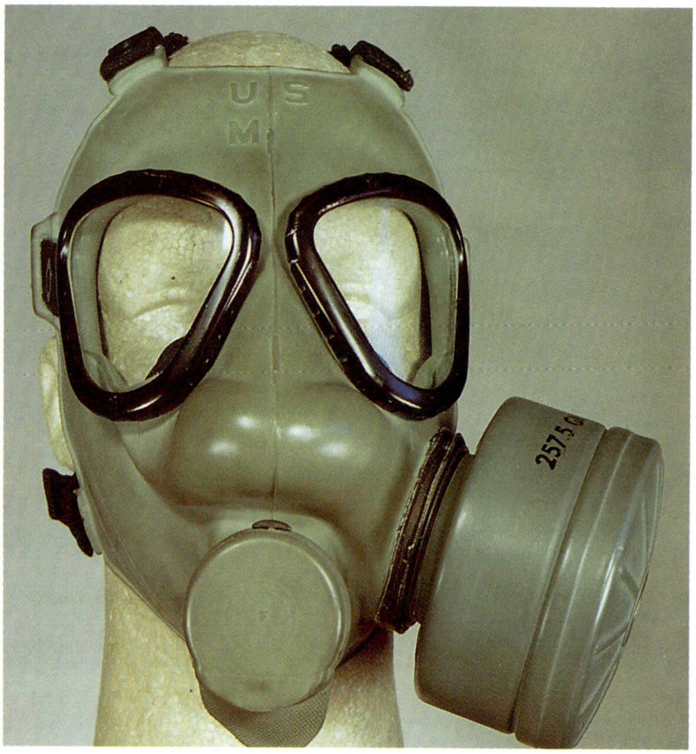

U.S. Army Field Protective Mask M9, 1952. One of the most successful and copied NBC respirators in the world, the M9 was developed in the late 40s, was the principal U.S. service respirator until the 60s, and continued to serve for many more years in 'special applications' alongside the later M17 which was meant to replace it. This is the direct descendent of the unsuccessful WWII M5-11-7 Assault Gas Mask.

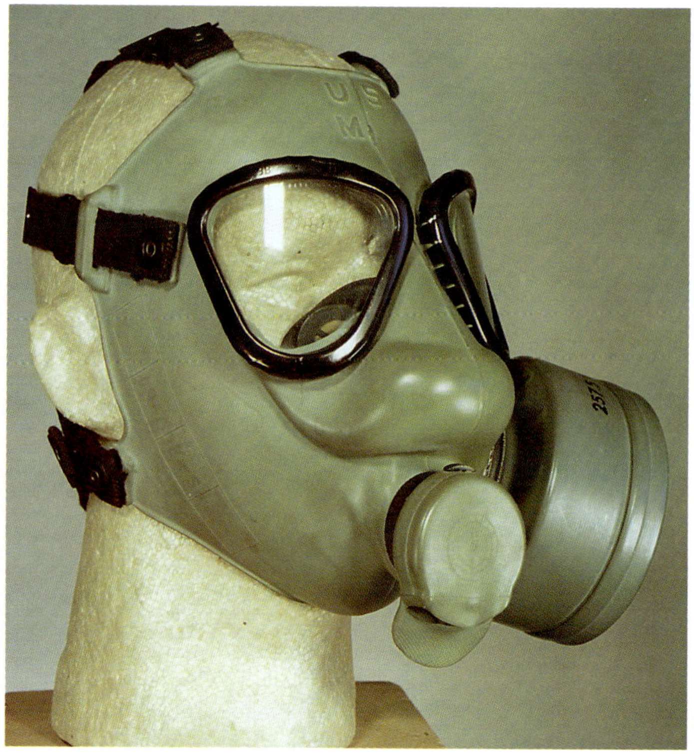

U.S. Army Field Protective Mask M9, 1952. View of the right oblique aspect shows molding on edge of facepiece for lot number and ID markings (stamped on). The C15 type exhalation valve was fitted. Some detail of the air flow control valve fitted to the internal oronasal cup may be seen through the right lens.

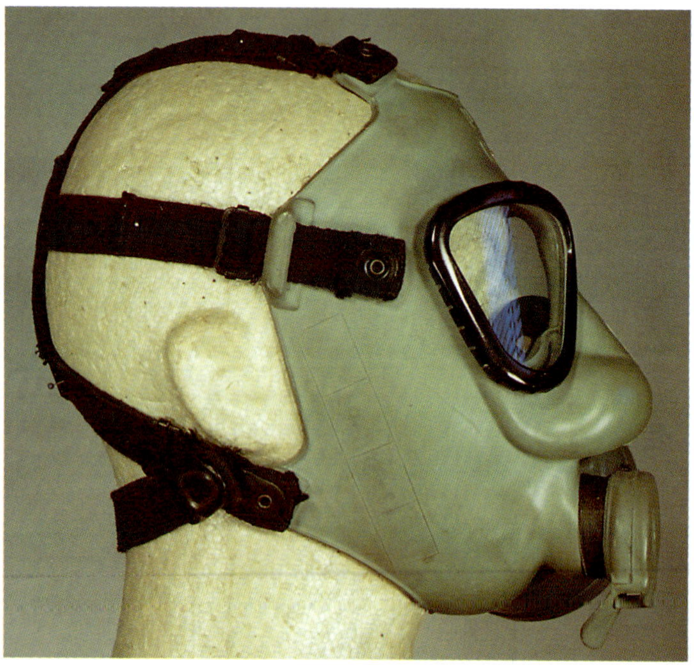

U.S. Army Field Protective Mask M9, 1952. The M9 mask was produced in both left and right hand filter mount versions, both taking the standard axial flow M11 with its screw thread fitting. Right side versions are somewhat scarce, having been produced for left-handed soldiers. Standard left-mount M9 masks are very common today.

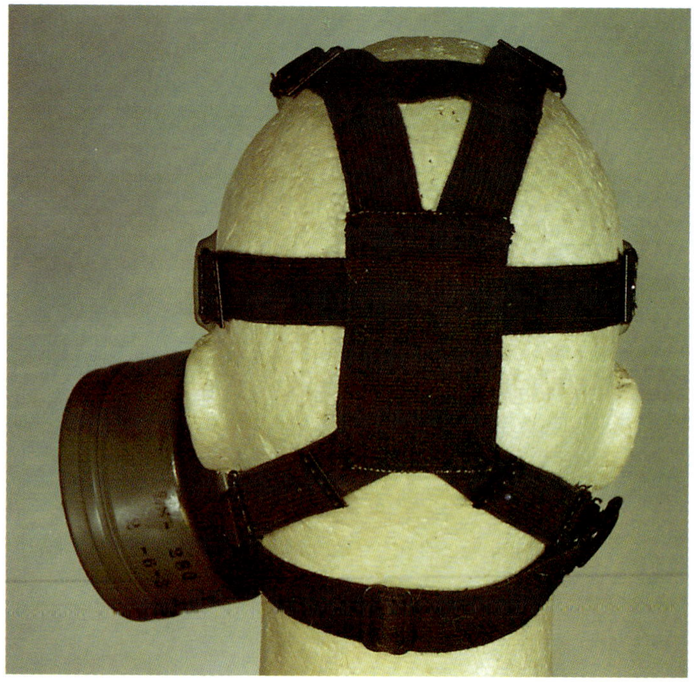

U.S. Army Field Protective Mask M9, 1952. View of the C8 type head harness and neck strap. The M9 and the M9A1 masks themselves are absolutely identical to each other; the change in designation was due to the substitution of the M11 carrier (M9A1) for the earlier C15R1 carrier (M9).

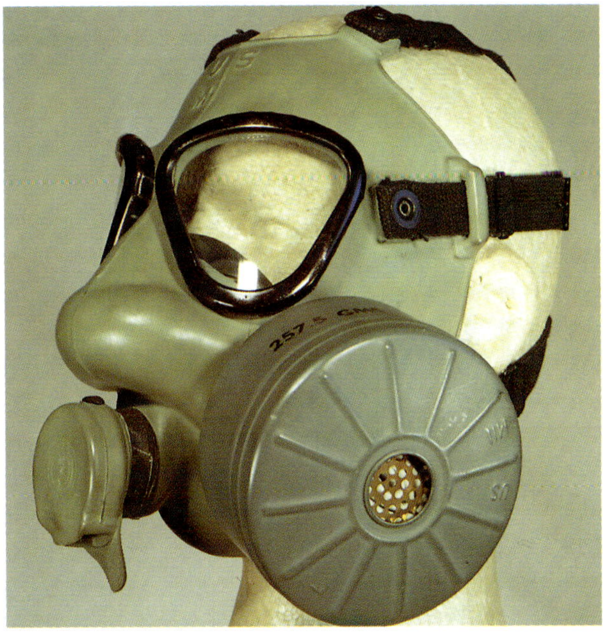

U.S. Army Field Protective Mask M9, 1952. View of the left oblique aspect., and fitted M11 axial flow filter. This example is in 'very good' condition, having all components but being a bit dirty. M9 masks are almost as commonly found today as the later M17 series. Small dents in the aluminum M11 canister are common, due to rough handling.

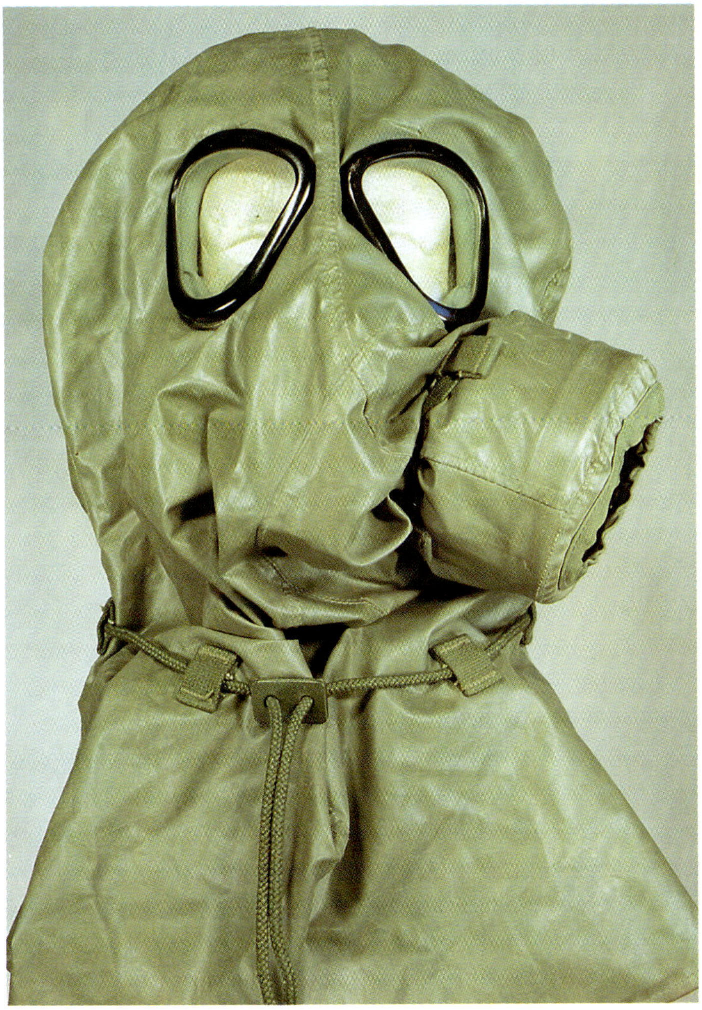

U.S. Army M9 mask fitted with M4 hood. The M4 hood was a butyl-coated fabric (cotton) protective hood which was used more often as part of the complete U.S. Army NBC protection ensemble. It could be used with the older Lightweight type service masks as well as the M8 Snout-type mask, through rearrangement of the filter tie-cords.

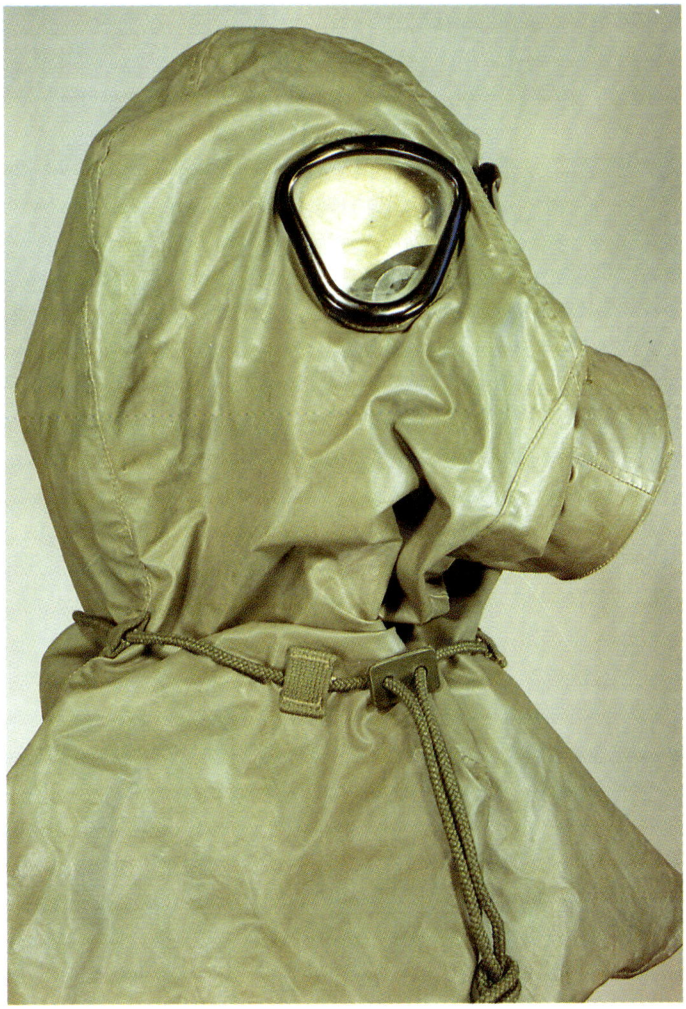

U.S. Army M9 mask fitted with M4 hood. The hood had no zipper, as do current chemical/biological protective hoods, but was fitted and rolled into the "ready" configuration in the same manner as on modern M40 series masks.

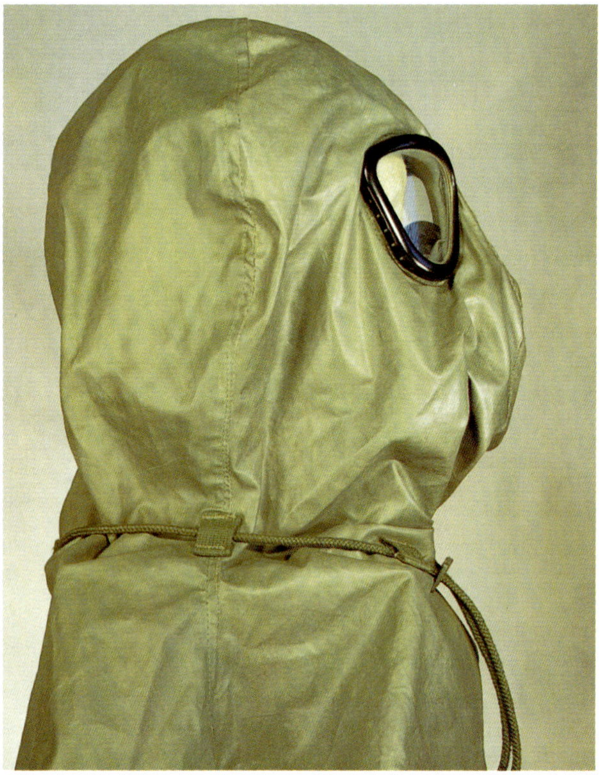

U.S. Army M9 mask fitted with M4 hood. The M4 hood provided excellent additional protection for the wearer against vessicant / mustard type agents.

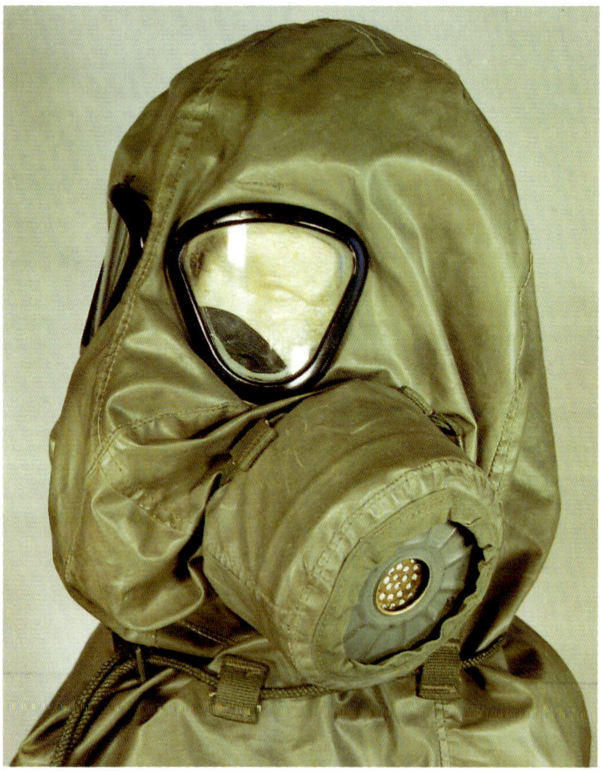

U.S. Army M9 mask fitted with M4 hood. Left oblique view shows complete coverage of M4 hood that extended to the M11 filter as well. Tie cord fitted between the filter and the mask, for adjusting purposes. This hood was an example of a well designed article which could not really be significantly improved upon.

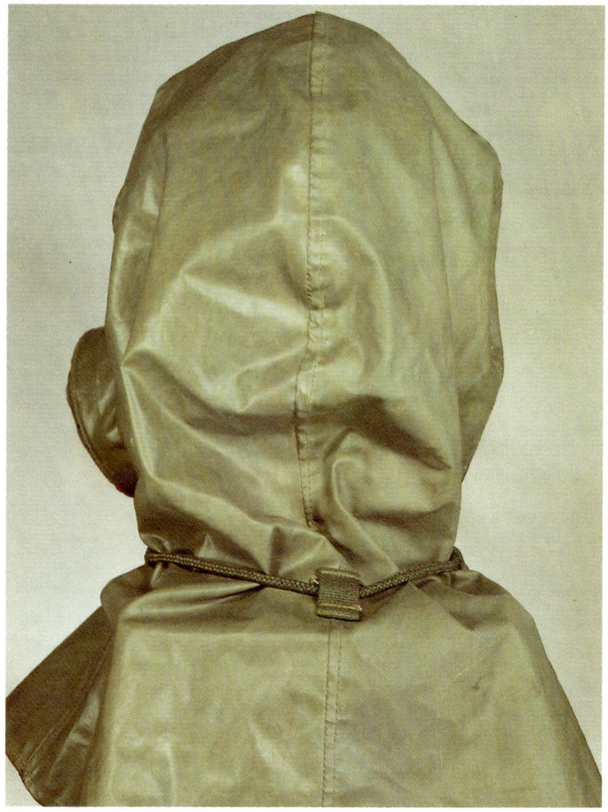

U.S. Army M9 mask fitted with M4 hoof. Rear view of the M4 hood in use.

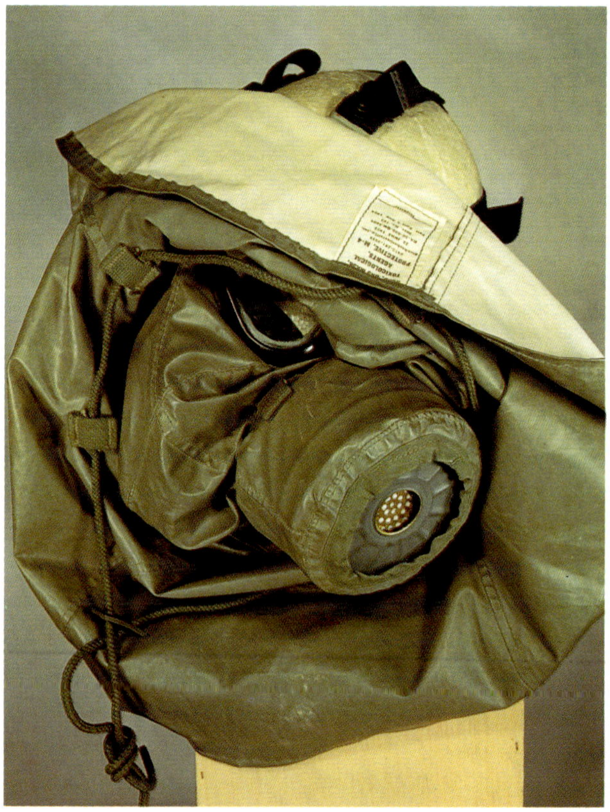

U.S. Army M9 mask fitted with M4 hood. Hood is partly pulled over forehead, showing ID label and some of the internal fabric detail.

U.S. Army M10 Special Purpose Gas Mask, 1950s

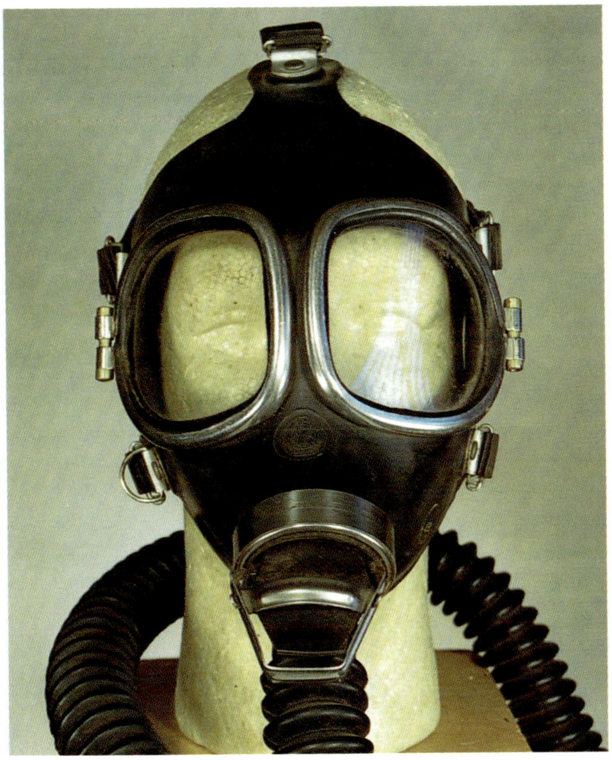

U.S. Army M10 Special Purpose Gas Mask, 1950s. The M10, M11, M11A1 and M12 gas masks all used the same facepiece and hose combination, shown here. Different filters were used for each special application.

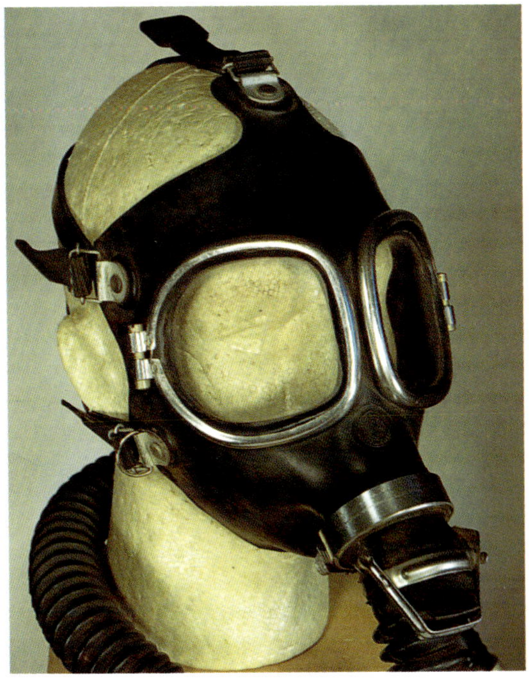

U.S. Army M10 Special Purpose Gas Mask, 1950s. The M10 type facepiece was a commercially available (MSA) molded rubber mask with twin glass lenses. Interestingly, the Japanese produced a model very similar to this in the same period, but molded from gray rubber and fitted with a canister directly on the facepiece's chin.

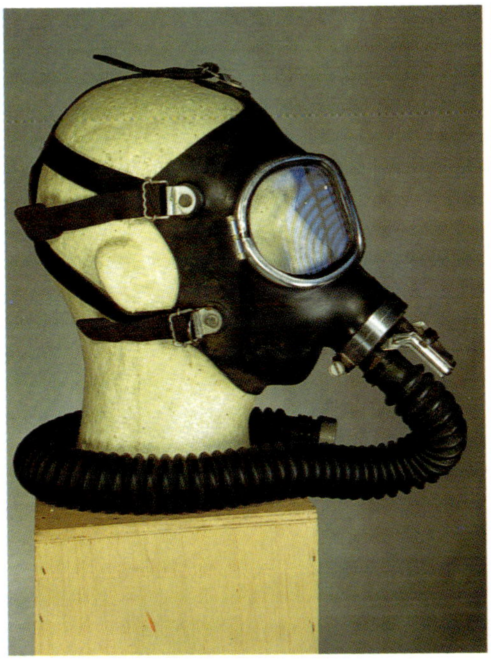

U.S. Army M10 Special Purpose Gas Mask, 1950s. Detail of the hose inlet and exhalation valve assembly is discernible. A later commercial version of this mask featured a more modern exhalation valve assembly (not a flapper type protected by a metal guard, which is little changed from the earliest WWI concepts).

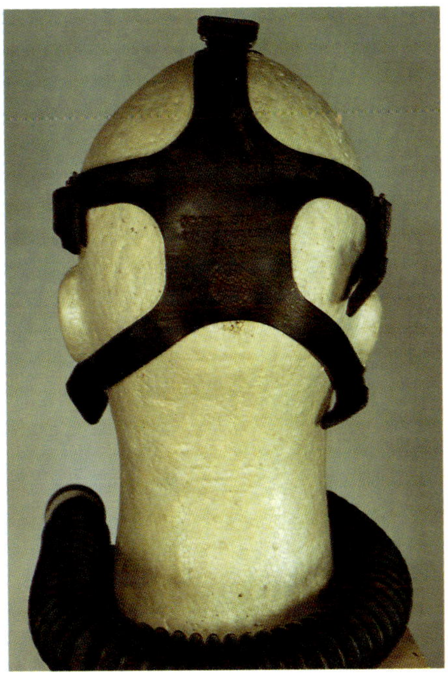

U.S. Army M10 Special Purpose Gas Mask, 1950s. Details of the rubber head harness are observable; the harness is very similar in design and appearance to that used on the Navy Mark V, and also on the British AVON S10.

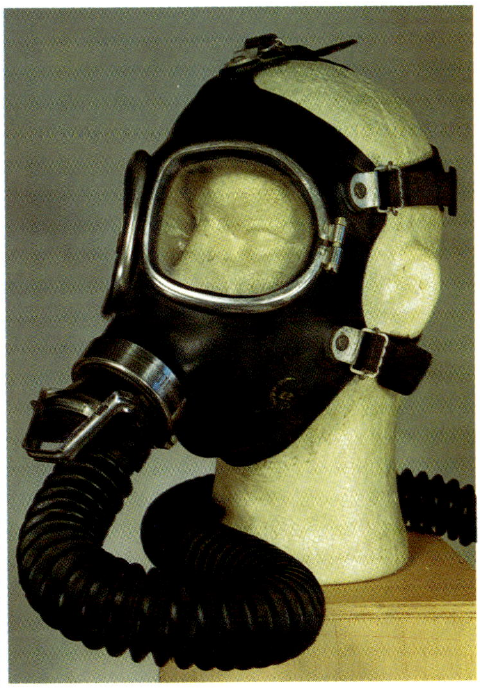

U.S. Army M10 Special Purpose Gas Mask, 1950s. Very good oblique view of this mask, clearly showing the inlet hose and exhalation valve assembly, as well as mold markings on the facepiece. A specially adapted version of this facepiece was used on the Army M13 Oxygen Breathing Gas Mask, which is not illustrated in this book.

U.S. Army Field Protective Mask M17, early 60s

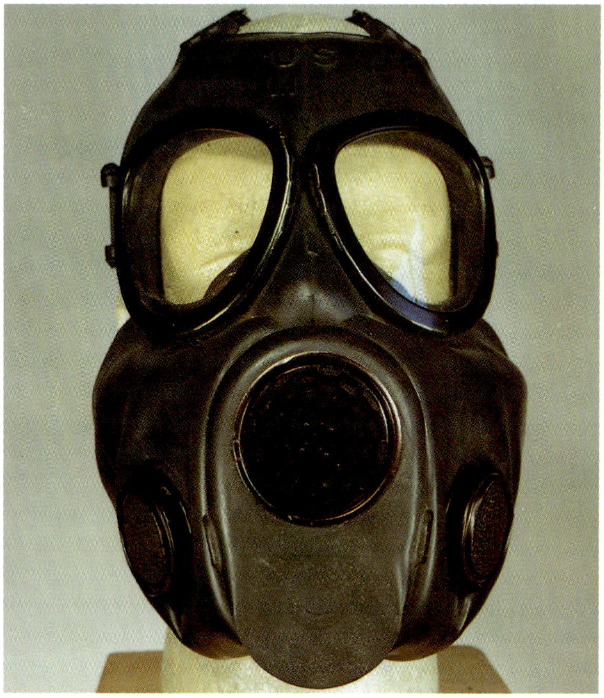

U.S. Army Field Protective Mask M17, early 60s. The original version of the tripartite M17 series, the M13 type filters were fitted into each side of the mask from within, after the oronasal cup was 'unbuttoned' and moved, to allow access. Prominent voicemitter and protected exhalation valve are directly up front, under C13 rubber cover.

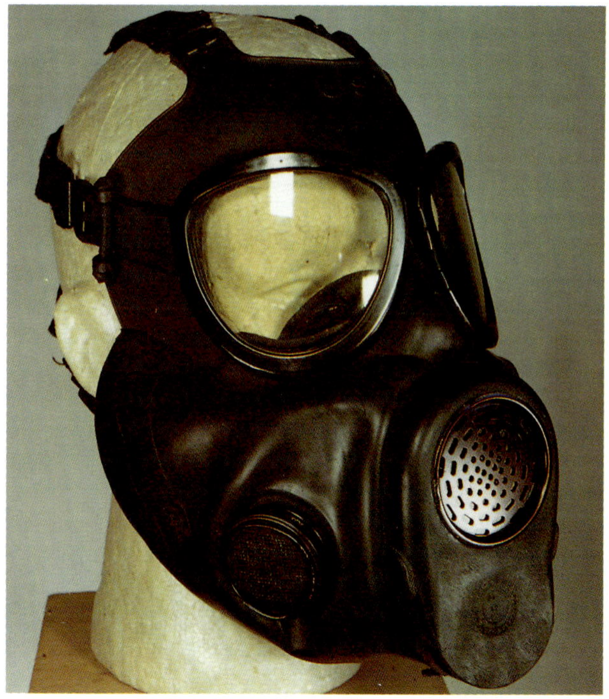

U.S. Army Field Protective Mask M17, early 60s. Mold marks are seen on right mask cheek edge (lot number) and on C13 exhalation valve cover (date of mfg.). Internal oronasal cup was identical in function to that used in M9 series. Filter inlet check-valve on right side may be seen here.

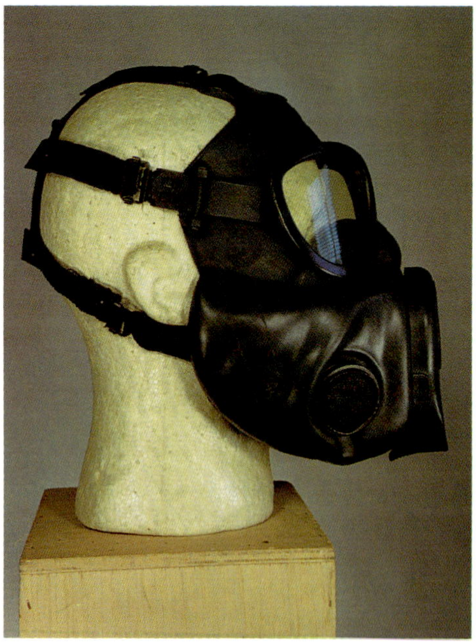

U.S. Army Field Protective Mask M17, early 60s. The protrusive bilateral filters (M13 series) were referred to commonly as 'pork-chop filters,' owing to their distinctive shape, and the M17 was occasionally termed the "Porky Pig mask," for obvious reasons. While a good overall protective respirator, the difficulty which changing the internally accessed filters posed was a possible liability in the event of a determined, sustained CBW attack.

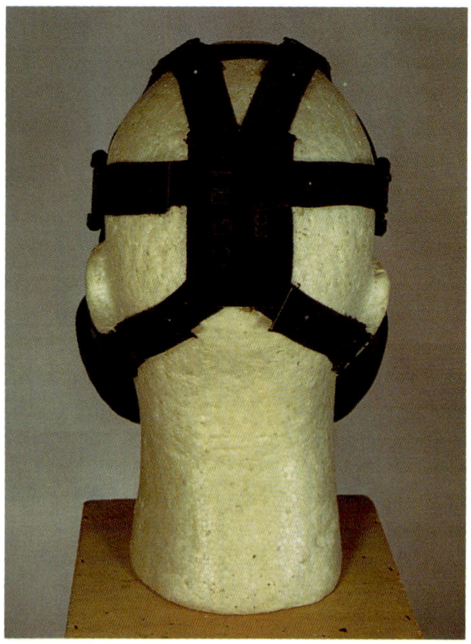

U.S. Army Field Protective Mask M17, early 60s. Detail of the C8R1 type harness is shown. Several respirators around the world have been based on or inspired by the M17, including the Czech M10M (a near look-alike), a Taiwanese carbon-copy, the PRC M-65, and the CIS (Russian) PMG-2 (which is an optical type mask).

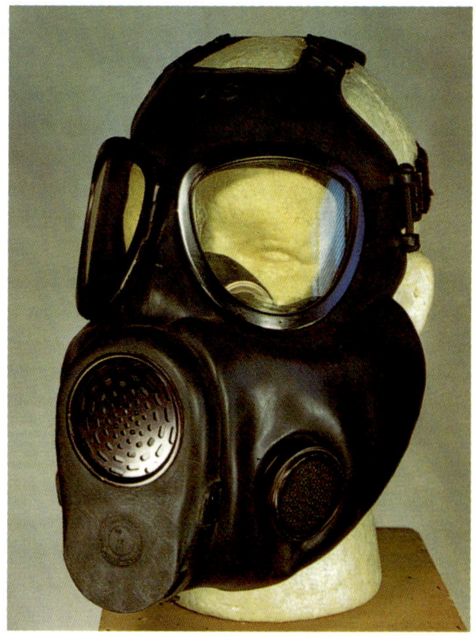

U.S. Army Field Protective Mask M17, early 60s. Good oblique left view, showing exhalation valve cover (C13) attachment button, and detail of left filter inlet check-valve.

U.S. Army Field Protective Mask M17A1, late 60s

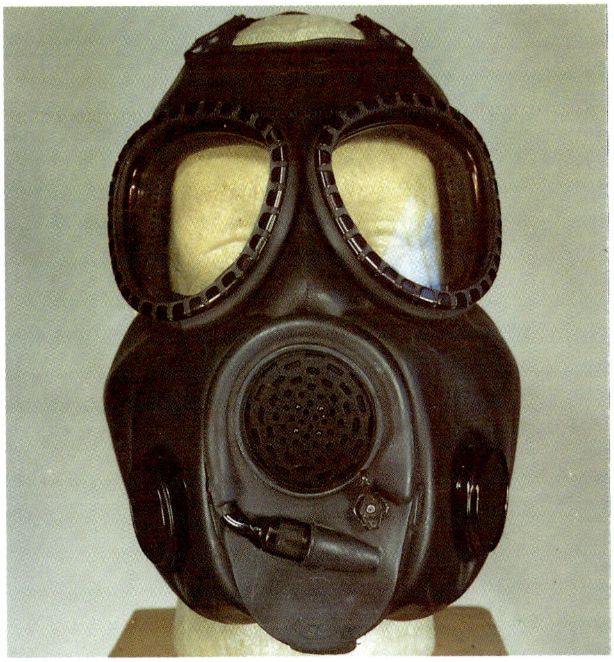

U.S. Army Field Protective Mask M17A1, late 60s. Virtually identical to M17 in appearance except for the new drink tube assembly configured into the exhalation valve assembly (and cover). The M17A1 also featured a special internal oral valve which could be used for resuscitation purposes, using a separate M1 tube and mouthpiece accessory. The M17A2 (not illustrated in this book) was identical in external appearance to the M17A1 mask but lacked the resuscitation assembly.

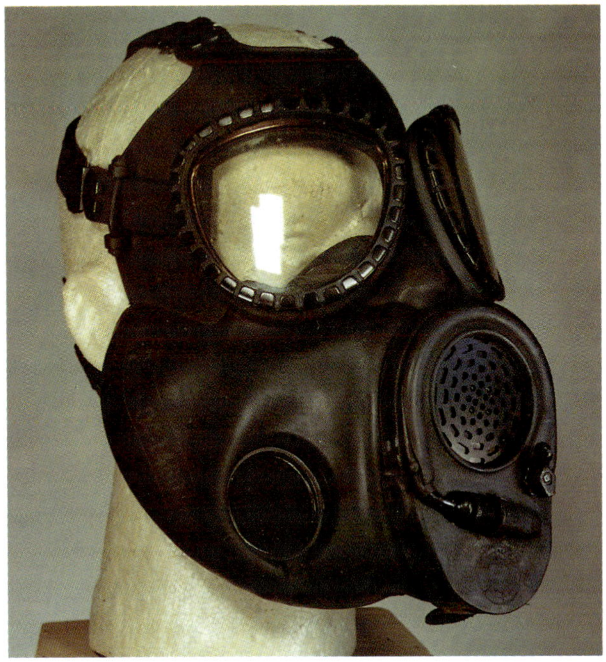

U.S. Army Field Protective Mask M17A1, late 60s. The example shown has the protective "outsert" accessory lenses fitted, which were normally used after the M6 type hood had been fitted. Lot number may be seen on right filter housing edge. Many M17A1s later had their internal resuscitation valve component removed or rendered inoperable, in compliance with M17A2 standards.

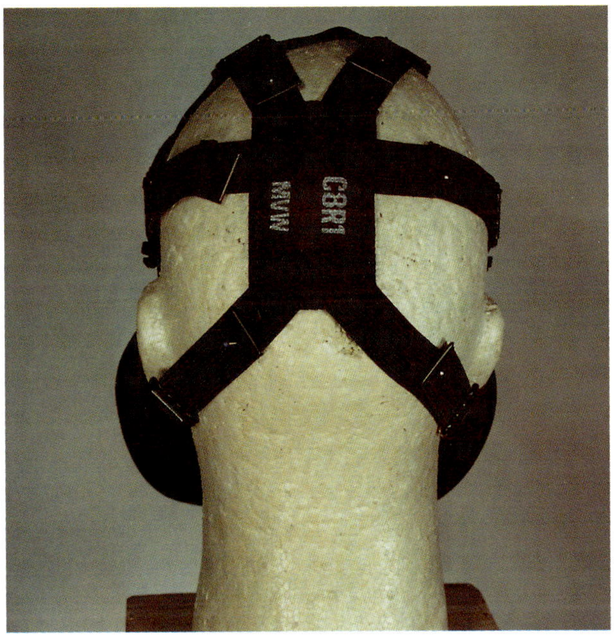

U.S. Army Field Protective Mask M17A1, late 60s. C8R1 harness illustrated. As the M17A1 model came into use, the earlier M17s were relegated to training and secondary, or reserve, status. When the M17A2 began being issued in the early 70s, some M17A1s remained in use (altered, as described), but the M17 model then used only for NBC training. M17A2 masks were the primary U.S. NBC respirators in use by all American armed forces at the time of the 1991 Gulf War.

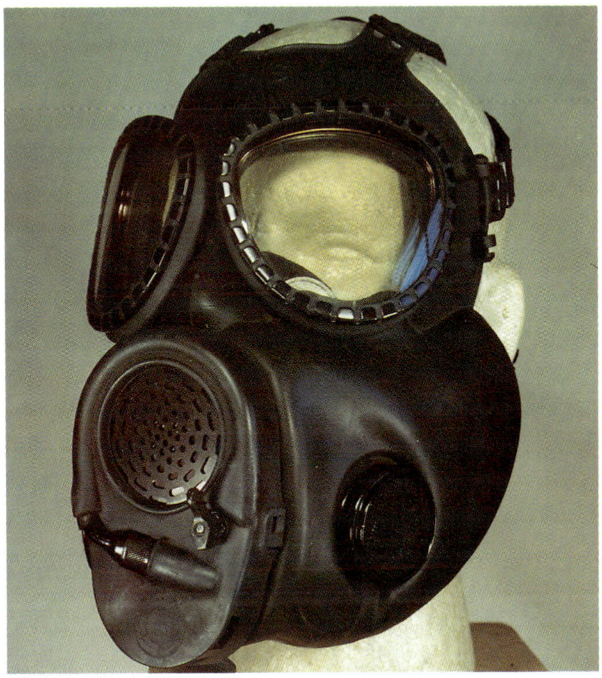

U.S. Army Field Protective Mask M17A1, late 60s. The last M17A2 type masks were manufactured in the mid 80s (about 1986 or 87), and all M17 series masks used the M13A2 filter sets as standard war filters. The original M13 and M13A1 filter sets were superseded by the M13A2 type, the last lots of which were produced in the late 1980s.

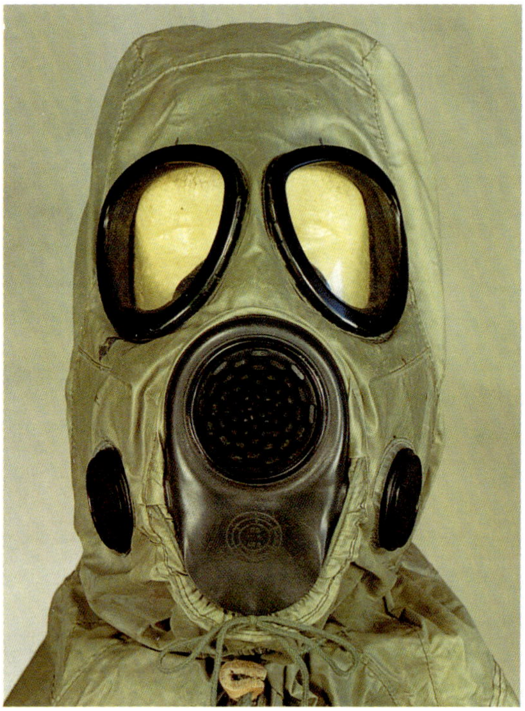

U.S. Army M17 mask fitted with M6A2 hood. The M6 series hoods were used with all M17 masks. The last version of the M6 hood series (the M6A2) featured a zippered front and was fabricated from butyl proofed nylon. Despite the protrusion of the voicemitter and exhalation valve assembly, the M17 faceblank provided far better protection against penetrating vessicant (mustard) type agents than the current silicone M40/M42 type (which must be used with an EPDM 'second-skin' facepiece protector).

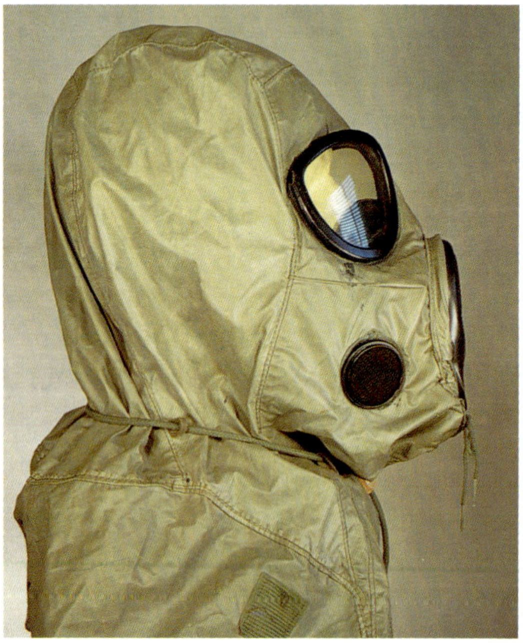

U.S. Army M17 mask fitted with M6A2 hood. When well worn, the hoods could have 'thin' areas in the butyl coating. This could be detected by holding the hood in front of a strong light source, and repaired by application of more butyl coating material. Velcro patches were used to secure straps, fitted under the arms, which held hood skirt down.

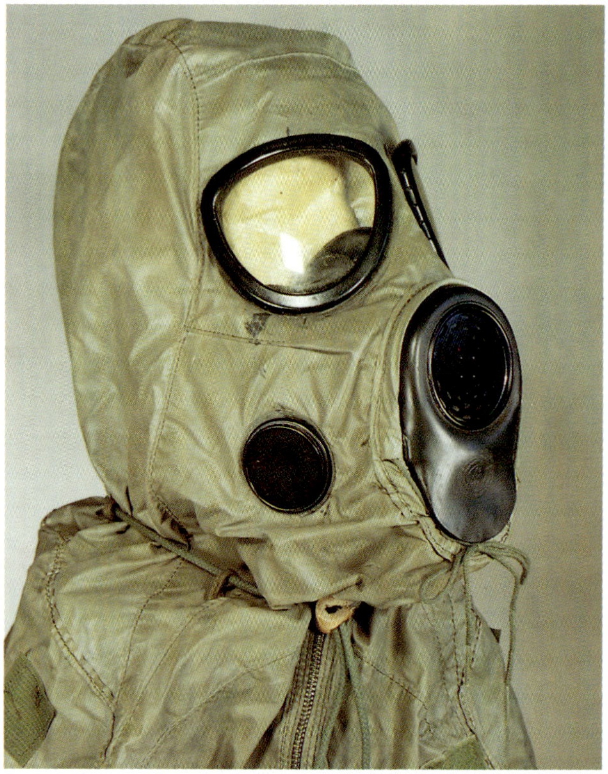

U.S. Army M17 mask fitted with M6A2 hood. The filter inlet check-valves protruded through the fabric of the hood, but were fitted with downward positioned vanes which provided some protection from entrainment of larger aerial spray droplets.

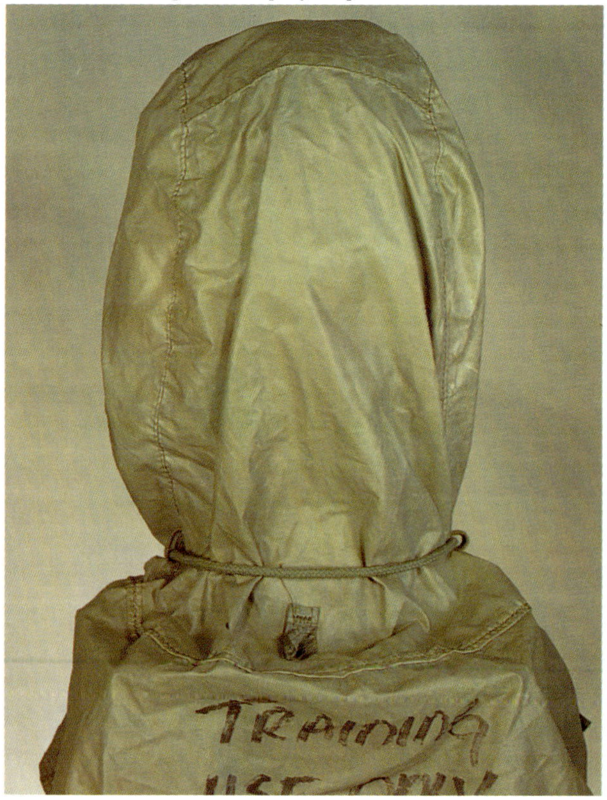

U.S. Army M17 mask fitted with M6A2 hood. Rear view of M6A2 hood; this specimen was used with the M17 mask to train recruits in basic NBC defense.

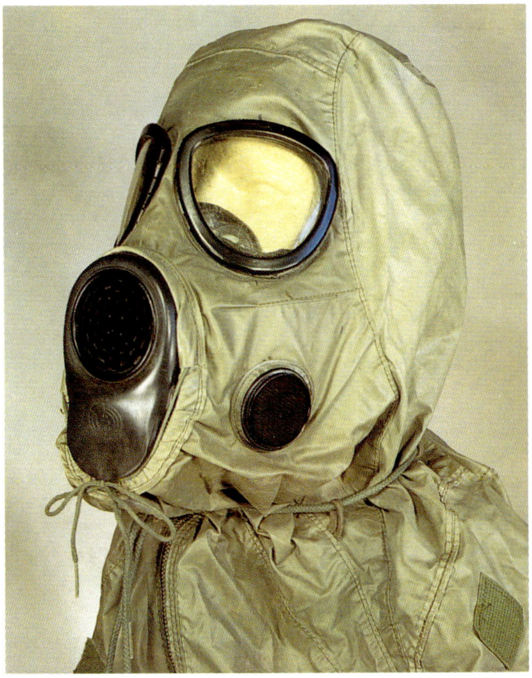

U.S. Army M17 mask fitted with M6A2 hood. Good oblique left view, showing details of mask components and hood fitting cord used to secure hood around exhalation valve cover. An alternative fitting had the hood being tied over the lower half of the C13 voicemitter/exhalation valve cover, so that exhaled air was vented down through the hood's skirt (further protecting the exhalation valve).

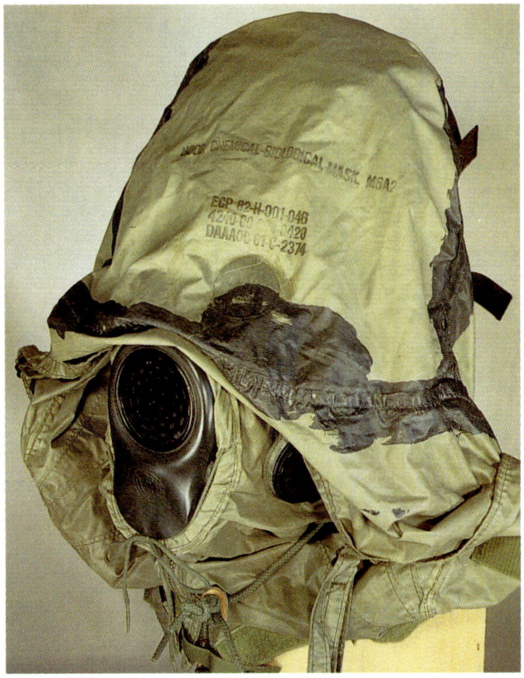

U.S. Army M17 mask fitted with M6A2 hood. The hood is partly drawn over the top of the mask, showing stamped identification nomenclature and reinforcing sealing of seams (black liquid butyl rubber).

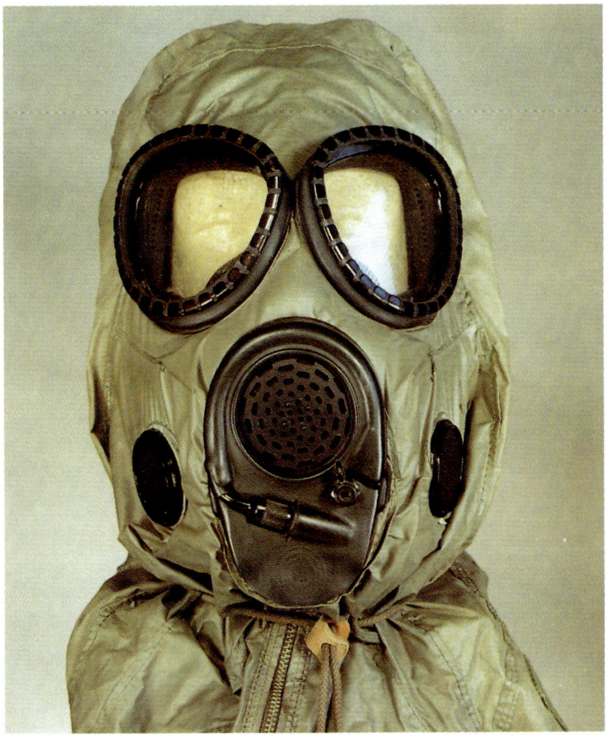

U.S. Army M17A1 mask fitted with M6A2 hood. This view shows the accessory "outsert" lenses in place. A second set were provided with dark shaded lenses. Front zipper was to enhance donning and doffing, and neck cord helped fit hood to head.

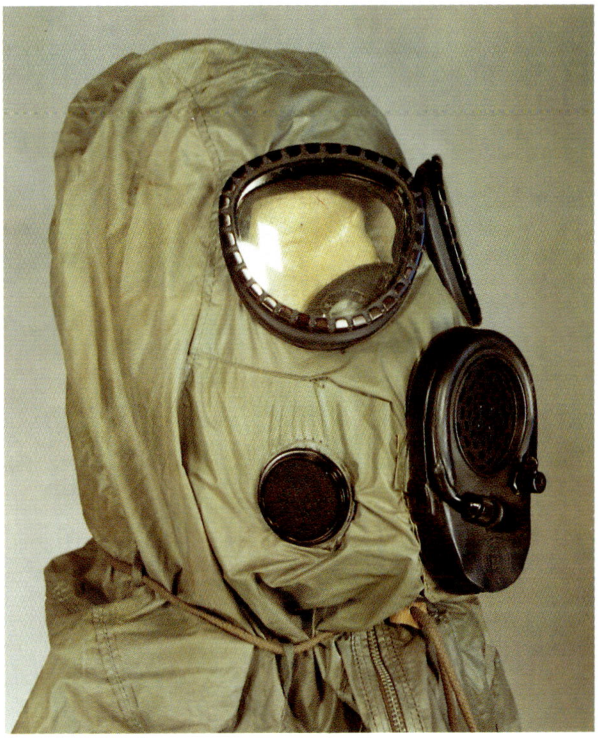

U.S. Army M17A1 mask fitted with M6A2 hood. Right oblique view shows details of hood and valve areas.

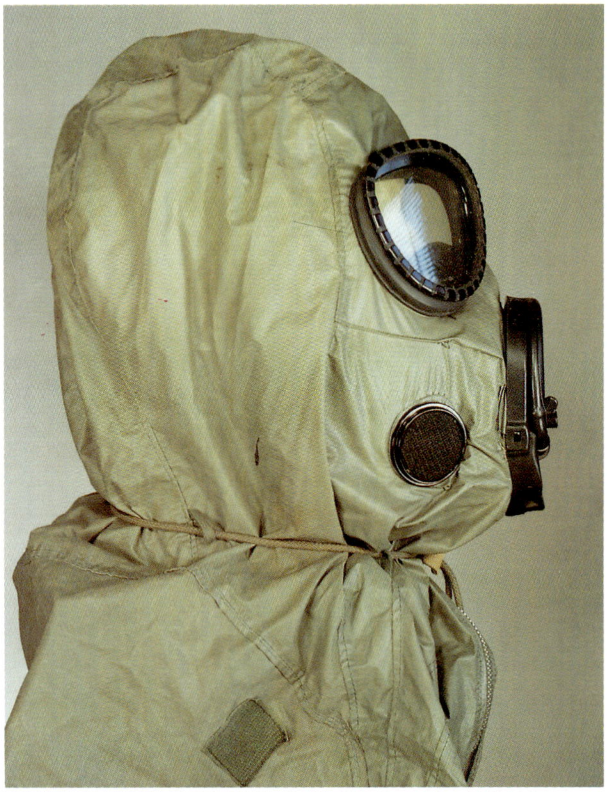

U.S. Army M17A1 mask fitted with M6A2 hood. Very little difference between M17 and M17A1/M17A2 type masks is discernible in profile, either with or without hood. Only visual clues to model are drink tube components on C13R1 voicemitter/valve cover (M17 mask used the C13 cover).

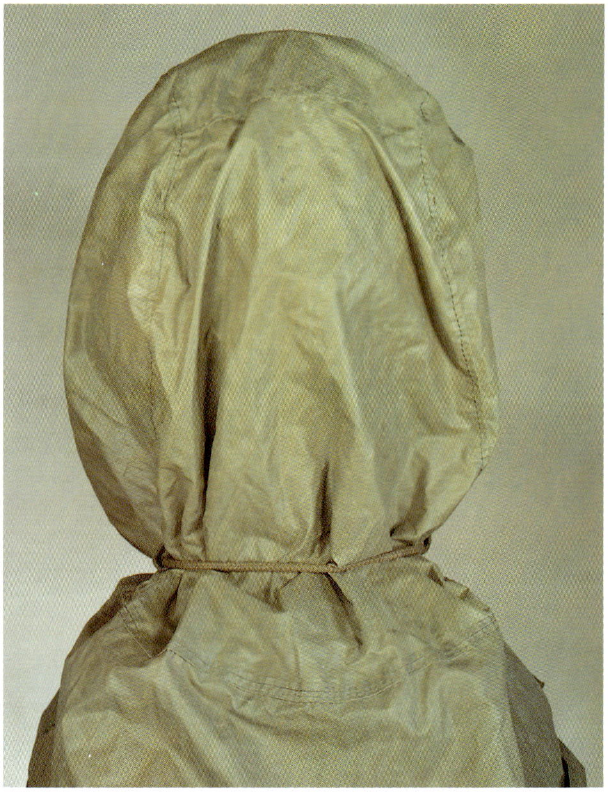

U.S. Army M17A1 mask fitted M6A2 hood. Rear view of hood. No distinguishing or identifying characteristics viewable from this angle.

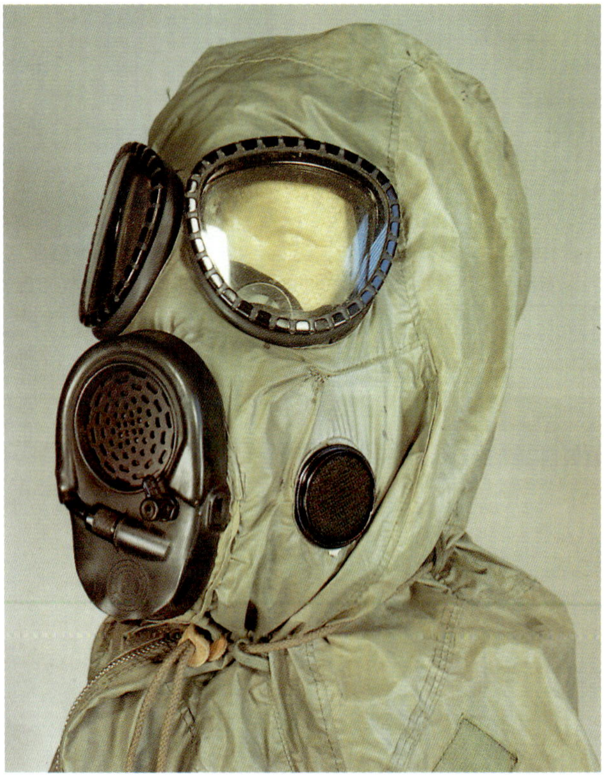

U.S. Army M17A1 mask fitted with M6A2 hood. Good left oblique view of mask and hood details.

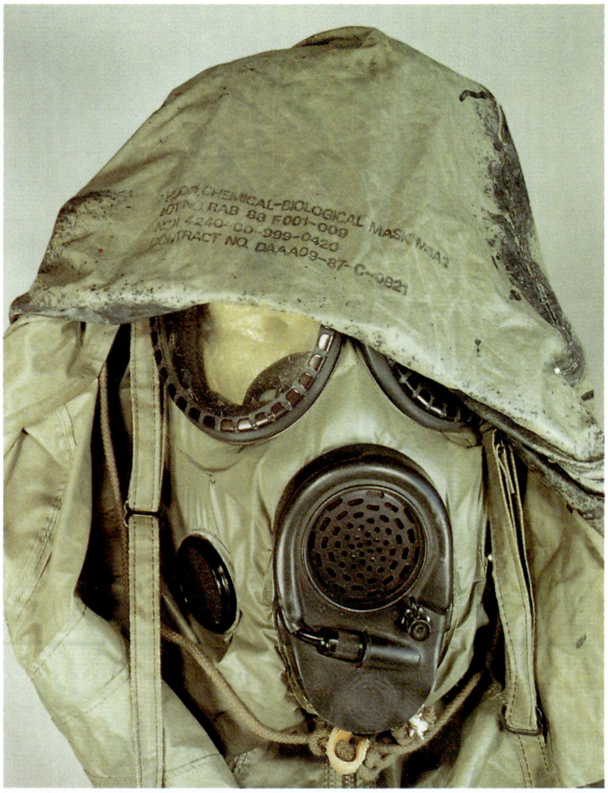

U.S. Army M17A1 mask fitted with M6A2 hood. Hood is partly drawn over top of head to reveal ID lettering, designation and seam sealing details. The drink tube was used with the M1B canteen cap.

U.S. Army Protective Mask, Armored Vehicle, M25A1, 1960s/70s

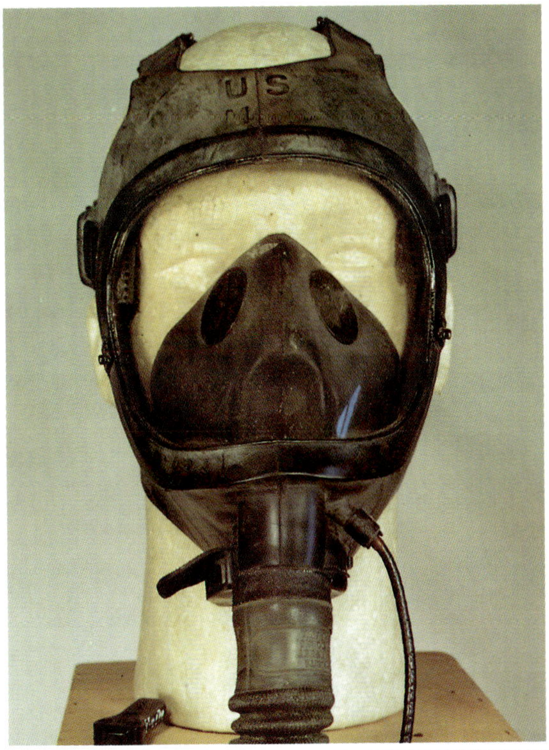

U.S. Army Protective Mask, Armored Vehicle, M25A1, 1960s/70s. A development of the earlier M14 armored vehicle mask (not illustrated), which looked substantially similar, the M25 series masks had a large, flexible plastic visor which provided a substantial field of view (were it not for the large internal oronasal cup). The aircraft version of this mask varied hardly at all in appearance, but featured a different carrier, differing filter connection components, and a head harness modification (along with alternate microphones and connectors). The M24 used the M7 aircraft NBC hood and the M25 and M25A1 used the M5 tank NBC hood, additionally. Both hoods looked very much like the M6 series hood used on the M17 masks.

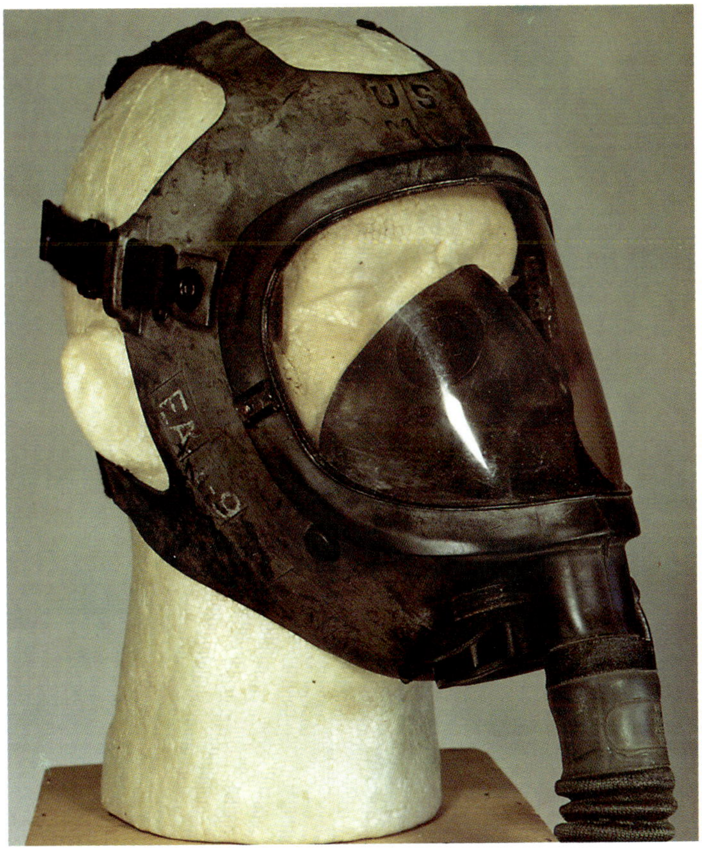

U.S. Army Protective Mask, Armored Vehicle, M25A1, 1960s/70s. This specimen is in 'very good' condition, although some general dirtiness is evident. The exhalation valve was located behind the inlet hose, which connected to the M10A1 type filter, where a further tie in to either a tank collective protection system (M25 series) or an aircraft system (M24) was possible.

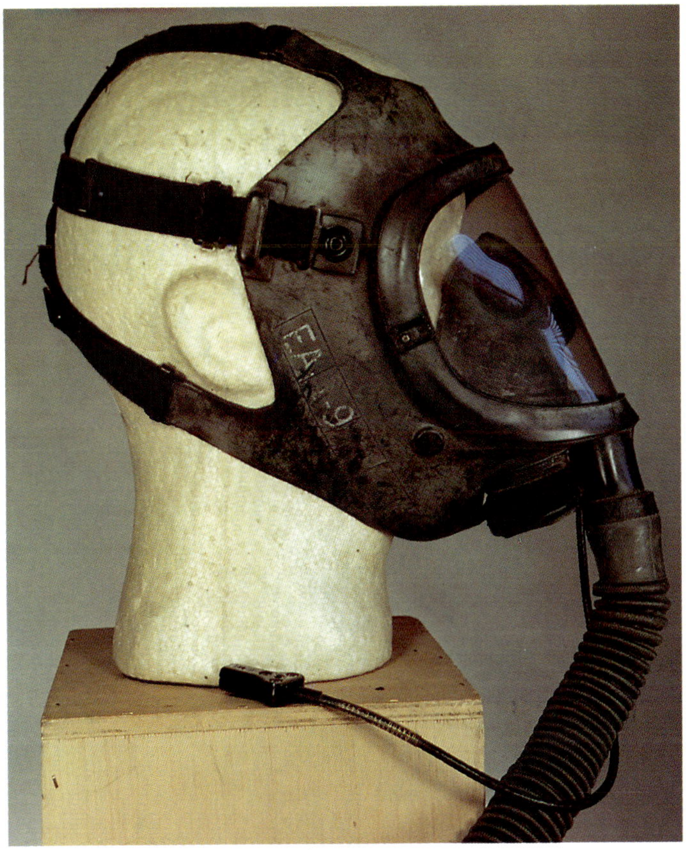

U.S. Army Protective Mask, Armored Vehicle, M25A1, 1960s/70s. Shown in profile are the nylon wrapped, internally reinforced (metal) hose and the microphone connector cable. Both the M24 and M25/M25A1 series masks used the C15 exhalation valve.

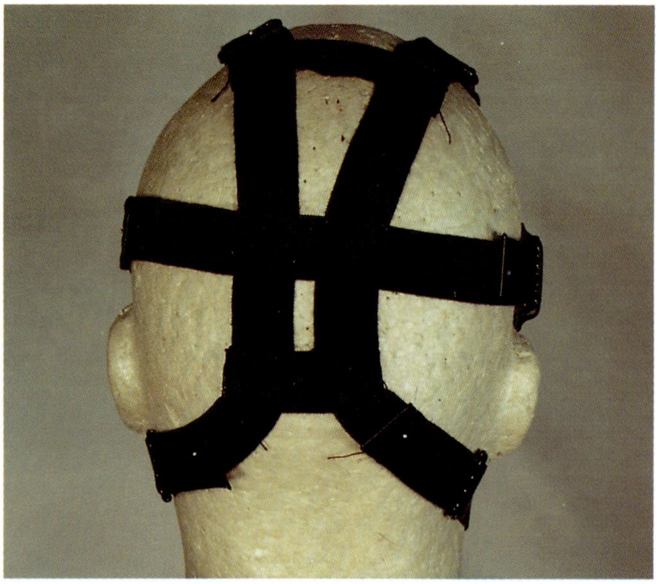

U.S. Army Protective Mask, Armored Vehicle, M25A1, 1960s/70s. Shown is the tank style elasticized head harness.

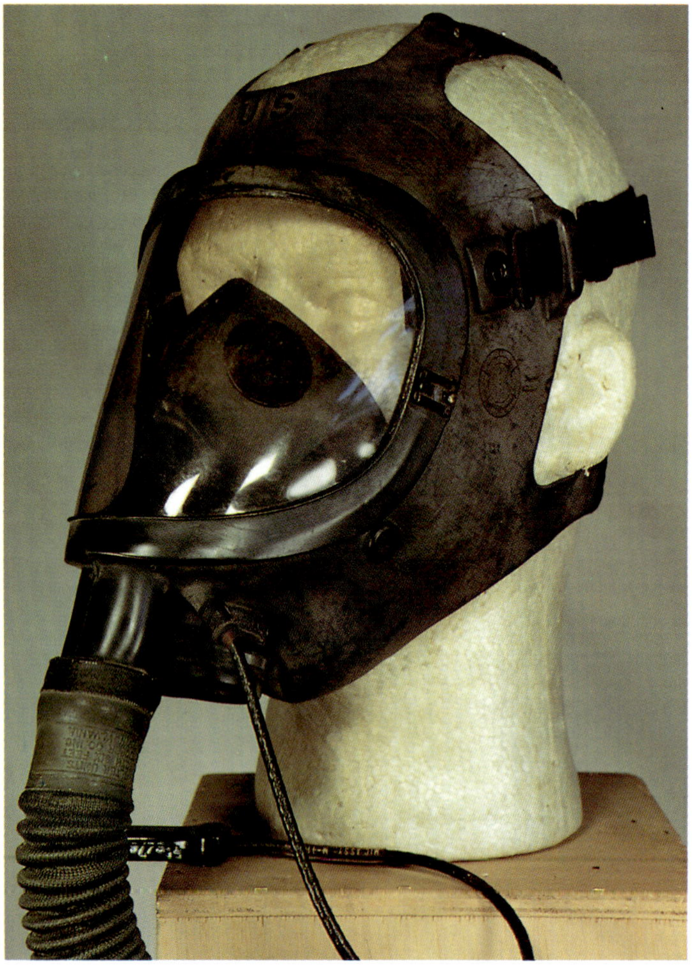

U.S. Army Protective Mask, Armored Vehicle, M25A1, 1960s/70s. Good view of the left oblique aspects of the mask, with microphone cable exit viewable. Note ID and dating mold mark on left side of facepiece.

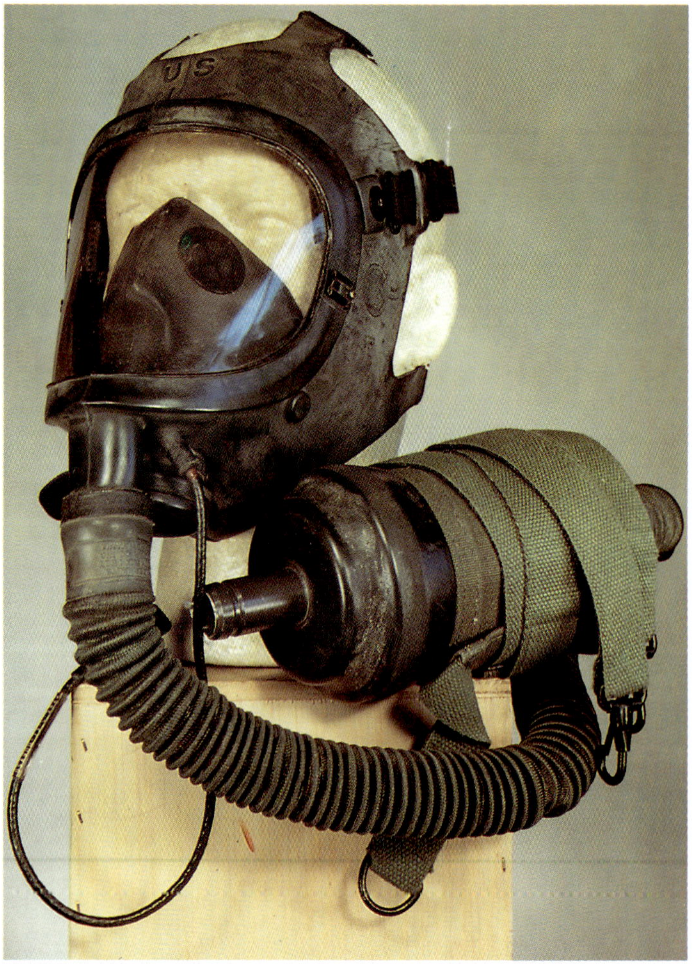

U.S. Army Protective Mask, Armored Vehicle, M25A1, 1960s/70s. Complete mask assembly shown with hose, filter canister (and M1 canister coupling connector), along with securing straps. The aircraft version (M24) came with an M8 aircraft oxygen to CB mask connector, which permitted use of the mask with both standard fixed wing oxygen systems and a personal bail-out bottle.

U.S. Army Protective Mask, Riot Control Agent, M28, late 1960s

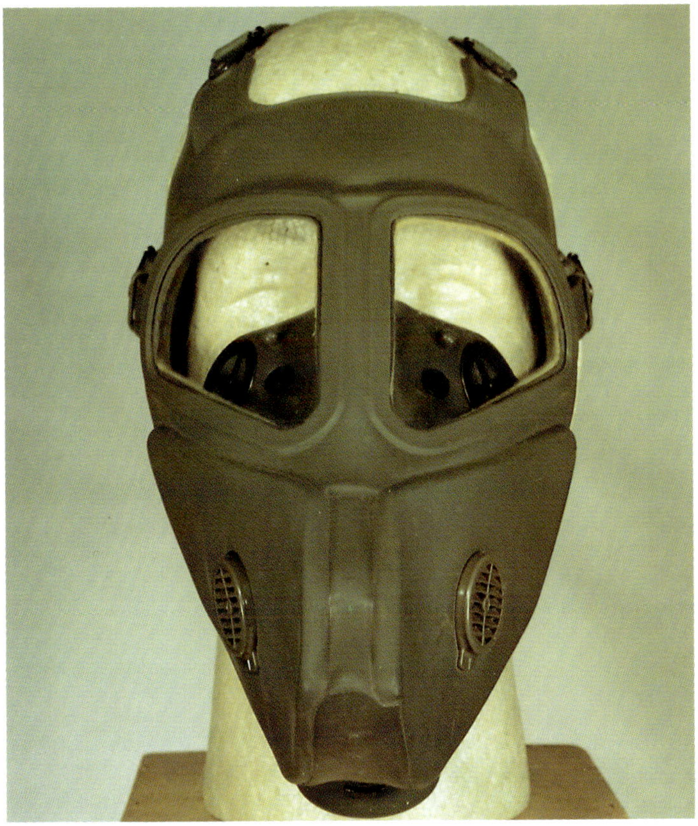

U.S. Army Protective Mask, Riot Control Agent, M28, late 60s. It is easy to see why this mask was called the "grasshopper mask," from this frontal aspect. Developed originally for use in Vietnam operations against Viet Cong tunnels, the former XM28E4 mask was also used against domestic rioting, and later by police departments.

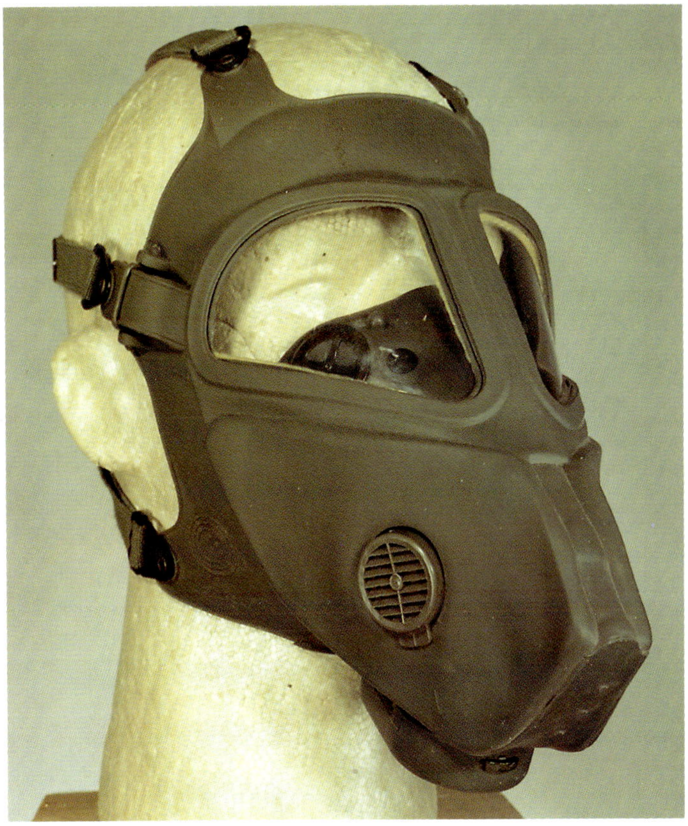

U.S. Army Protective Mask, Riot Control Agent, M28, late 60s. Compare this mask with the M22 / CD V-805 civilian mask for similarities in appearance. The M28 mask folded back upon itself, along the crease lines immediately below the lenses, and could be stowed in a carrier half its unfolded length and width.

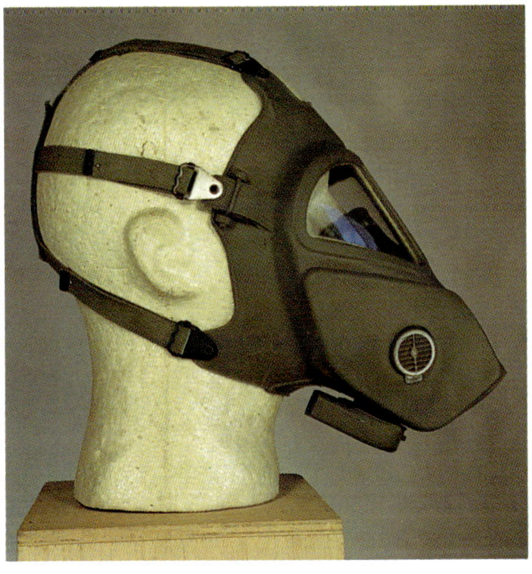

U.S. Army Protective Mask, Riot Control Agent, M28, late 60s. Good view of the right profile, showing internal oronasal cup, details of harness, right filter inlet valve and exhalation valve, below chin. This specimen is in 'excellent' condition, having neither been issued nor used.

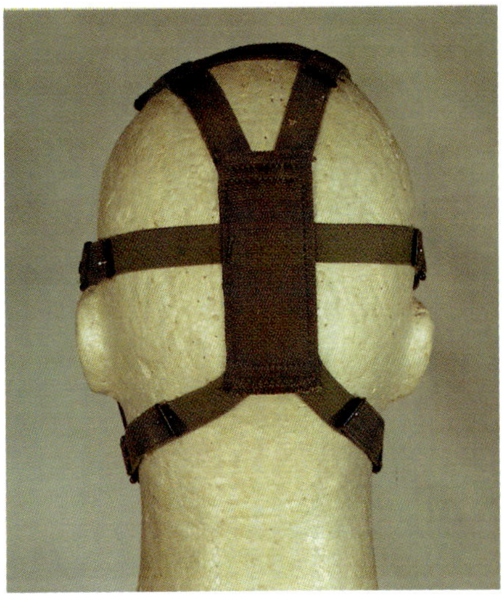

U.S. Army Protective Mask, Riot Control Agent, M28, late 60s. Elasticized head harness similar to C8R1 type harness (M17 series).

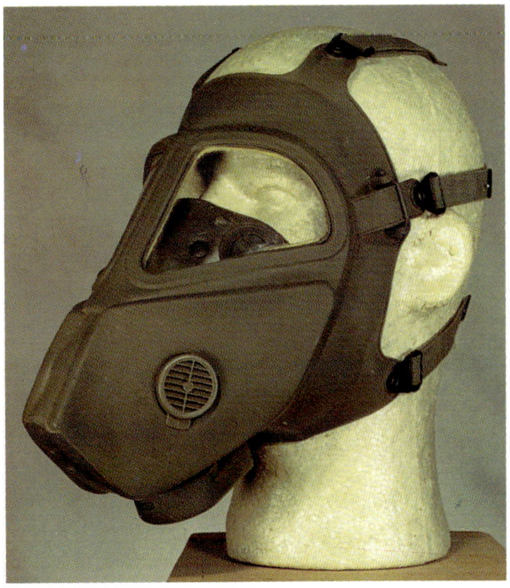

U.S. Army protective Mask, Riot Control Agent, M28, late 60s. The mask was small, compact and relatively nonobtrusive, with good field of vision, making it especially suitable for use in flushing Viet Cong from their labyrinthine subterranean tunnel complexes. In their own defense against harassing agents, the Viet Cong devised home-made protective masks using sections of plastic shower curtain, and wood charcoal wrapped in gauze pads (they were very ineffectual).

USAF/USN Chemical and Biological Protective Mask MCU-2/P

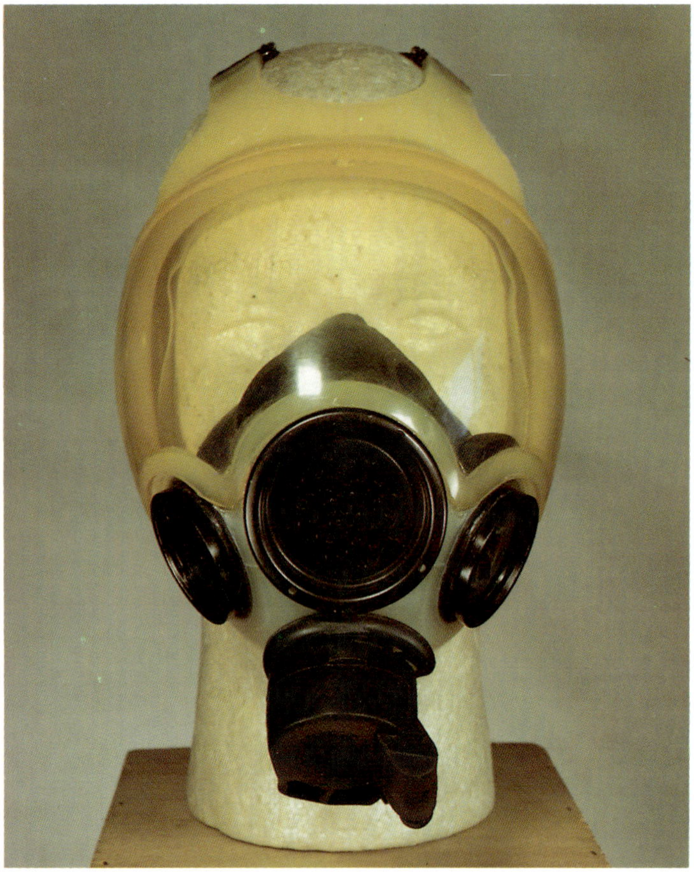

USAF/USN Chemical and Biological Protective Mask MCU-2/P (Scott Aviation), late 80s. This specimen shows the very early, limited production Scott Aviation manufactured model with its translucent silicone facepiece. The clear silicone was shown to take on a yellowish tinge with age and effects of sun & heat. Clear protective outer visor shield is not fitted, nor is C2 type filter. Very similar in appearance to original XM-30 developmental prototypes.

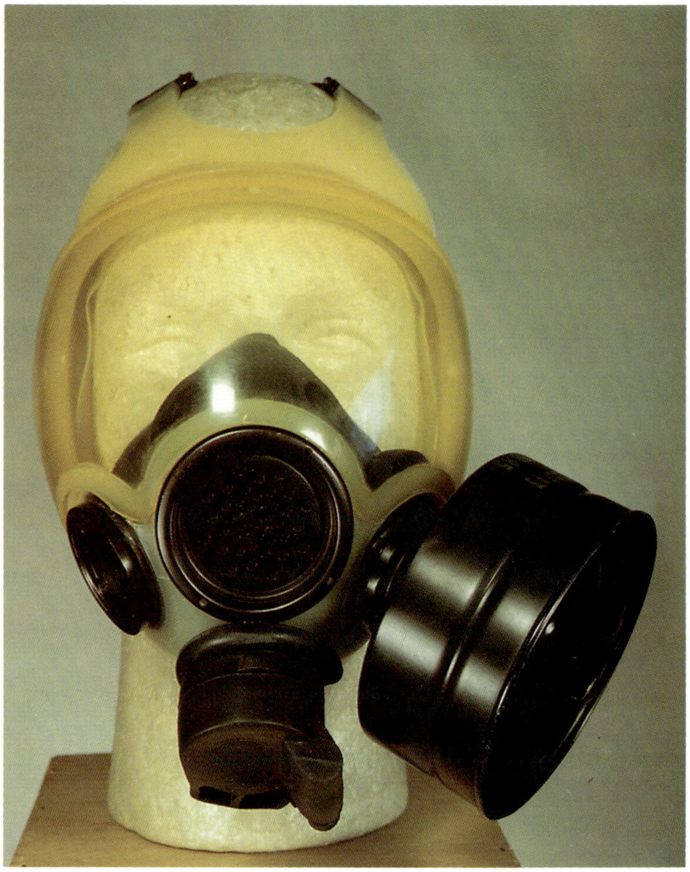

USAF/USN Chemical and Biological Protective Mask MCU-2/P (Scott Aviation), late 80s. C-2 filter is attached in this view. Note that facepiece silicone molding does not fit flush with inlet (left side) and secondary voicemitter fitting (right side). Later production runs had flush fit (compare with later MCU-2/P and MCU-2A/P examples). Clear hard shell visor protector is not fitted here.

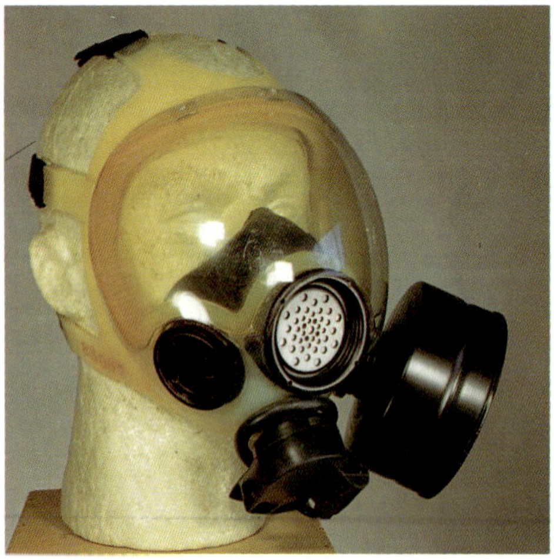

USAF/USN Chemical and Biological Protective Mask MCU-2/P (Scott Aviation), late 80s. Good right oblique view, which shows clear hardshell visor protector fitted, and lot number on lower right margin of facepiece. Silicone offers excellent face-seal qualities but abysmal penetration resistance to vessicant (mustard type) agents, hence the controversy over its continued use.

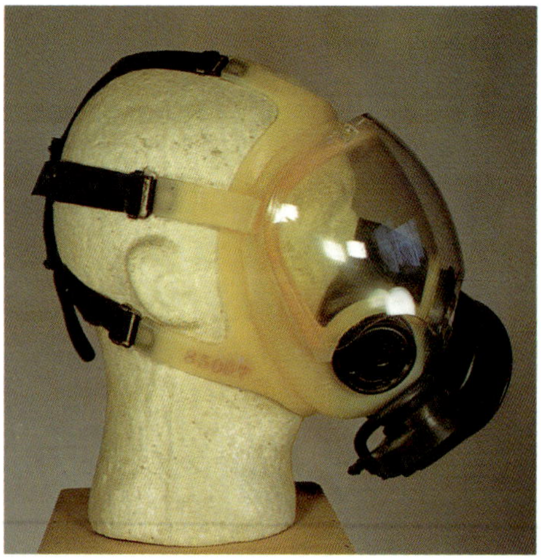

USAF/USN Chemical and Biological Protective Mask MCU-2/P (Scott Aviation), late 80s. Yellowed clear silicone of facepiece discerned, along with molded-in harness buckle hardware detail. The clear hardshell visor is referred to as a face-form preserving feature but the primary function is to protect the soft, transparent clear plastic lens from damage.

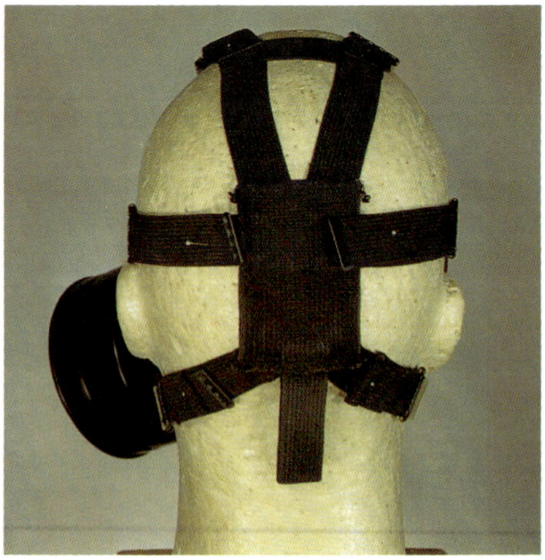

USAF/USN Chemical and Biological Protective Mask MCU-2/P (Scott Aviation), late 80s. Details of elasticized (C15R1 style) head harness are clear. Straps are pinned for clarity.

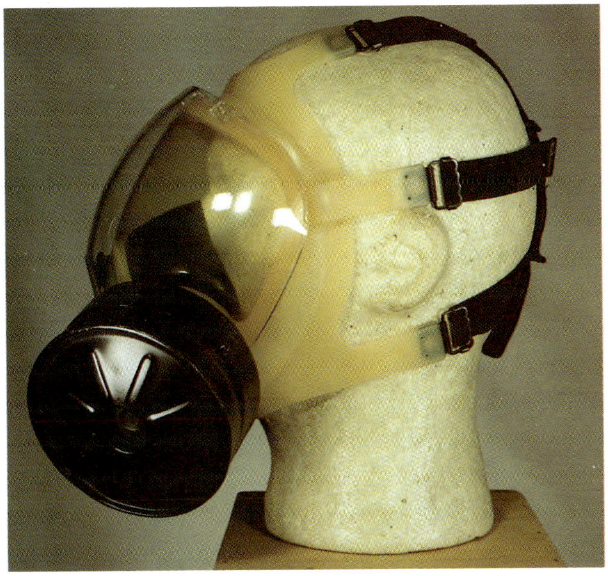

USAF/USN Chemical and Biological Protective Mask MCU-2/P (Scott Aviation), late 80s. Left profile of mask, showing C-2 filter (black body—latest C2A1 filter has dark metallic green body) mounted, with protective clear hardshell visor assembly fitted.

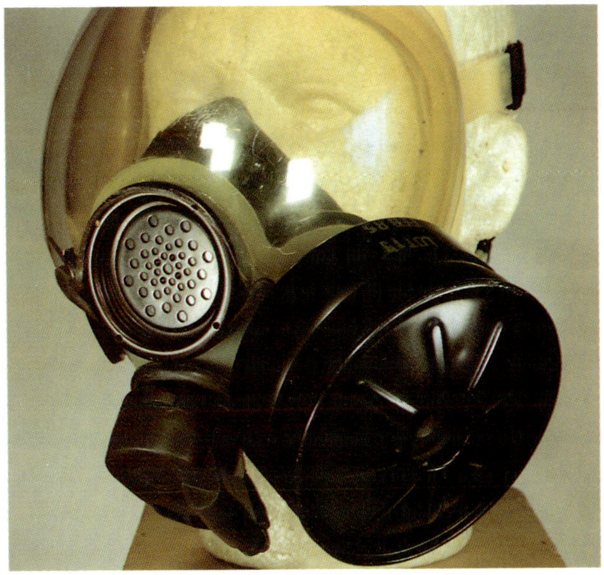

USAF/USN Chemical and Biological Protective Mask MCU-2/P (Scott Aviation), late 80s. Good view of early style voicemitter, and exhalation/drink valve cover. Later style voicemitter (MCU-2A/P) had smaller voicemitter and microphone connector both situated within annular ring shown.

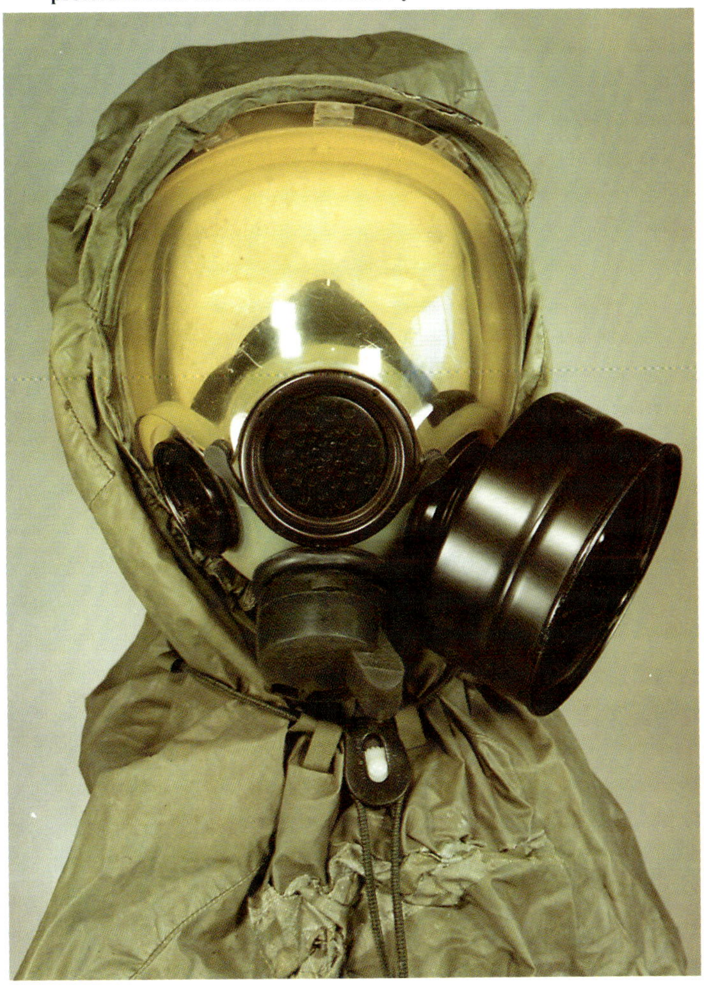

USAF/USN Chemical and Biological Protective Mask MCU-2/P (Scott Aviation), late 80s. Frontal view of early Scott Aviation manufactured mask fitted with clear hardshell visor protector, C-2 filter and "Hood, Chemical and Biological, MCU-2/P Series Masks."

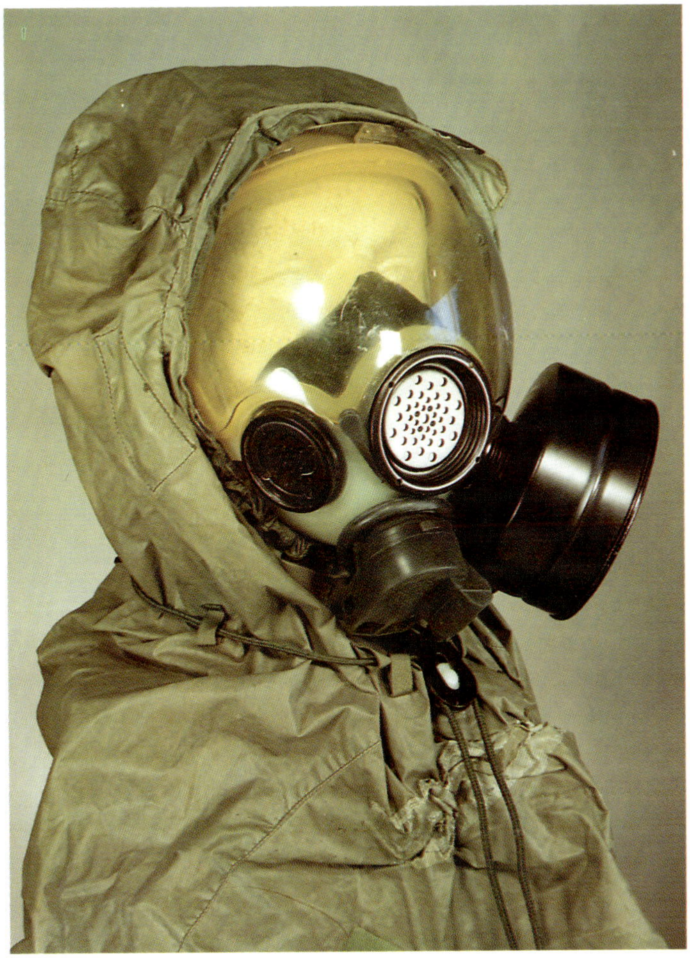

USAF/USN Chemical and Biological Protective Mask MCU-2/P (Scott Aviation), late 80s. Right oblique view shows lower part of silicone mask exposed to possible penetration by vessicant type agents.

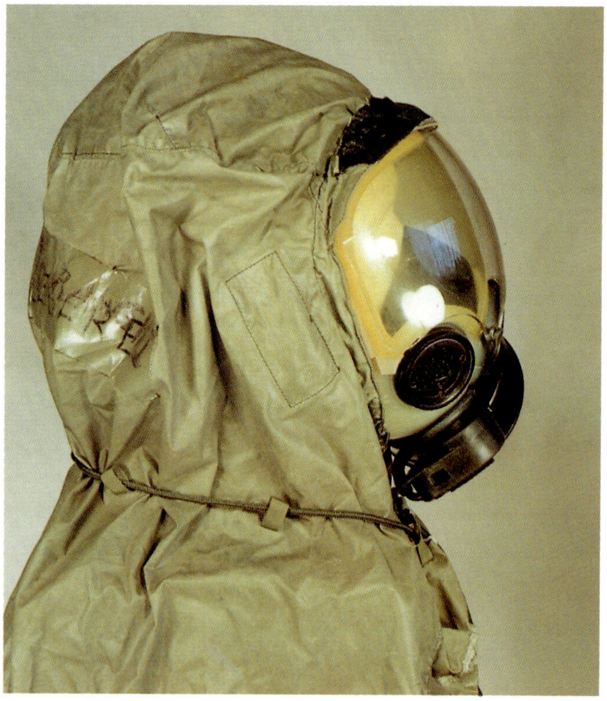

USAF/USN Chemical and Biological Protective Mask MCU-2/P (Scott Aviation), late 80s. Right profile shows black 'duct tape' which has been added to top of hood. The hood does not have a specific model designator, other than a FSN part identification, and the imprint "Hood, Chem/Bio, MCU-2/P Series Masks."

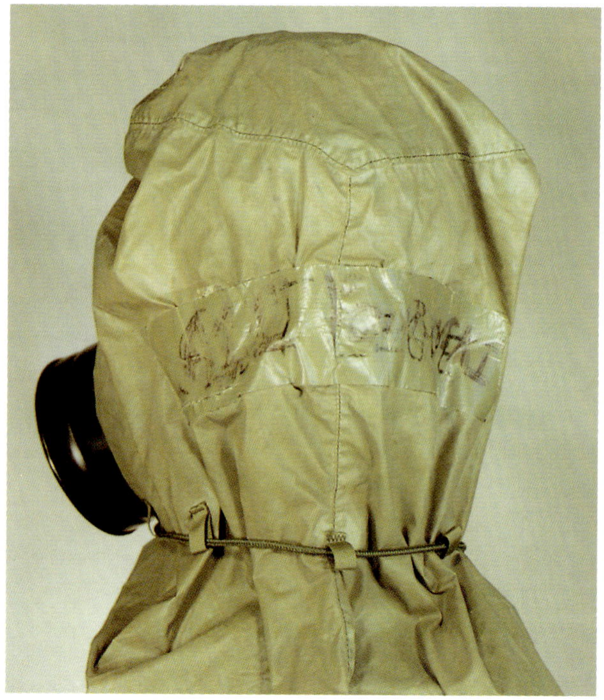

USAF/USN Chemical and Biological Protective Mask MCU-2/P (Scott Aviation), late 80s. Rear view of MCU-2/P type hood is unremarkable. The front of the hood has a small, soft visor which projects over the top of the face visor area. OD 'duct tape' strip across back of hood was imprinted with issuee's name.

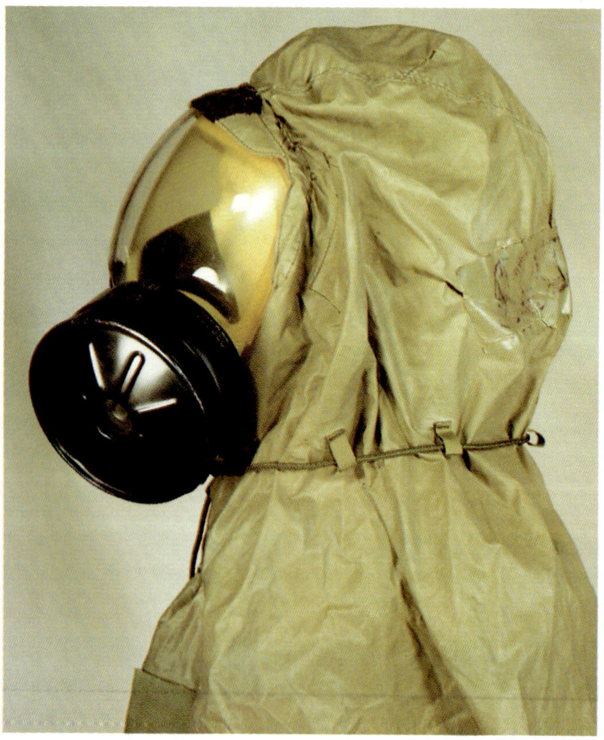

USAF/USN Chemical and Biological Protective Mask MCU-2/P (Scott Aviation), late 80s. Left profile of hood on mask shows soft bill projection over forehead of mask. The hood was secured via underarm straps and Velcro patches, similar to M6A2 hood used on M17 masks, but lacked a frontally located zipper.

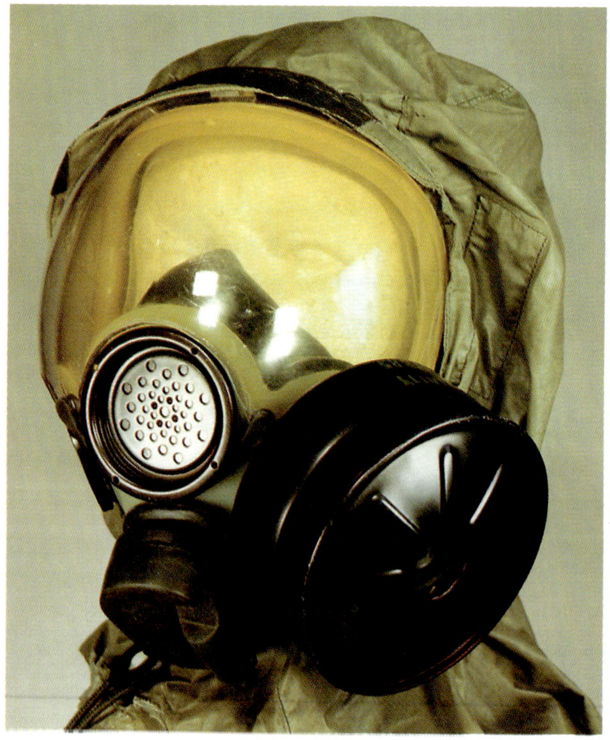

USAF/USN Chemical and Biological Protective Mask MCU-2/P (Scott Aviation), late 80s. Good left oblique view shows detail. Another hood that was used with the MCU-2/P series masks was designated "Hood, Antiflash, Flame Resistant" and was fabricated of light brown Aramide material (Nomex). It was fitted similarly to the regular butyl-proofed hood but was made of a soft, knitted fabric that had no straps for securing (not illustrated in this book).

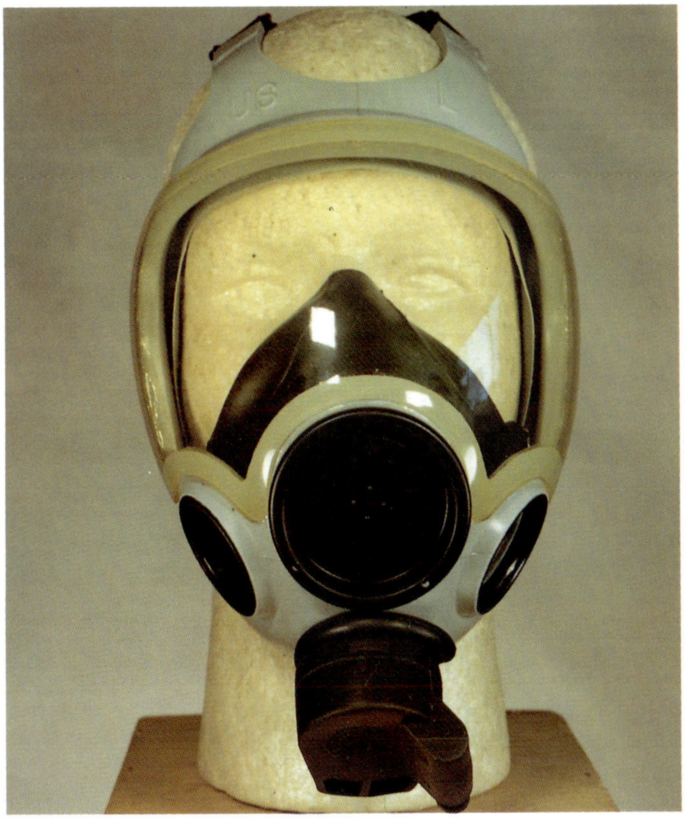

USAF/USN Chemical and Biological Protective Mask MCU-2/P (ILC, MSA), 1990. Later style MCU-2/P mask, shown without clear hardshell visor protector fitted. The MSA and ILC manufactured MCU-2/P masks featured light gray silicone facepieces, characterised by flush molding around filter inlet (left) and auxiliary voicemitter outlet (right).

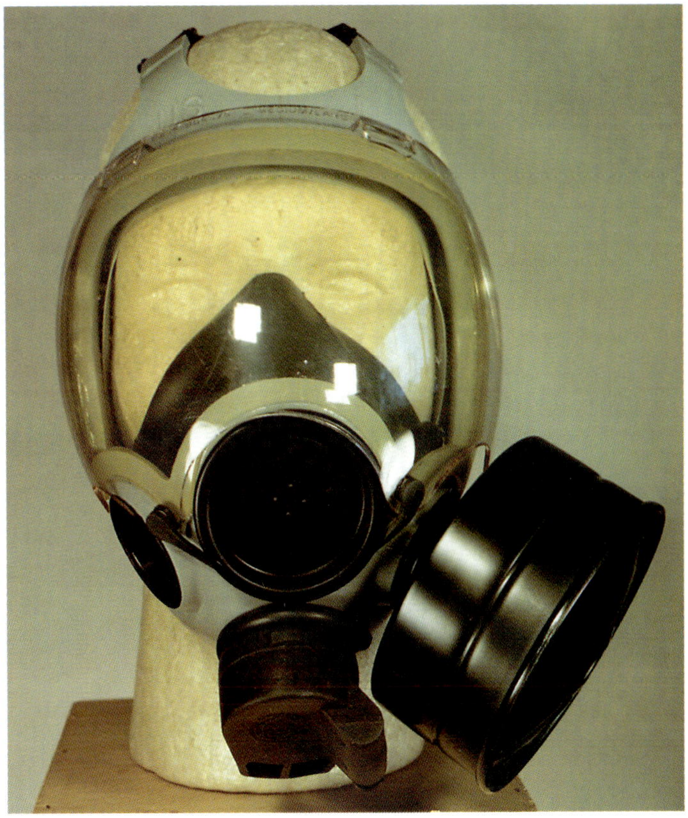

USAF/USN Chemical and Biological Protective Mask MCU-2/P (ILC, MSA), 1990. Clear hard visor protector has been fitted in this view. Early hardshell visor protectors had two slotted facepiece ridge grippers to hold in place, while later version had three. Three attachment points provided better protection against mask deformation while stowed in carrier, and also held clear hardshell in place more securely (the visor protector shown is an early model).

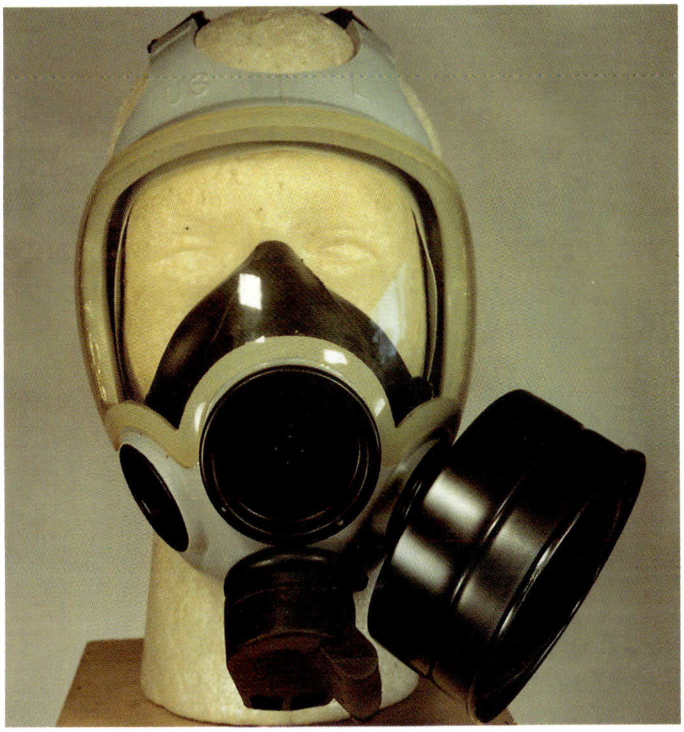

USAF/USN Chemical and Biological Protective Mask MCU-2/P (ILC, MSA), 1990. C-2 filter fitted to left inlet.

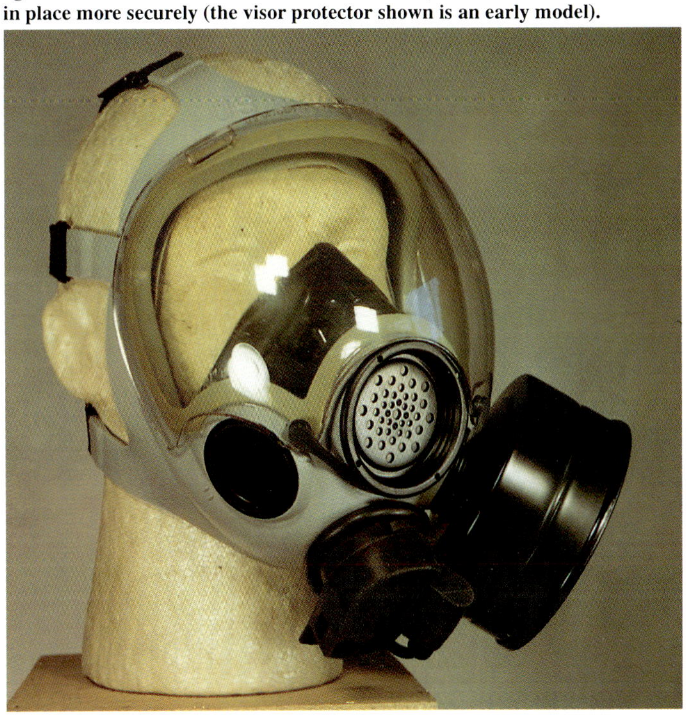

USAF/USN Chemical and Biological Protective Mask MCU-2/P (ILC, MSA), 1990. Good right oblique view shows black silicone strap which secures bottom part of clear visor protector to voicemitter housing. Molded "U.S." and size numeral viewable on forehead strap extrusions.

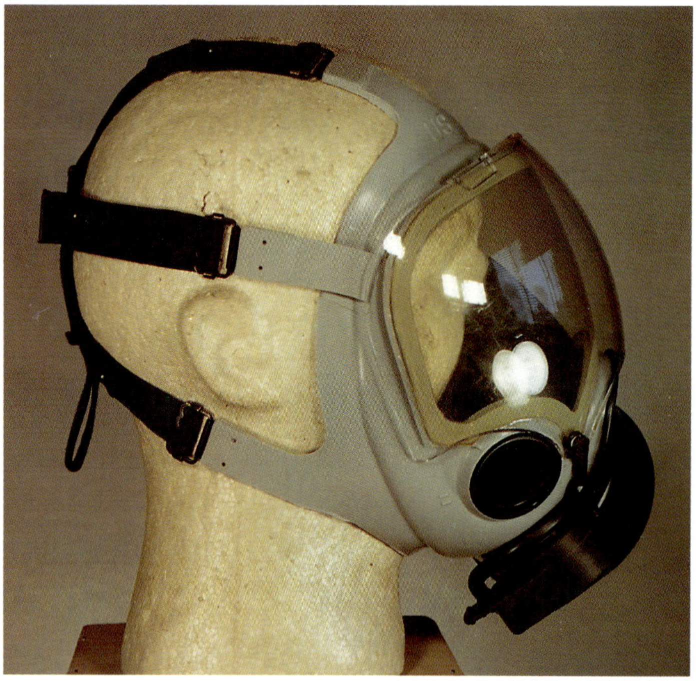

USAF/USN Chemical and Biological Protective Mask MCU-2/P (ILC, MSA), 1990. Right profile of later style MCU-2/P mask variant. The XM-30 prototype, from which the MCU-2/P derived, was rejected by the US Army, which went on to develop the XM40, immediate experimental predecessor to the M40 production mask.

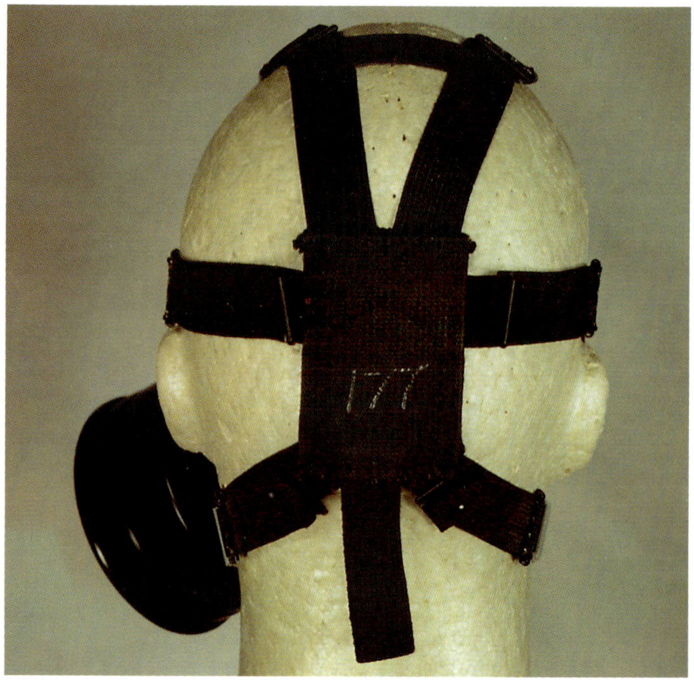

USAF/USN Chemical and Biological Protective mask MCU-2/P (ILC, MSA), 1990. View of the head harness, identical to that used in Scott Aviation produced, limited production model. The '177' numeral inscription is a user-added identification mark.

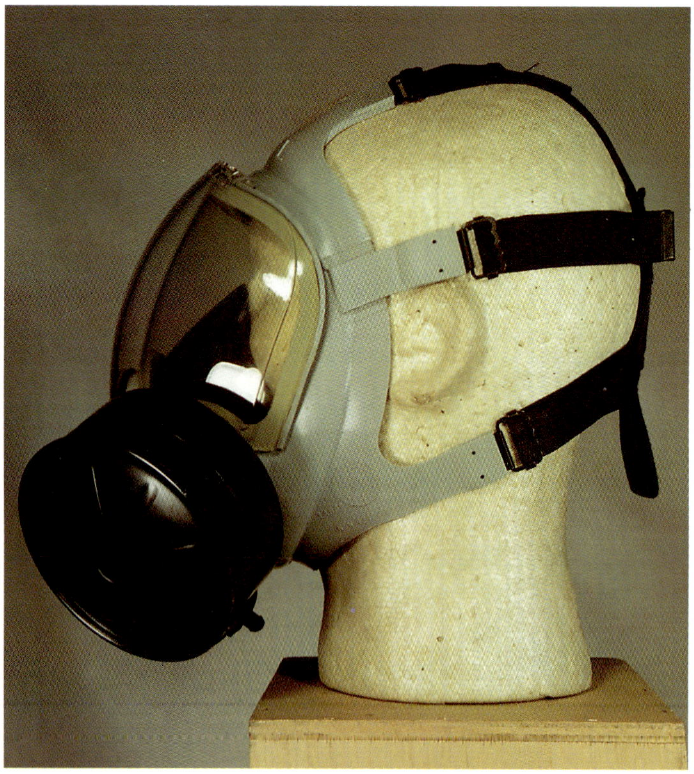

USAF/USN Chemical and Biological Protective Mask MCU-2/P (ILC/MSA), 1990. Left profile view of MSA/ILC manufactured '2/P' model. MSA/ILC mold marks conveying manufacturer ID and facepiece date are to be seen on the lower left part of the facepiece. The mask is sometimes referred to as the "Mickey-2," by military users, and was used by U.S. Navy personnel during the 1991 Gulf War.

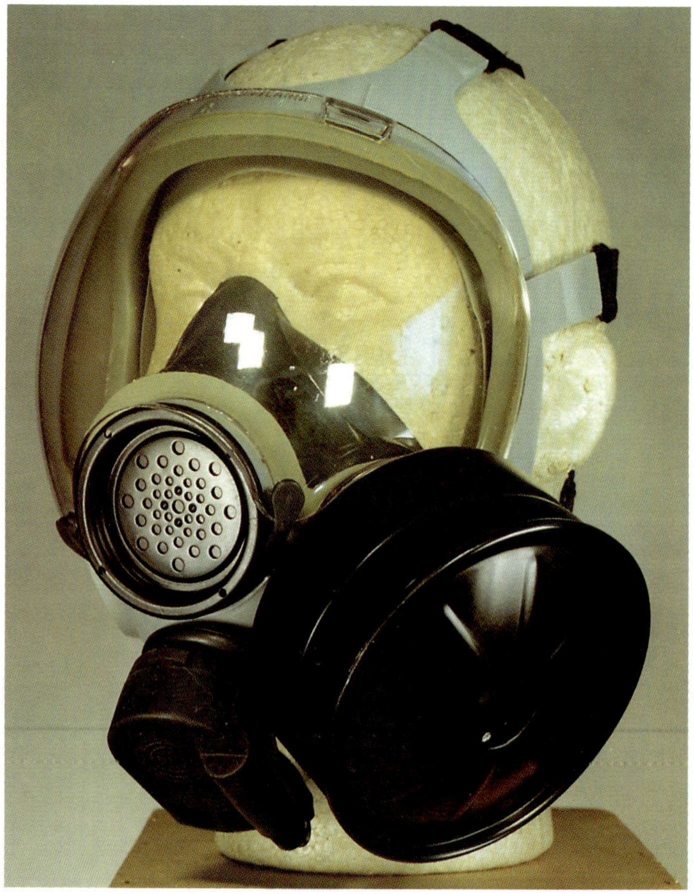

USAF/USN Chemical and Biological Protective Mask MCU-2/P (ILC/MSA), 1990. A good left oblique view of the mask shows the voicemitter detail clearly.

USAF/USN Chemical and Biological Protective Mask MCU-2A/P (ILC,MSA)

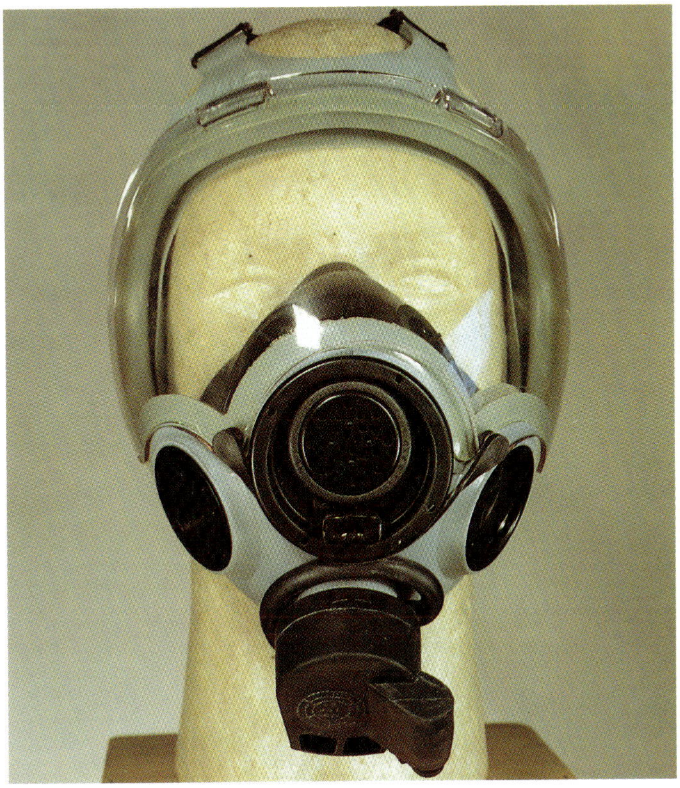

USAF/USN Chemical and Biological Protective Mask MCU-2A/P (ILC, MSA), 1991. The last variant "2A/P" model, shown in frontal aspect with clear hardshell visor protector (early style) fitted. Clearly viewed is the new style annular voicemitter and microphone connector block (below diaphragm). Note flush molding around left and right ports. Other changes were internal.

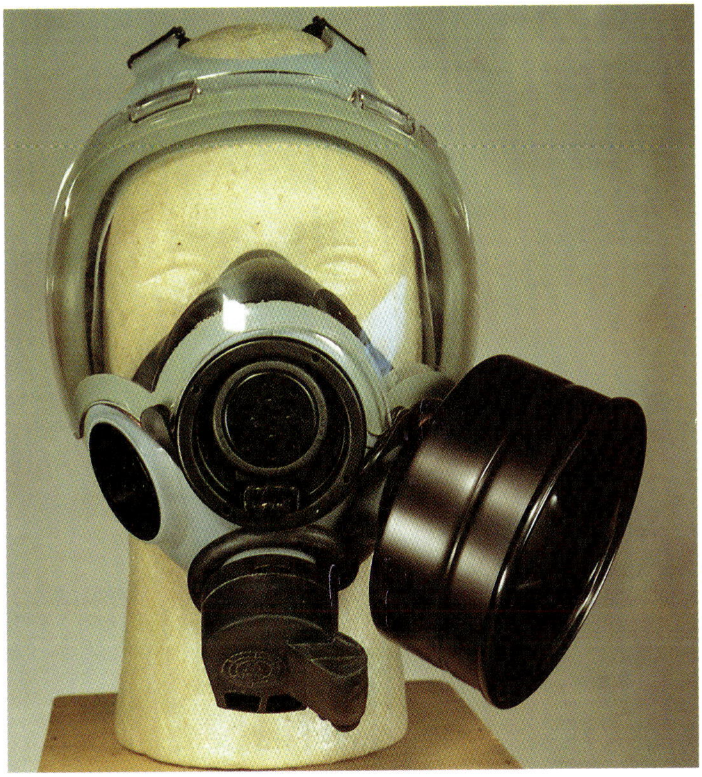

USAF/USN Chemical and Biological Protective Mask MCU-2A/P (ILC, MSA), 1991. C-2 filter fitted to left side inlet port. Other users of the Mickey-2 were the U.S. Coast Guard, FBI, CIA and various other Federal agencies. ID and date mold mark may be seen on exhalation valve cover.

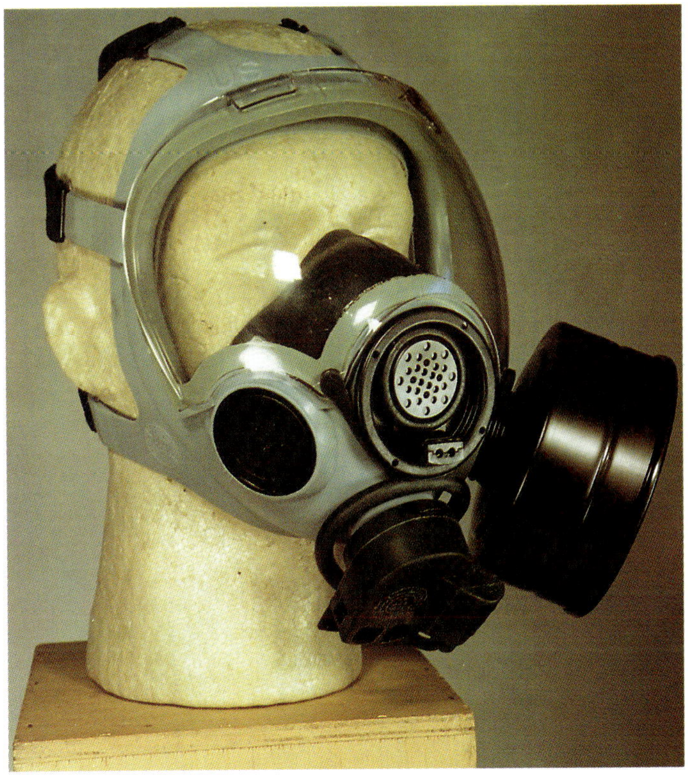

USAF/USN Chemical and Biological Protective Mask MCU-2A/P (ILC/MSA), 1991. Excellent right oblique view clearly shows new style voicemitter and microphone connection detail. A dark hardshell visor was issued with the Mickey-2, which would be used in place of the clear model.

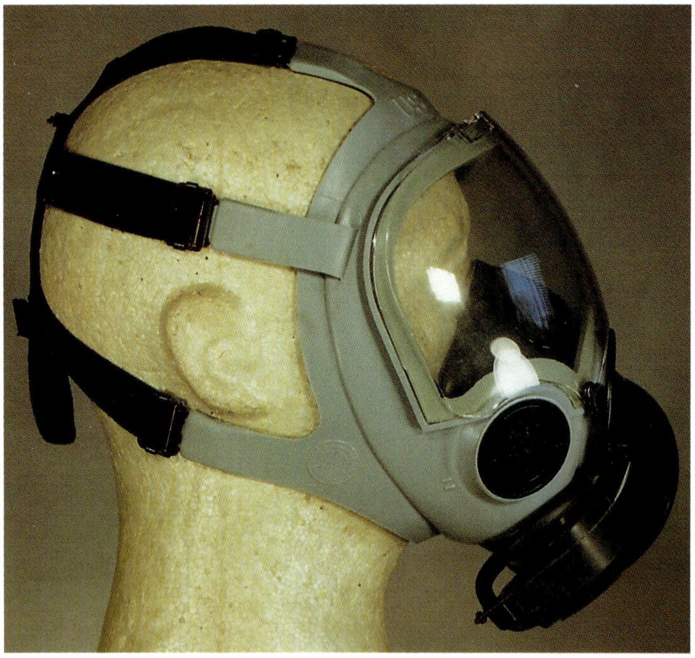

USAF/USN Chemical and Biological Protective Mask MCU-2A/P (ILC/MSA), 1991. Right profile view shows ID and date of manufacture molding on lower edge of gray silicone facepiece. A major modification occurred late in the mask's production, when the poorly designed exhalation valve/drink tube former was finally redesigned. Various "quick fixes" were tried, prior to the complete redesign of this part, including a small circular screen insert between the valve disc and the support annulus which may be found on some earlier production numbers

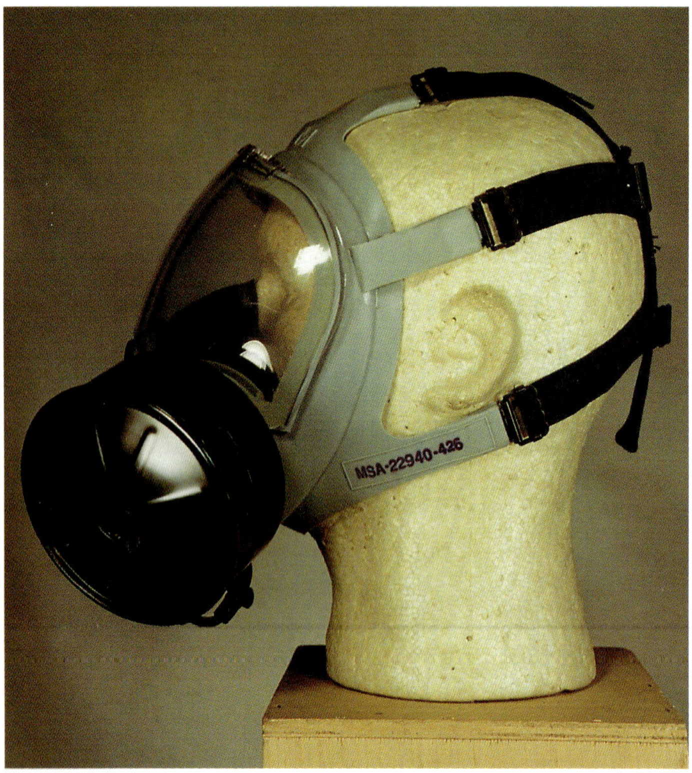

USAF/USN Chemical and Biological Protective Mask MCU-2A/P (ILC, MSA), 1991. Left profile of MSA manufactured mask clearly identifies contractor and lot number.

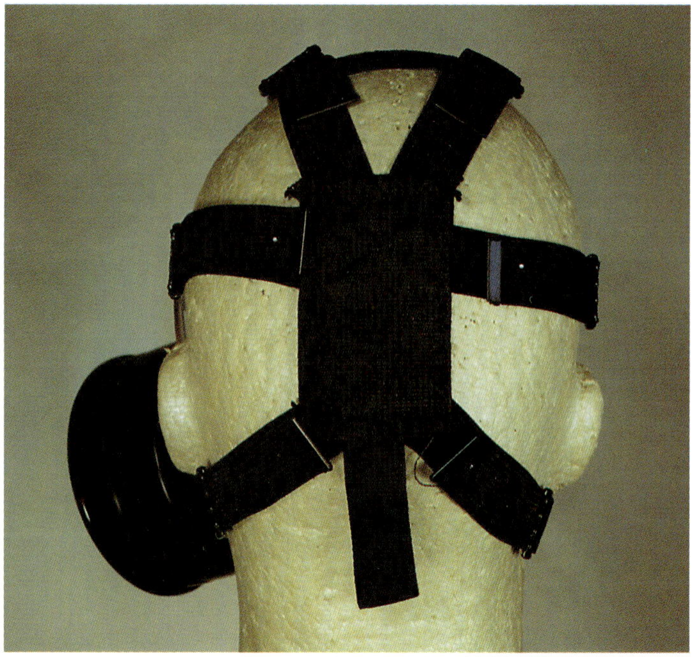

USAF/USN Chemical and Biological Protective Mask MCU-2A/P (ILC, MSA), 1991. Rear view of head harness—identical to earlier versions. Straps pinned for clarity.

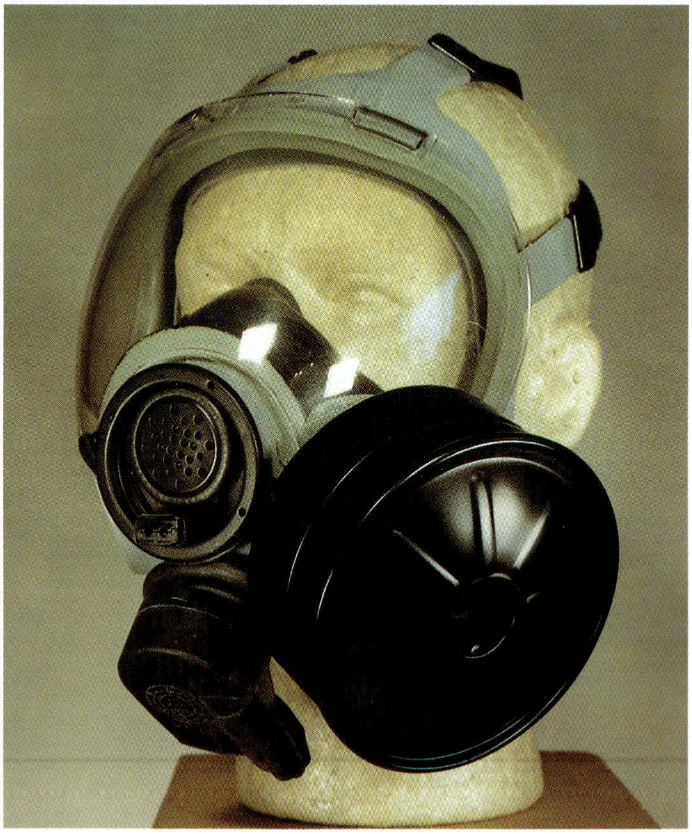

USAF/USN Chemical and Biological Protective Mask MCU-2A/P (ILC, MSA), 1991. Good left oblique view shows voicemitter and microphone connector block details. This example is in issued but 'excellent' condition, as are most later-model Mickey-2s. In this condition, current average cost is about $75, while specimens still new in issue packaging can command about $120-150. Two C-2 filters sealed in cans are initially issued with each Mickey-2 mask.

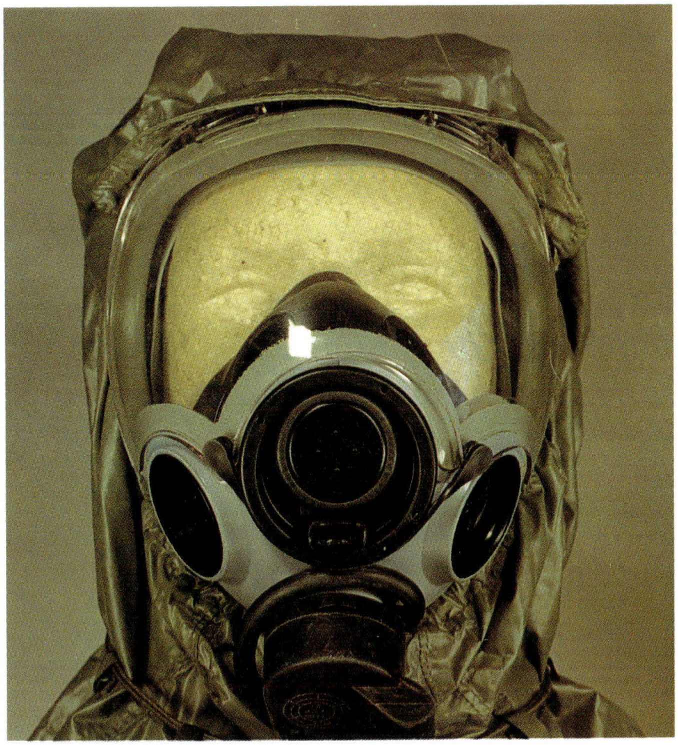

USAF/USN MCU-2A/P mask fitted with hood. Essentially identical to MCU-2/P and hood.

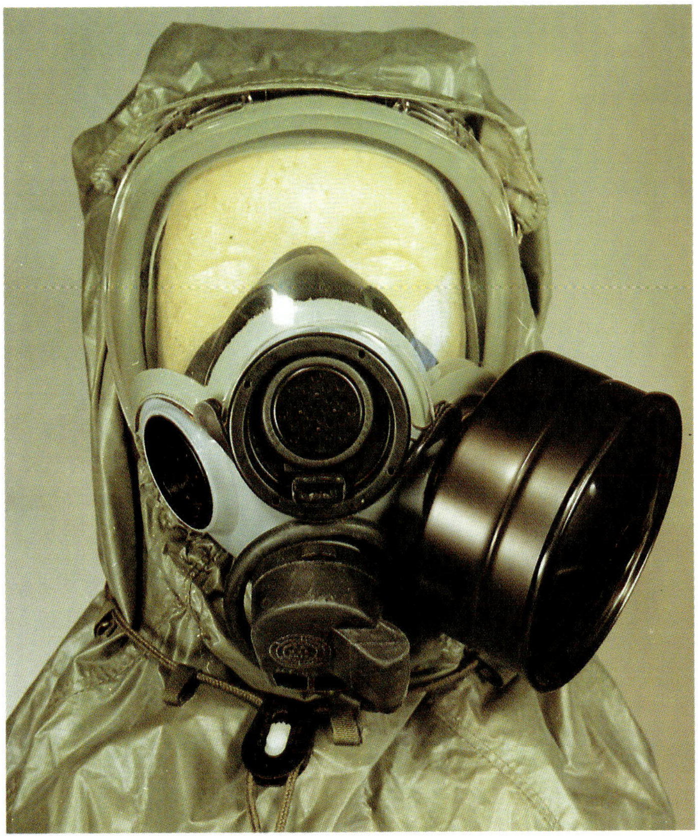

USAF/USN MCU-2A/P mask fitted with hood. Detail of voicemitter and exhalation valve cover mold marks viewable. Filter is C2; newer (currently being issued) C2A1 filter uses slightly different type of charcoal and seams of canister are sealed with different (non environmentally hazardous) material.

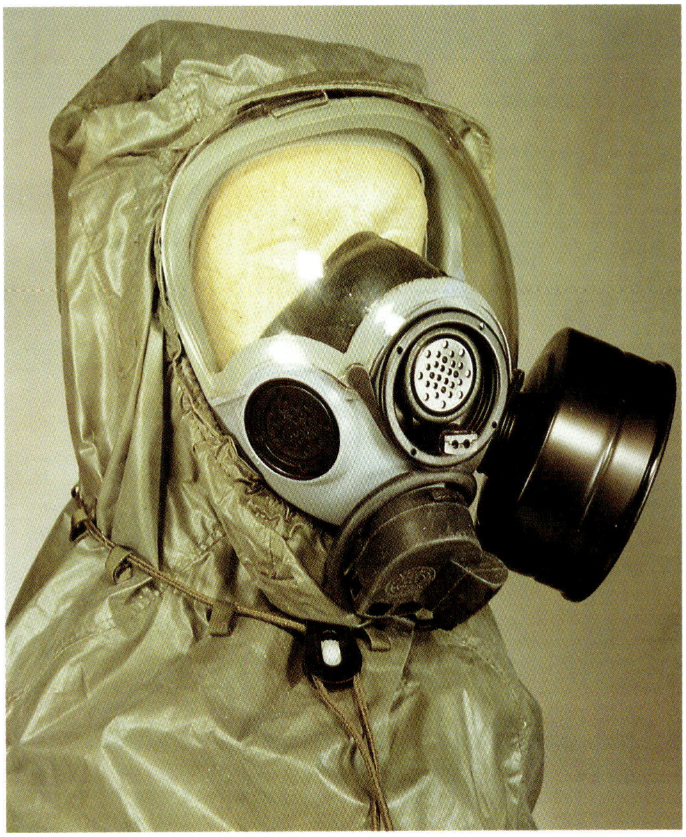

USAF/USN MCU-2A/P mask fitted with hood. Comparison of the Mickey-2 is invited with the Canadian C-4, which uses Bromobutyl rubber compound for its facepiece. The Canadian C-4 mask would probably have been adopted by U.S. forces if the U.S./Canadian cooperation of the 70s to develop a common respirator had been successful. Bromobutyl rubber has a substantially higher resistance to penetration by vessicant agents than silicone rubber, and also confers a high degree of user comfort.

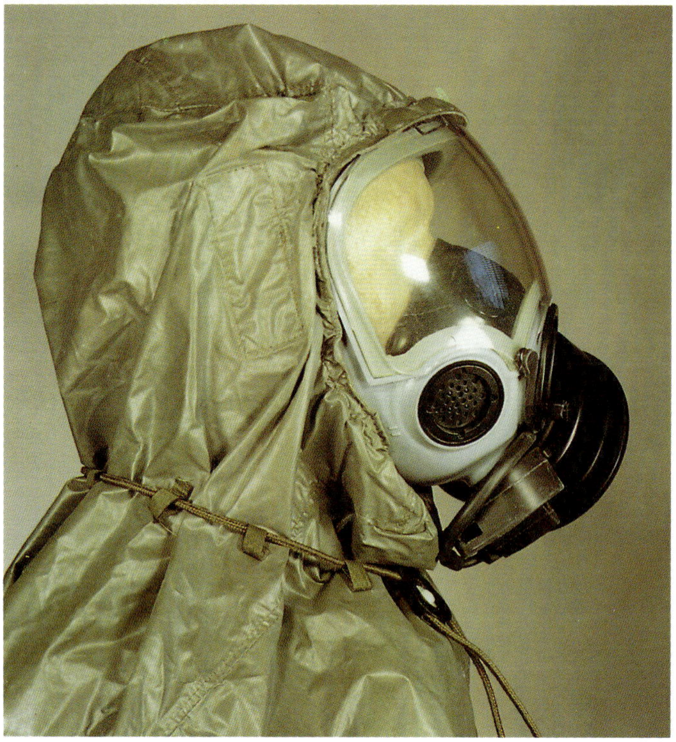

USAF/USN MCU-2A/P mask fitted with hood. Snap fitted straps stitched inside the hood mate with the mask's head harness temple pieces to securely hold the hood to the mask. Reinforced areas where the straps are sewn may be seen in this profile view, in the area where the ears would be.

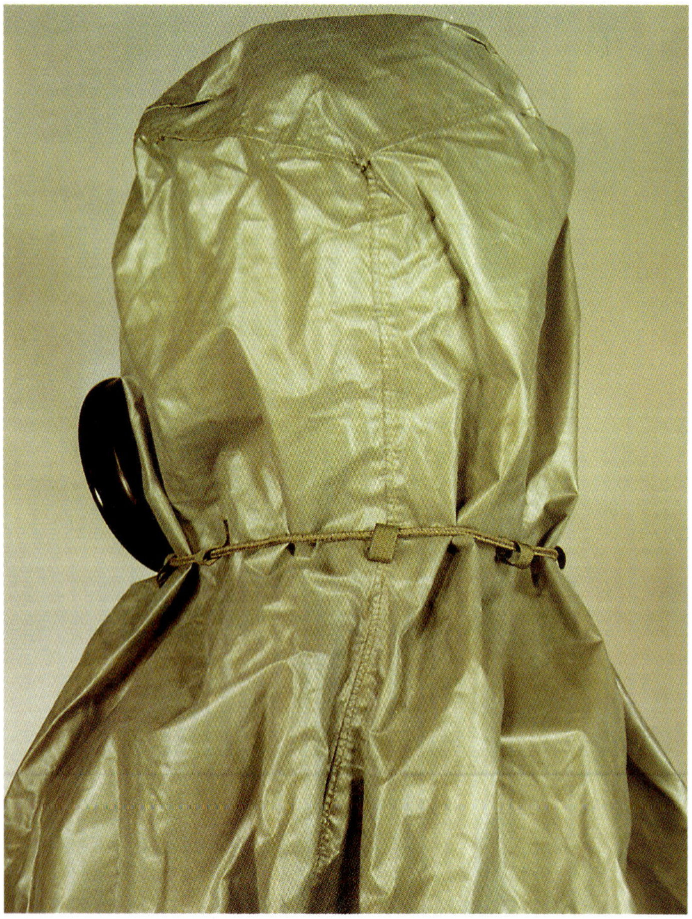

USAF/USN MCU-2A/P mask fitted with hood. Rear view of hood is unremarkable and identical to hood used with MCU-2/P model.

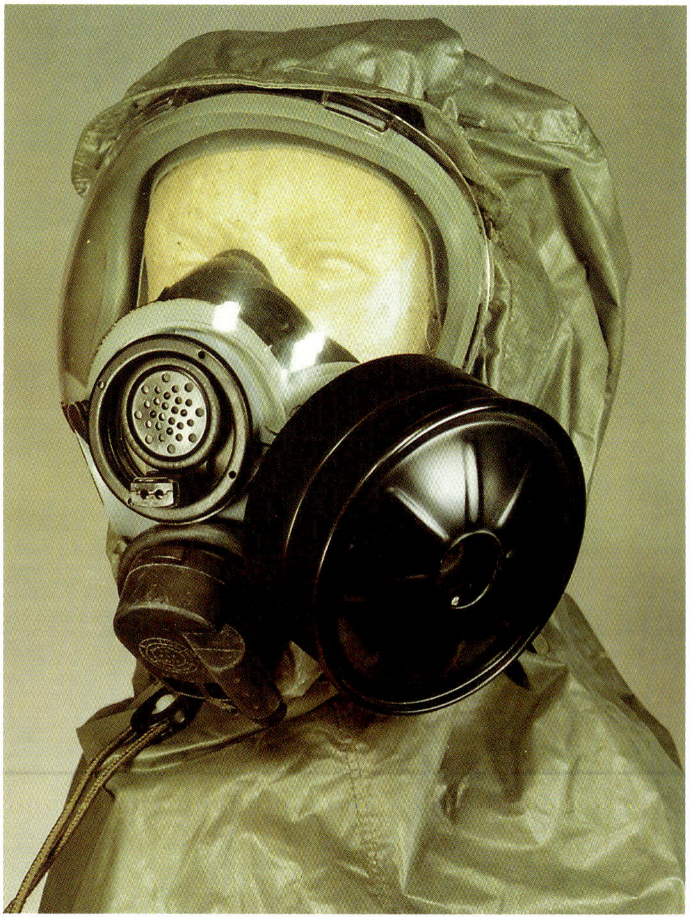

USAF/USN MCU-2A/P mask fitted with hood. Good left oblique view of mask/hood assembly. Clear hardshell visor is older version (two upper points of attachment to facepiece lens ridge).

U.S. Army Field Protective Mask M40, 1990

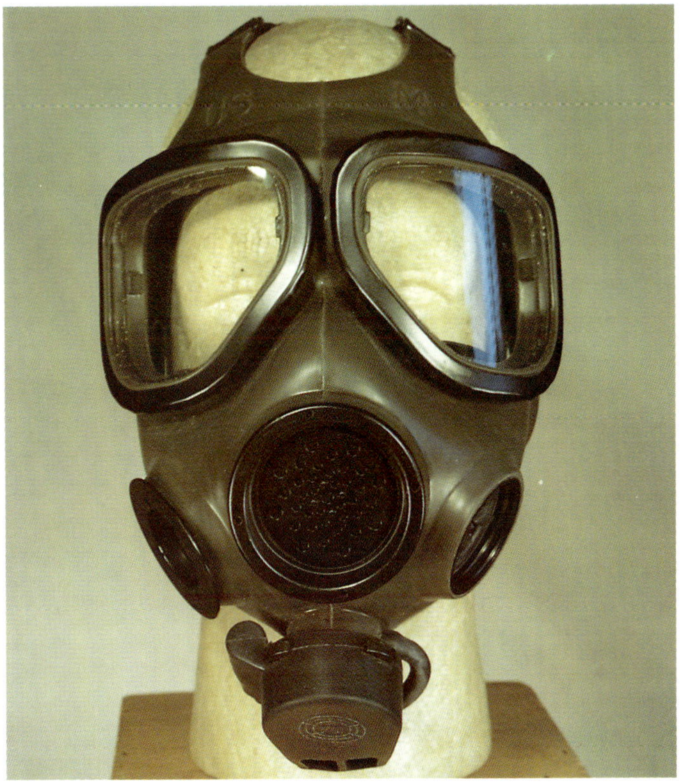

U.S. Army Field Protective Mask M40, 1990. A redesigned and substantially reworked version of the XM-30 developmental model which used a conventional ("low-risk") twin-lens design. Voicemitter is similar to Mickey-2 "2/P" model, but exhalation valve is redesigned to eliminate the problem experienced with the Mickey-2 version. Both masks feature internal oronasal cup and reversed peripheral seal on facepiece.

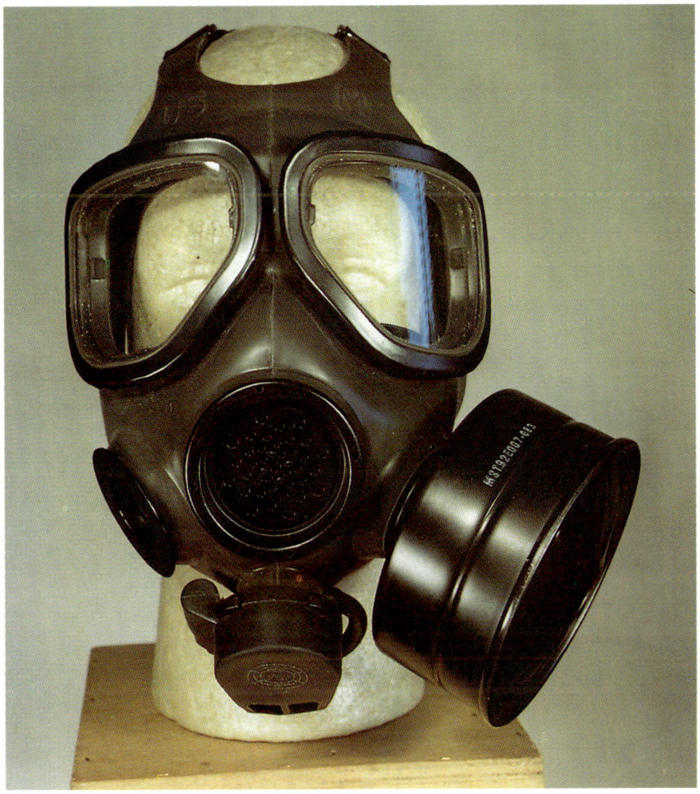

U.S. Army Field Protective Mask M40, 1990. Only a limited number of these were available at the start of the Gulf War and initiation of a crash program for widespread production was decided against so as to sidestep possible 'problems' relating to distribution and supply of the new mask. Black C2 filter is shown fitted.

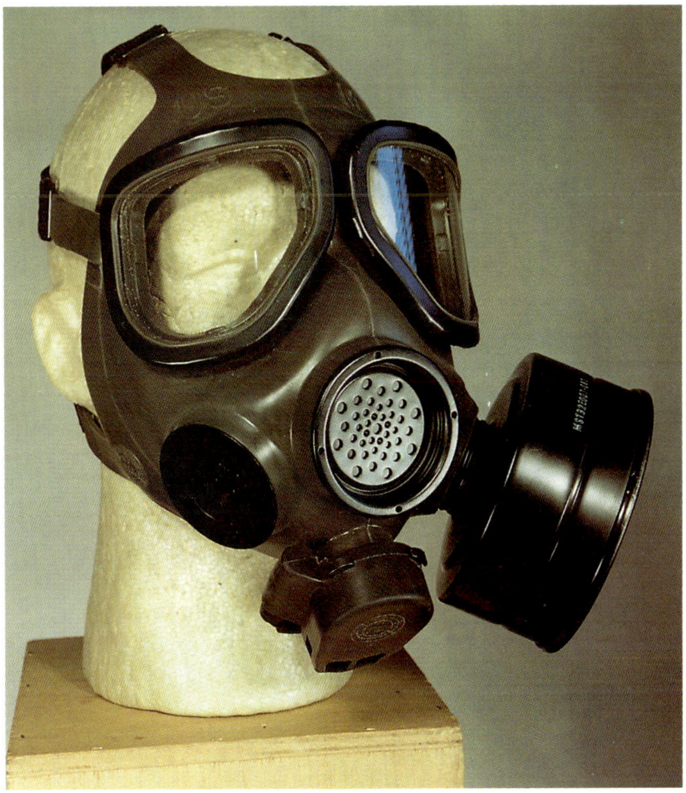

U.S. Army Field Protective Mask M40, 1990. Good right oblique view of the M40, showing voicemitter detail. Drink tube assembly and valve cover was different than that on Mickey-2. Internal oronasal cup was made of (black) silicone rubber, as was rest of facepiece.

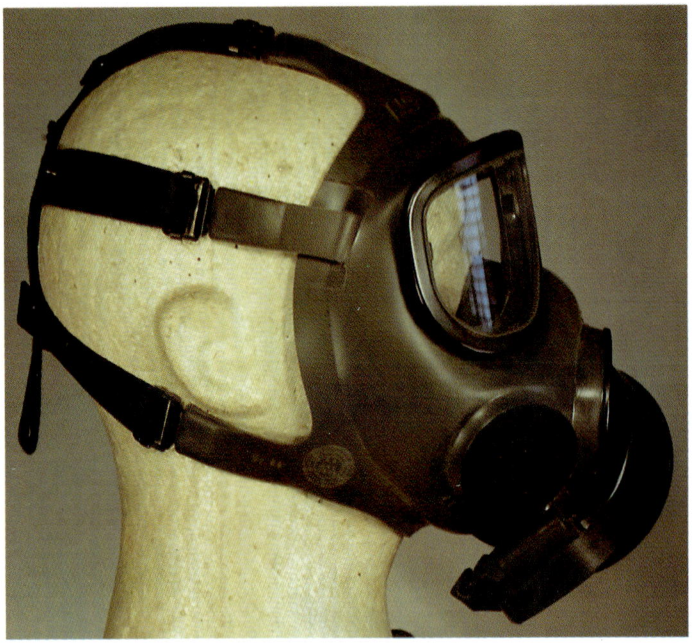

U.S. Army Field Protective Mask M40, 1990. Comparison of this view with similar aspects of Mickey-2 and Canadian C-4 masks is invited. General style concept of twin-lens eye pieces is similar to that used in previous U.S. Army masks, although reconfigured to obtain better field of vision. One piece, soft thermoplastic molded lenses, such as that used on Mickey-2, presented new challenges in fabrication and manufacturing technology, which delayed resolution of problems encountered and application of solutions to achieve production requirements.

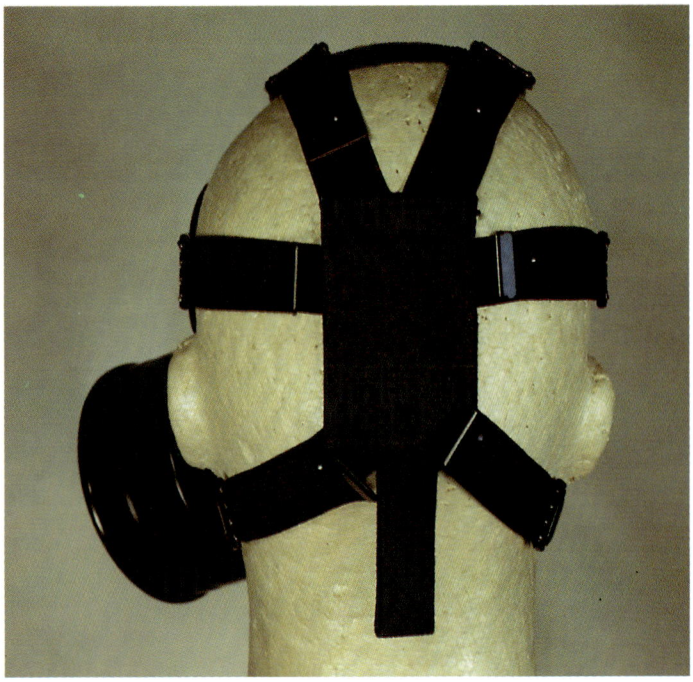

U.S. Army Field Protective Mask M40, 1990. View of elasticized head harness is unremarkable. Straps are pinned for clarity.

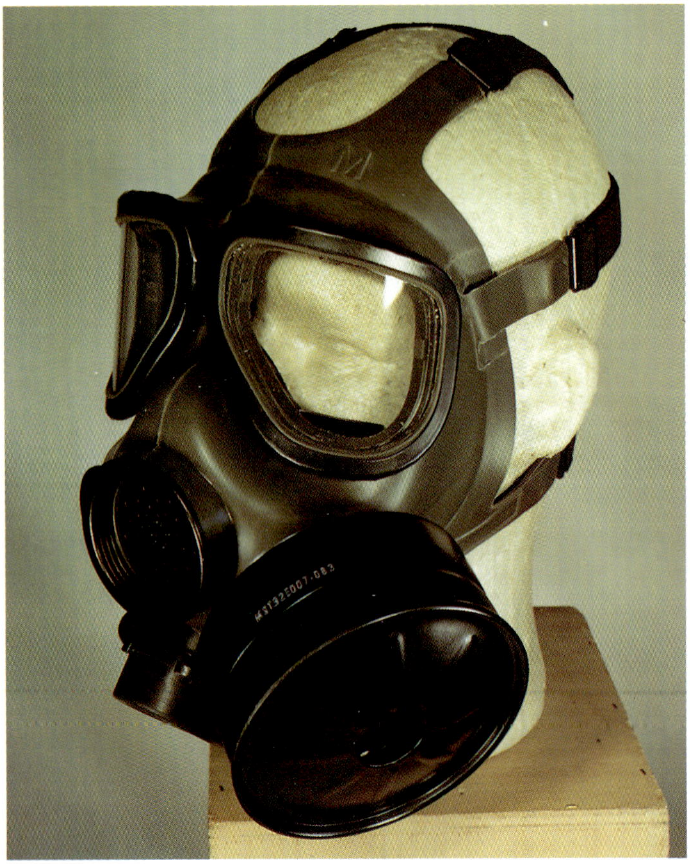

U.S. Army Field Protective Mask M40, 1990. High angle left oblique view shows some strap and lens frame detail.

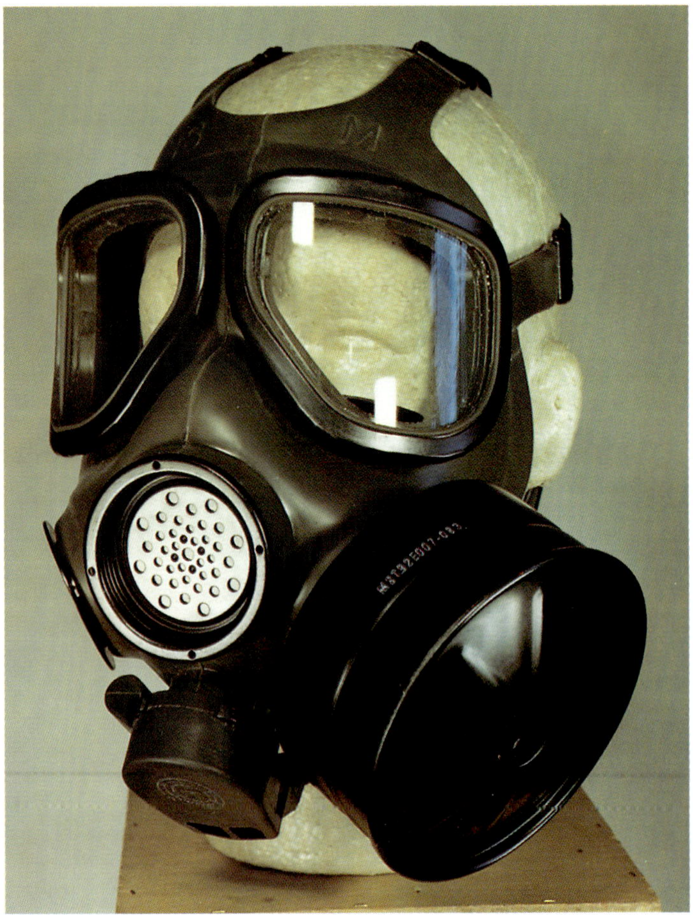

U.S. Army Field Protective Mask M40, 1990. Low angle left oblique view shows detail of voicemitter filter lot markings, right side auxiliary voicemitter flange and exhalation valve cover (with date mold mark).

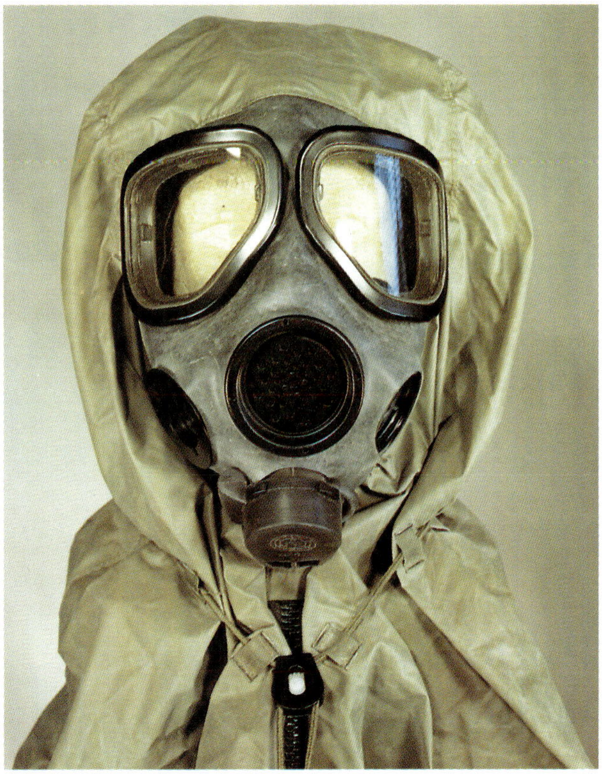

U.S. Army M40 mask fitted with (original) protective hood. Frontal view of M40 mask fitted with butyl-coated nylon hood (with integrated black EPDM facepiece cover): the immediate solution to the problem of silicone rubber's vulnerability to vessicant penetrating agents. The EPDM component fitted over the left and right ports and voicemitter annulus to secure under the exhalation valve with Velcro. As can be seen, it was always not a very tight or secure fit.

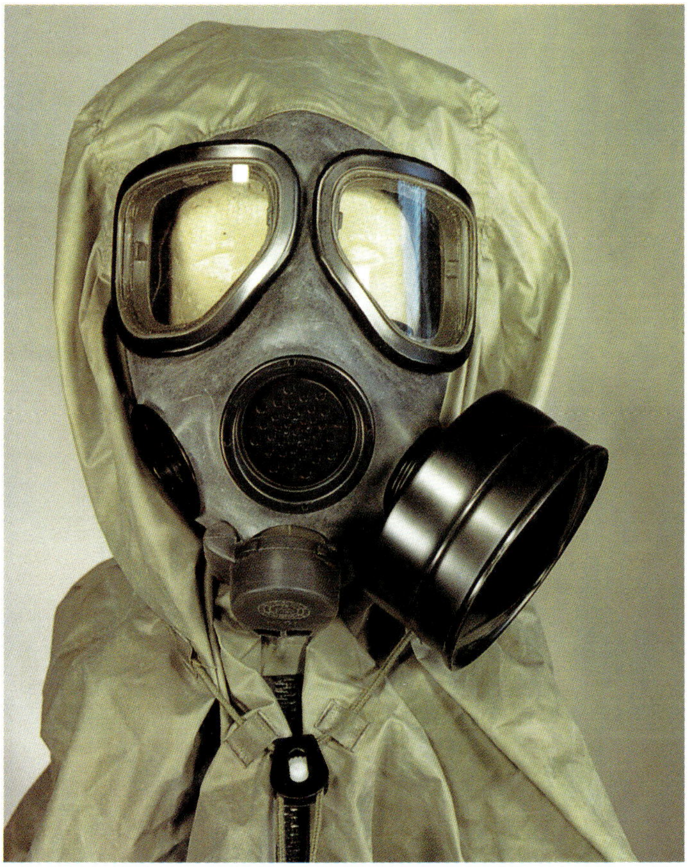

U.S. Army M40 mask fitted with (original) protective hood. Frontal view, with C2 canister in place. The M40 style butyl proofed and EPDM hood was fitted with a centrally located zipper, as well as a neck draw-cord. Accessory clear "outsert" lenses are not fitted.

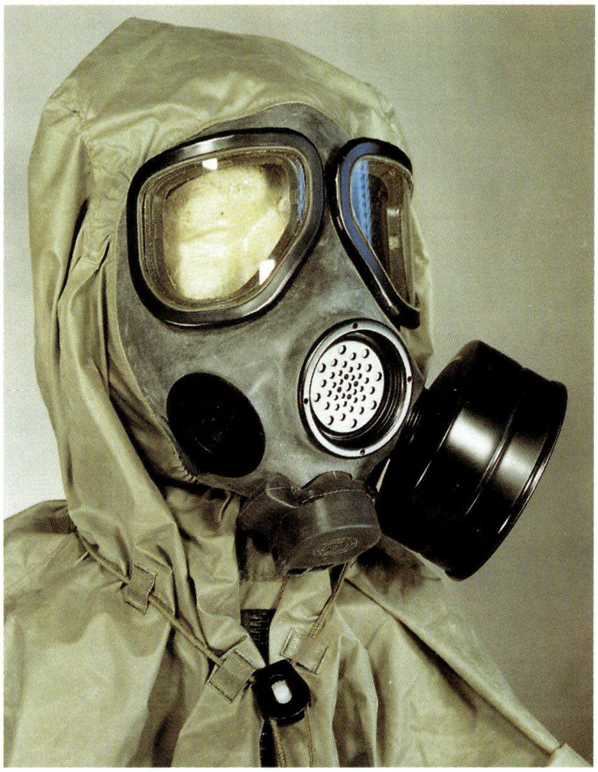

U.S. Army M40 mask fitted with (original)protective hood. Right oblique view shows voicemitter and exhalation valve detail.. Auxiliary voicemitter port on right side of mask has flanged edge which helps hold the EPDM section on the mask; EPDM is partly secured to other side of mask by filter canister on left inlet port. Section of exposed OD colored silicone rubber may be seen just above exhalation valve cover, where EPDM material does not fit tightly.

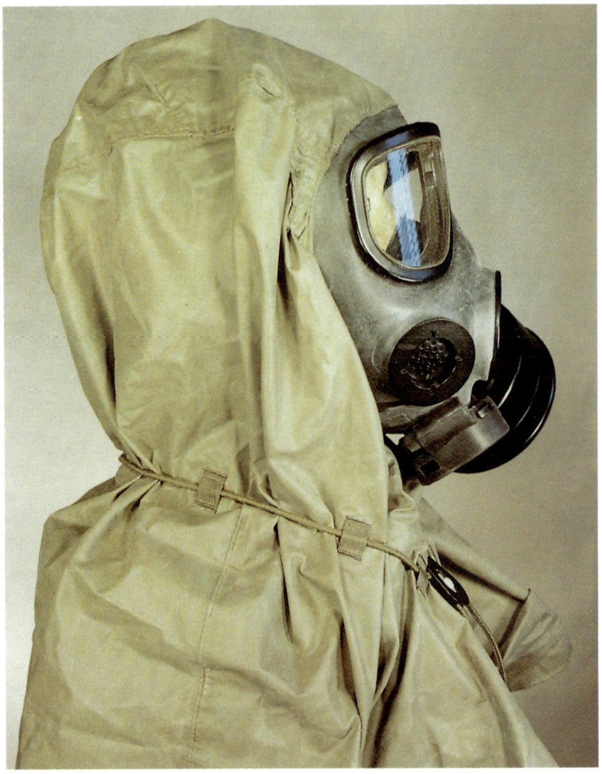

U.S. Army M40 mask fitted with (original) protective hood. The M40 and M40A1 mask facepieces are identical; only the hood has been changed, resulting in a new designation (M40A1). Right profile view show auxiliary voicemitter. All primary U.S. service masks from the M17 series onwards have incorporated a voicemitter, and most have a side or secondary voicemitter for telephone type communications, as well.

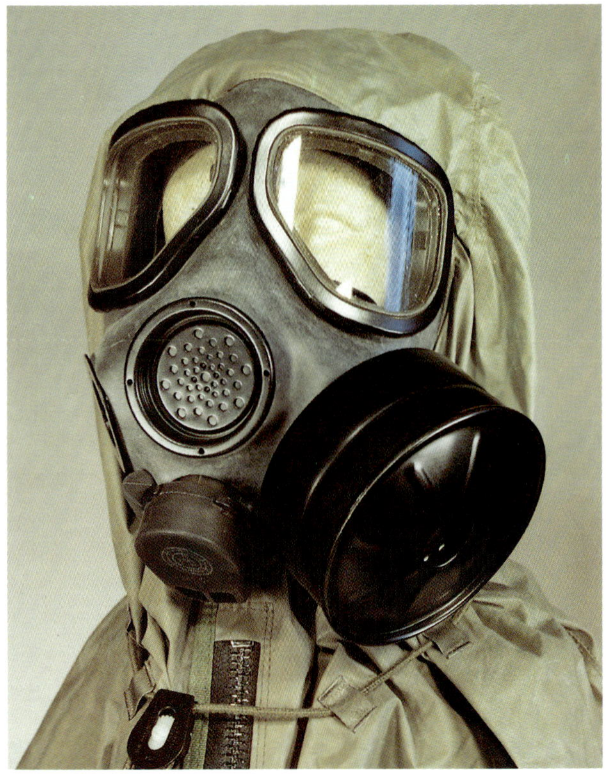

U.S. Army M40 mask fitted with (original) protective hood. Left oblique view shows uncertain security of fit around various protrusions through the EPDM material (inlets, voicemitters, eye lens frames, etc.). Decontamination of mask and hood after an attack with vessicants would be complicated and potentially hazardous. Although it is one of the oldest chemical agents in the modern chemical warfare arsenal, sulfur mustard (agent HD)is still considered one of the deadliest. Iraq maintained and used substantial quantities of HD against their Iranian enemies, during the 1984-88 war with Iran.

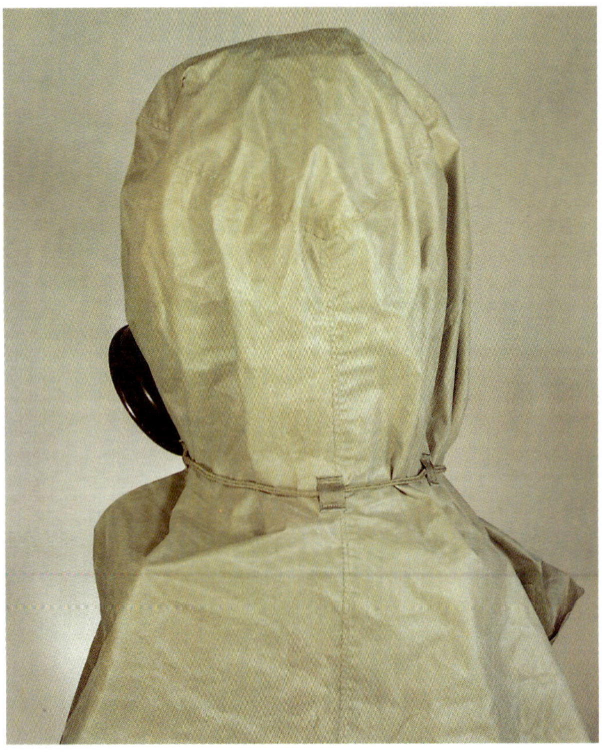

U.S. Army M40 mask fitted with (original) protective hood. View of rear aspect of hood is unremarkable.

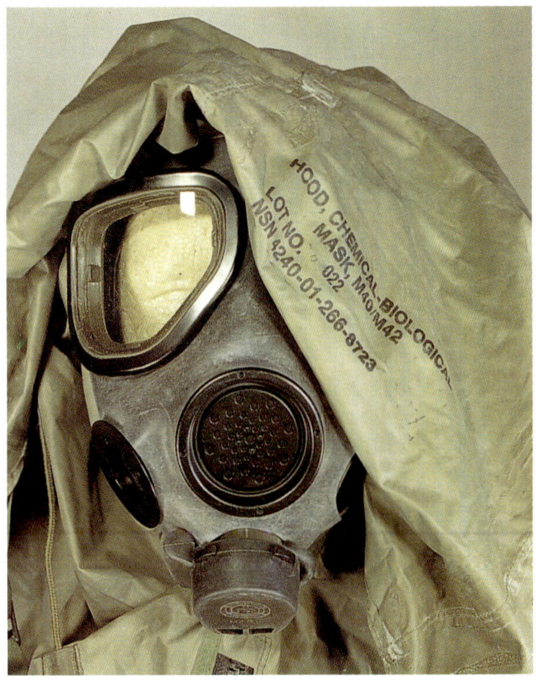

U.S. Army M40 mask fitted with (original protective hood. In this view, the hood is partly drawn over the top of the mask to show interior details and identification markings.

U.S. Army Field Protective Mask M40A1, 1994

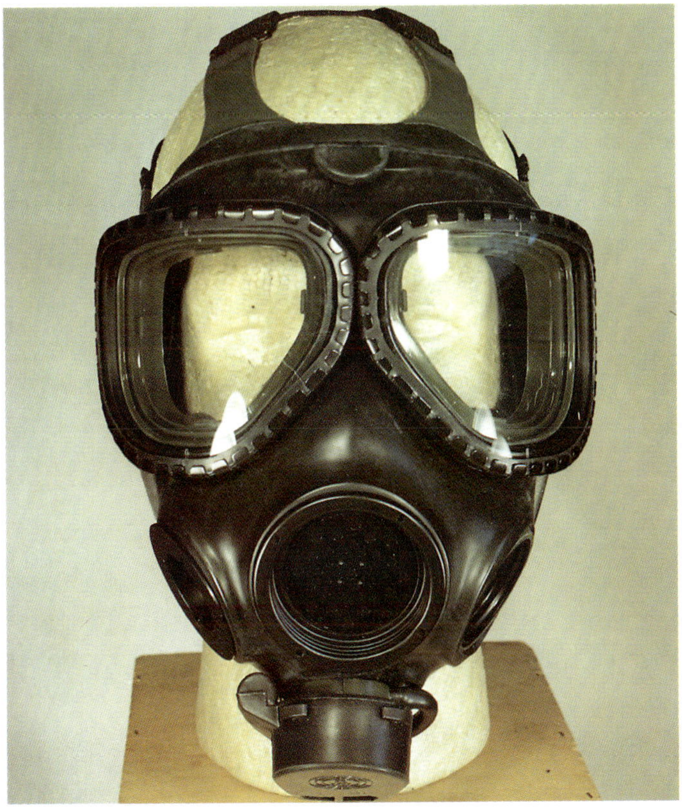

U.S. Army Field Protective Mask M40A1, 1994. Frontal view of M40A1. The facepiece of the M40A1 is identical to the M40, only the hood design has been changed. On the M40A1 the EPDM material has been molded into a fully conforming facepiece cover, referred to as a "second skin." The butyl proofed nylon hood is now a separate component, very much in the manner of the older M6A2 hood used on the M17 series masks. The EPDM second-skin, once installed, remains on the mask at all times. Accessory "outsert" lenses are installed in this view.

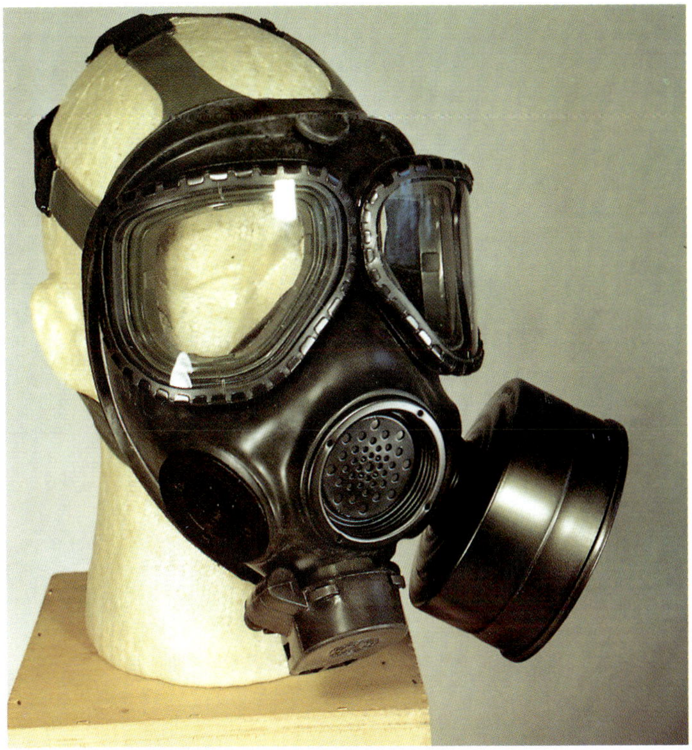

U.S. Army Field Protective Mask M40A1, 1994. Right oblique aspect reveals molded ridge protrusion about circumference of EPDM facepiece cover, with molded 'tab' directly over forehead section. It is obvious that the EPDM second-skin fits the facepiece far better and more securely than the original one-piece hood/EPDM design did.

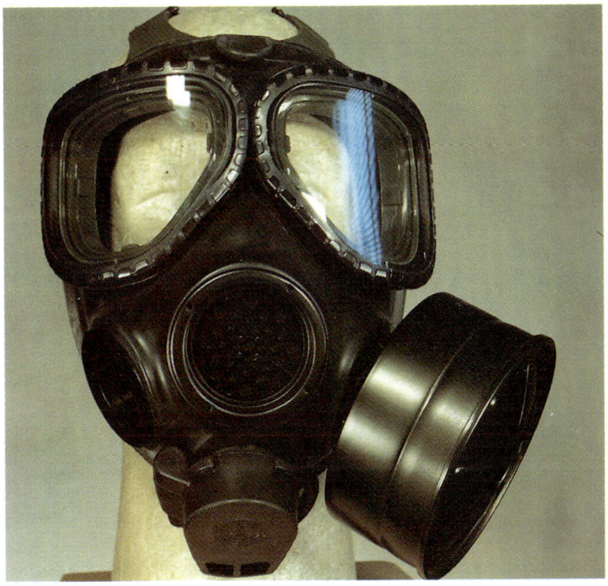

U.S. Army Field Protective Mask M40A1, 1994. Second generation C2A1 filter canister is installed, although green metallic color is so dark it is difficult to discern the difference. New M40A1 style EPDM second-skin gives the mask a very different appearance.

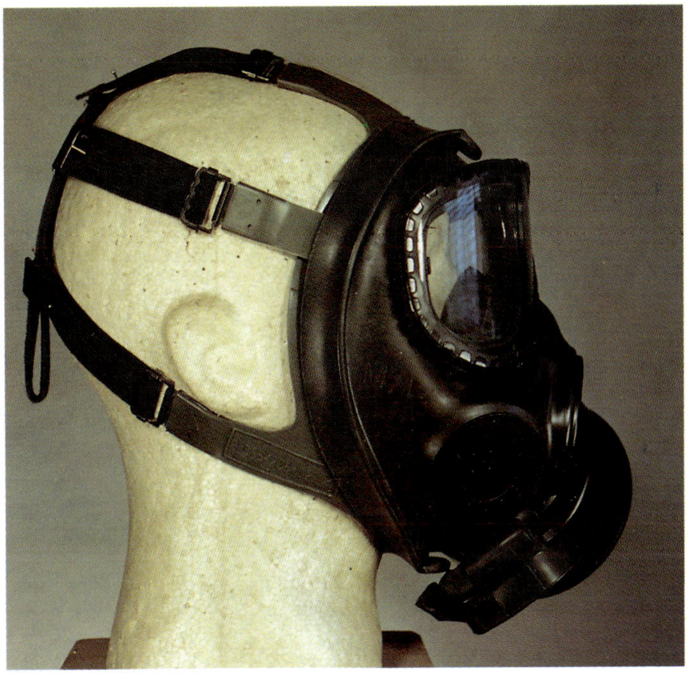

U.S. Army Field Protective Mask M40A1, 1994. Right profile view of A1 variant clearly shows molded circumferential ridge on EPDM second-skin, as well as protrusive tabs at top and bottom of cover, all of which help hold the butyl-proofed hood in place. Lens 'outserts' are installed in this view.

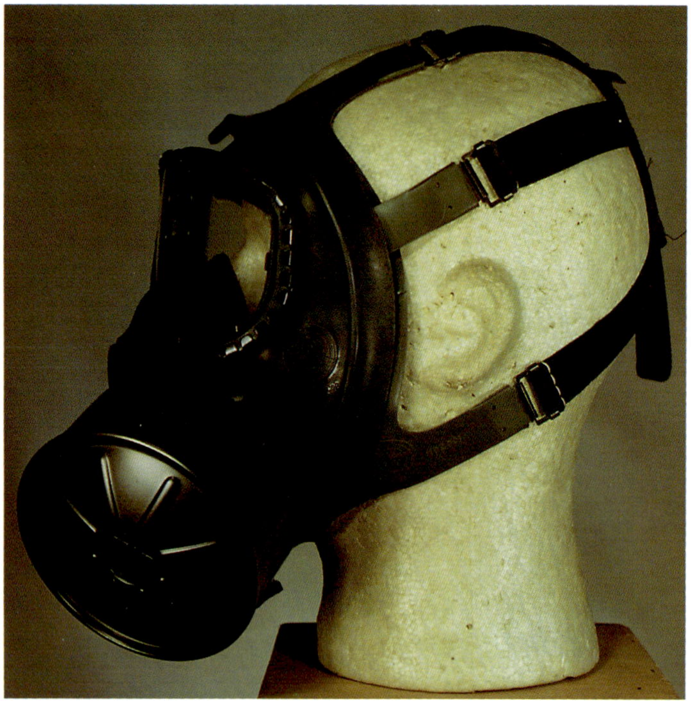

U.S. Army Field Protective Mask M40A1, 1994. Left profile view shows ID/ date molding mark on EPDM second-skin facepiece cover below and aft of left eye lens. Facepiece harness molded-in strap hardware is identical to that use on Mickey-2 masks.

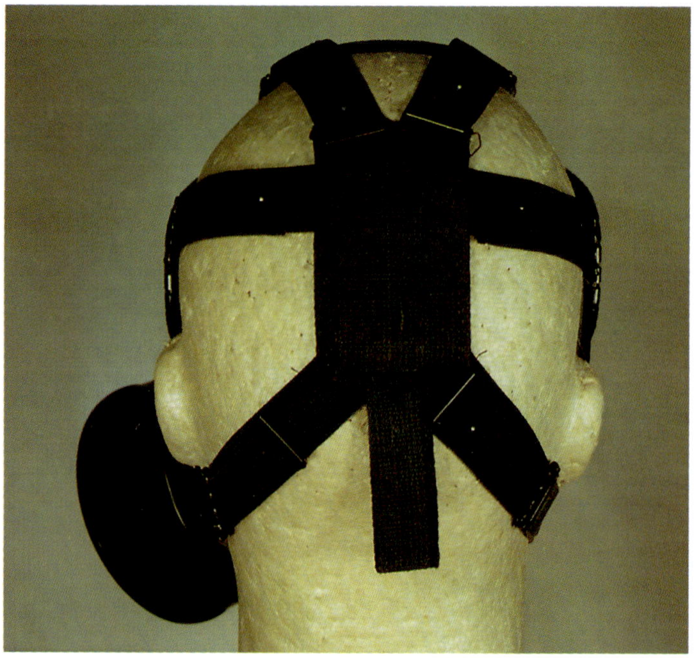

U.S. Army Field Protective Mask M40A1, 1994. View of elasticized head harness is unremarkable; identical to that used on M40 version.

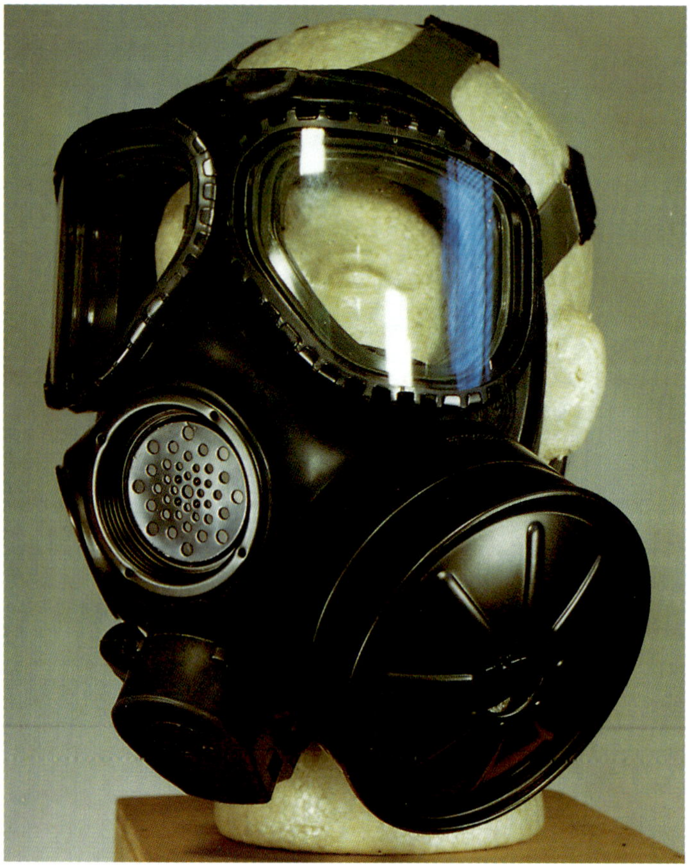

U.S. Army Field Protective Mask M40A1, 1994. Left oblique view shows voicemitter, filter and exhalation valve/drink device details. Accessory eye lens 'outserts' are installed.

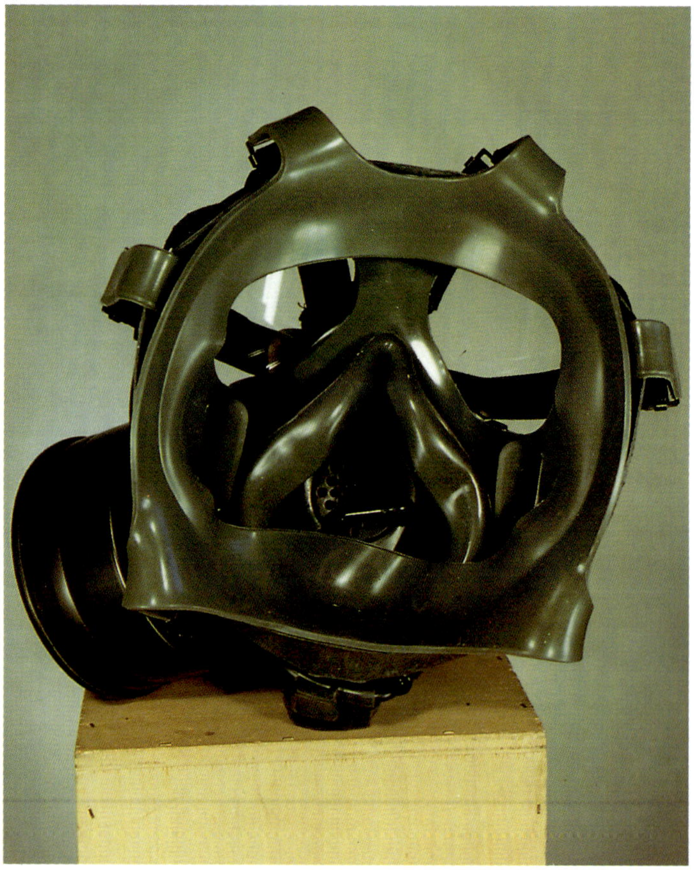

U.S. Army Field Protective Mask M40A1, 1994. View of the interior of M40 series mask. Clearly shown are the reversed peripheral face-seal, silicone oronasal cup, internal drink stem, left side air deflection guide, and internal voicemitter grill. The silicone rubber used in the M40 and M40A1 facepieces provides superior face-sealing qualities, which was a primary motivation in the material's selection.

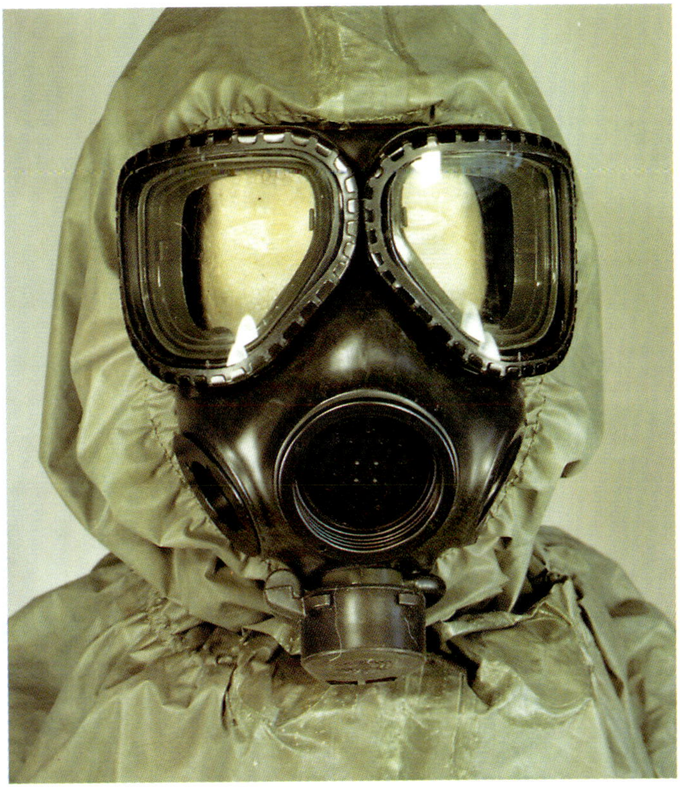

U.S. Army M40A1 mask fitted with EPDM second-skin facepiece cover and separate butyl-proofed hood. Good overall detail view. Note reinforced top seam on hood. The centrally situated zipper used on the M40 type hood has been eliminated. The section of silicone faceblank to which the exhalation valve is attached is still exposed, due to the complication of the drink-tube take-off juncture. This is a potentially vulnerable area to HD, consequently.

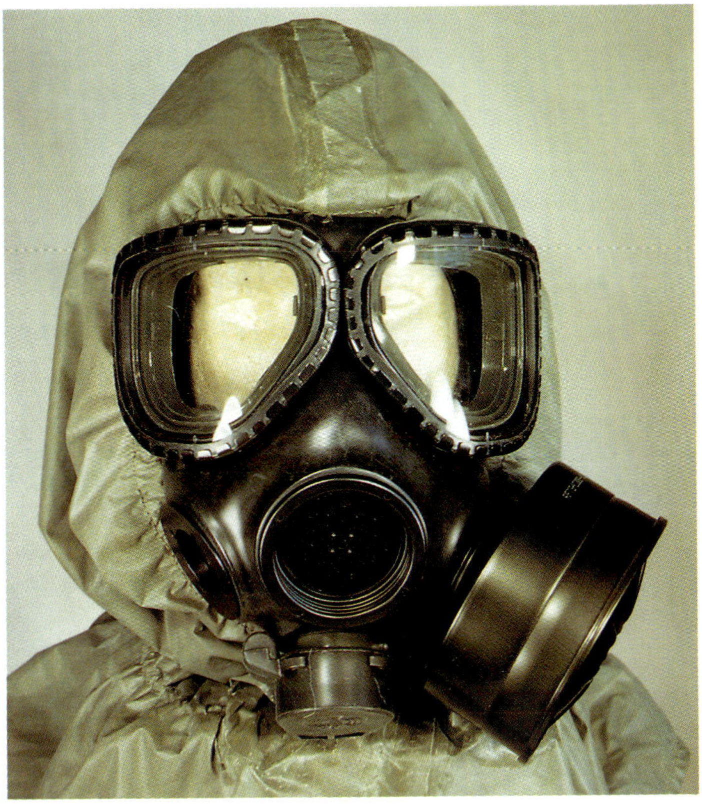

U.S. Army M40A1 mask fitted with EPDM second-skin facepiece cover and separate butyl-proofed hood. The C2A1 filter is fitted; its dark metallic color is more easily viewed in this photo. Lens 'outserts' are fitted. With the new hood and facepiece cover, the M40A1 variant is far more suitable for providing adequate protection against penetrating agents, although the ultimate solution would be to use a chlorobutyl or bromobutyl rubber compound for the facepiece, rather than silicone rubber.

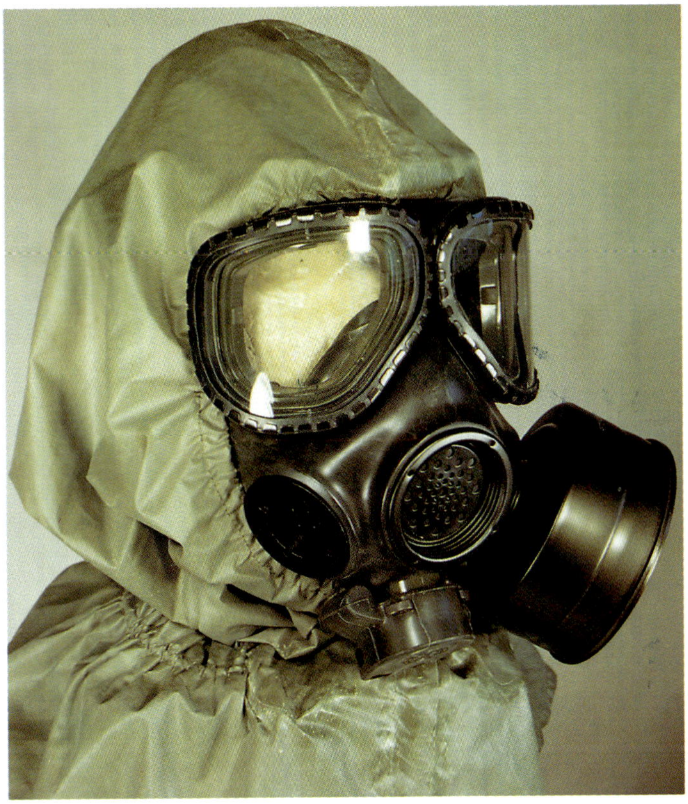

U.S. Army M40A1 mask fitted with EPDM second-skin facepiece cover and separate butyl-proofed hood. The C2A1 filter is manufactured by MSA (in the U.S.) under licensing agreement with Racal Industries of Canada, which originated the design as part of the limited U.S.-Canadian NBC cooperative interactions of the 70s.

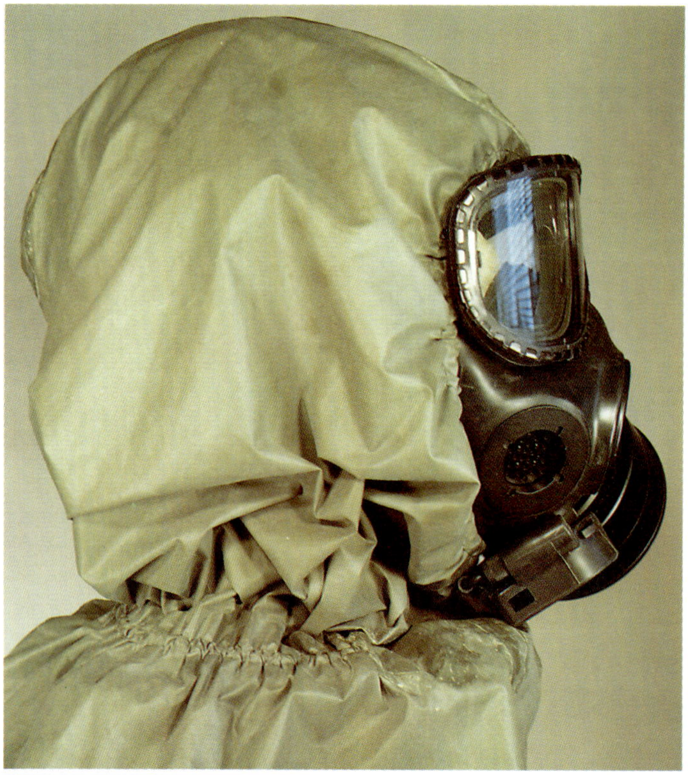

U.S. Army M40A1 mask fitted with EPDM second-skin facepiece cover and separate butyl-proofed hood. Right profile unremarkable.

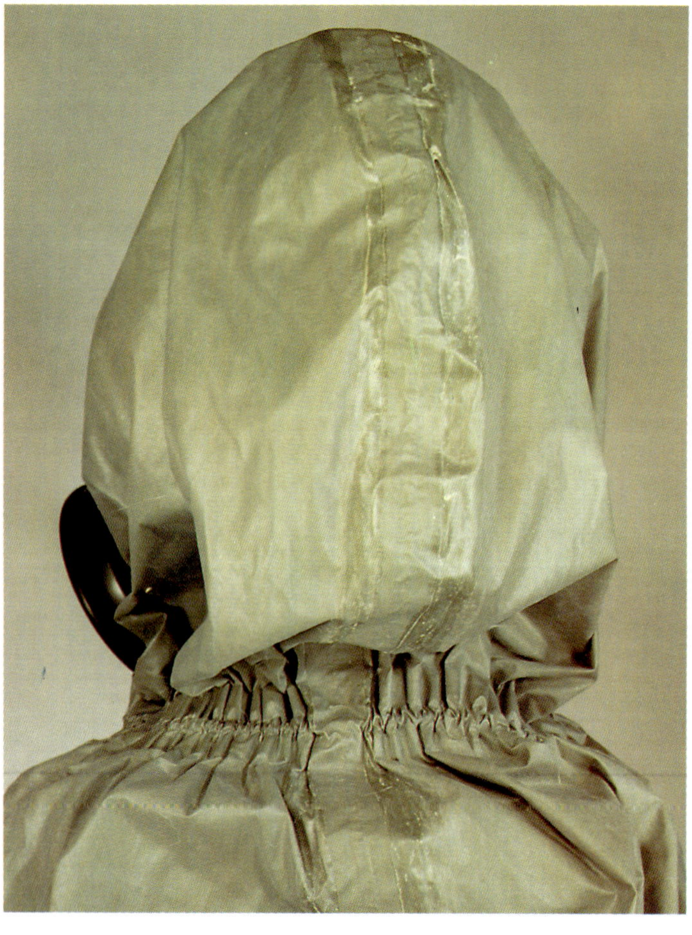

U.S. Army M40A1 mask fitted with EPDM second-skin facepiece cover and separate butyl-proofed hood. View of rear of hood is unremarkable except for the reinforced central seam visible, which runs from top to bottom of the skirt.

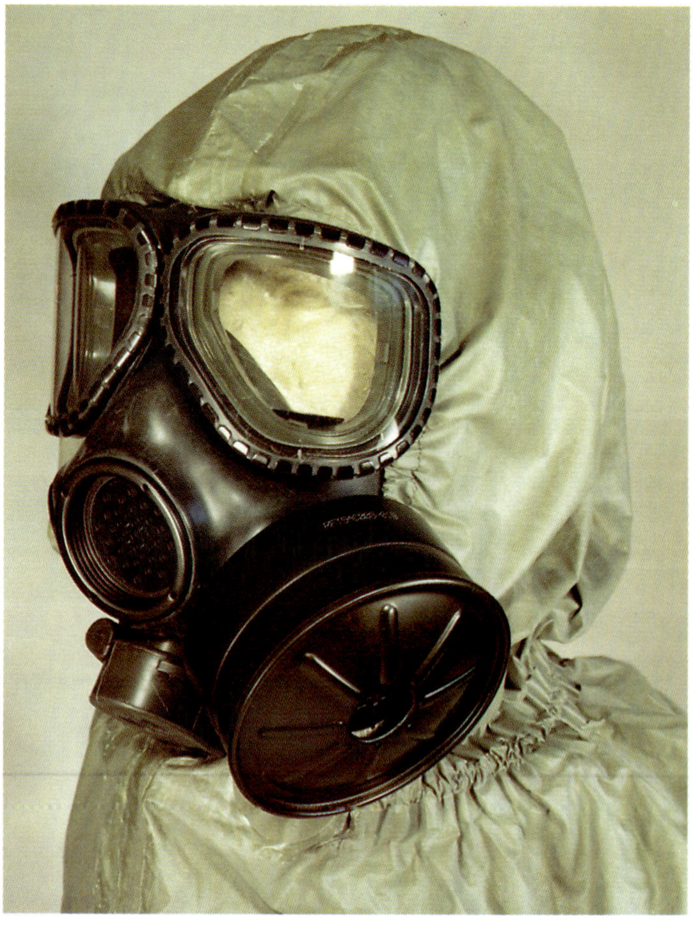

U.S. Army M40A1 mask fitted with EPDM second-skin facepiece cover and separate butyl-proofed hood. Excellent left oblique view of the mask and hood combination. Lens accessory 'outserts' are installed.

U.S. Army Protective Mask, Armored/Combat Vehicle, M42, 1990

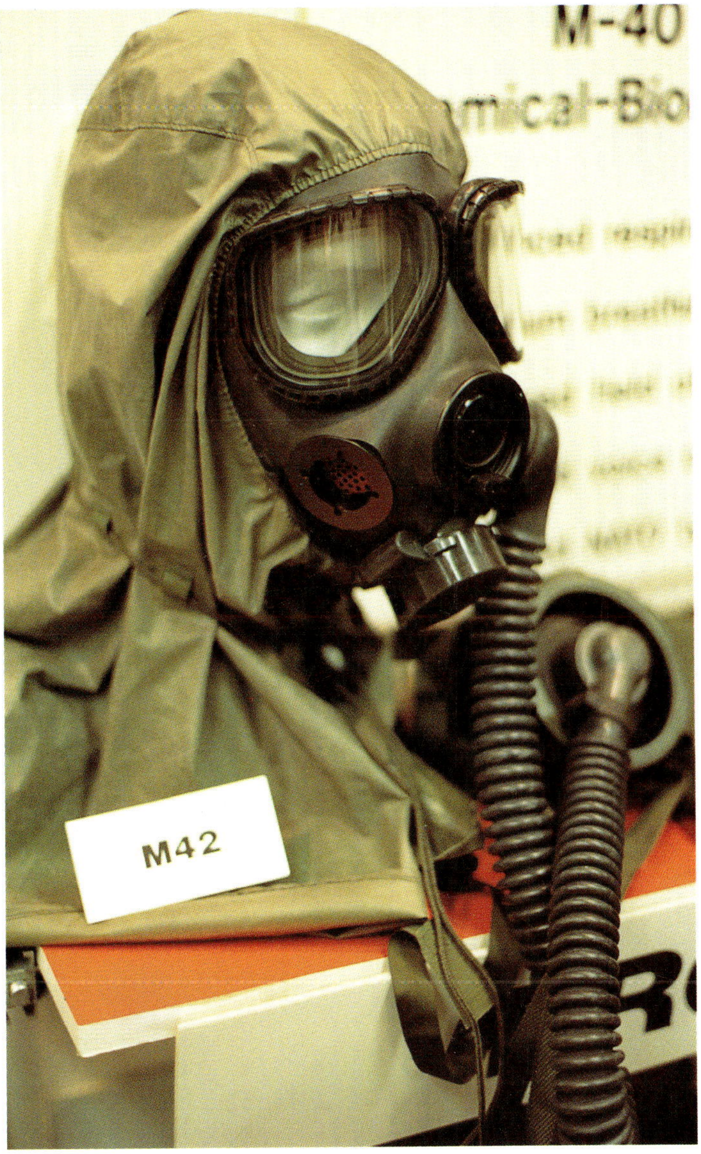

U.S. Army Protective Mask, Armored/Combat Vehicle, M42, 1990. Essentially identical to the original M40 mask, the M42 used a fixed hose connected to the left facepiece inlet port, which joined an M10A2 type filter, and could be used either independently or with a collective filtration system. The EPDM and butyl-proofed hood was one piece, as with the M40 design, and most components were interchangeable. Shown is the whole mask/hood/hose and canister assembly in right oblique angle.

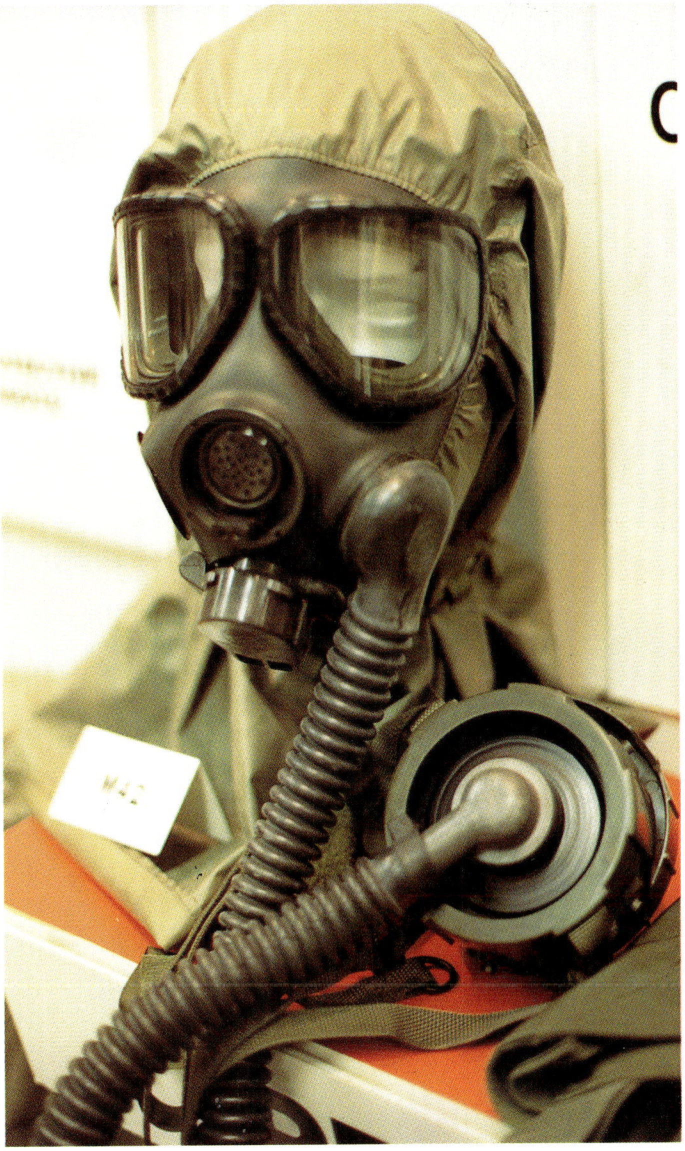

U.S. Army Protective Mask, Armored/Combat Vehicle, M42, 1990. Left oblique view of the original M42 assembly. The current M42A1 uses the same separated EPDM facepiece cover and butyl-proofed hood concept as the M40A1, and has undergone a few changes in components(consisting of use of a softer, more comfortable oronasal cup and a detachable hose connector on the left inlet port, allowing use with the C2A1 filter as an option to collective protection hook-up).

U.S. Army Protective Mask, NBC Aircrew, M43 Type I (AH 64 Helicopter)

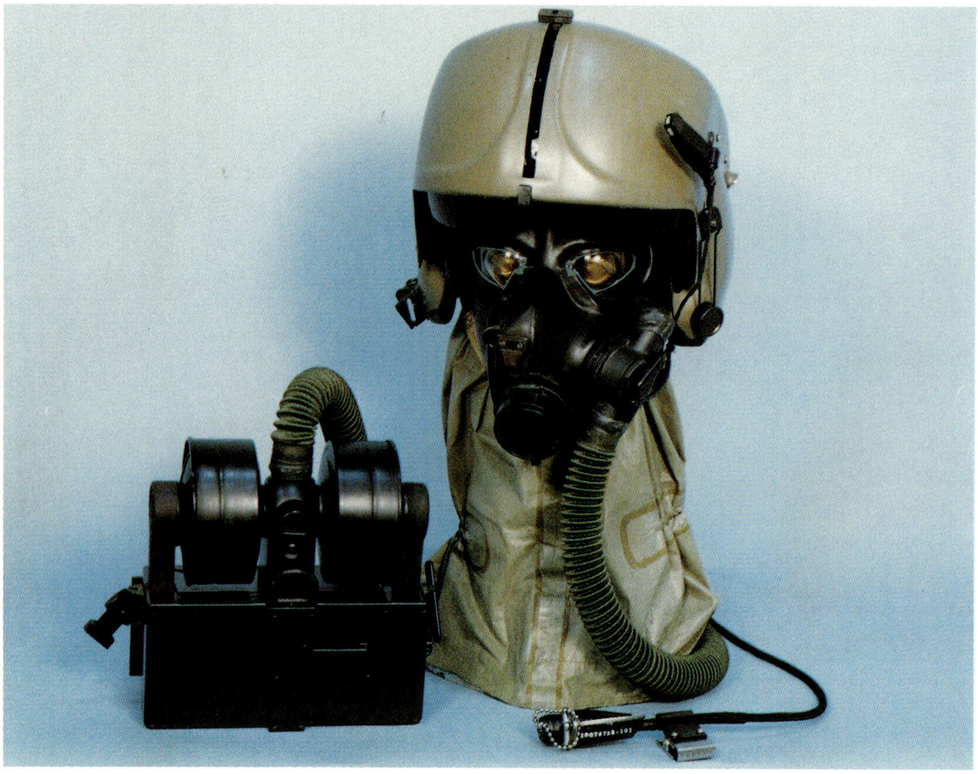

U.S. Army Protective Mask, NBC Aircrew, M43 Type I (AH-64 Helicopter), early 90s. View of respirator as worn, with blower/filter unit. The Type I version is used only on Apache helicopters, while Type II is used in all other U.S. Army aviation applications. (U.S. Army photograph, courtesy of Jane's Information Group).

U.S. Army Protective Mask, NBC Aircrew, M43E1 Type I (Apache Helicopter)

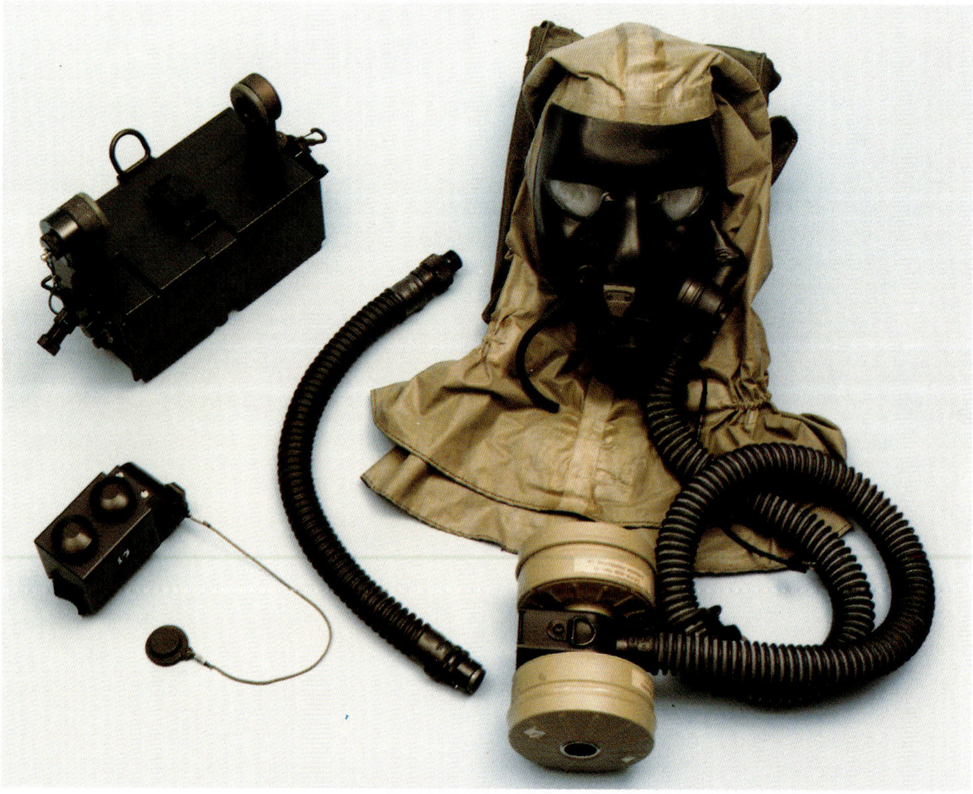

U.S. Army Protective Mask, NBC Aircrew, M43E1 Type I, (Apache Helicopter), mid 90s. Shown is the M43E1 developmental prototype which has now been standardized as the M43A1. Unique to the M43A1 model is the double skirted butyl-proofed hood and a modification of the blower system which allows standard batteries to be used (the M43 used a special battery). (Photograph courtesy of Jane's Information Group).

Italian SGE 1000 NBC Respirator, 1992

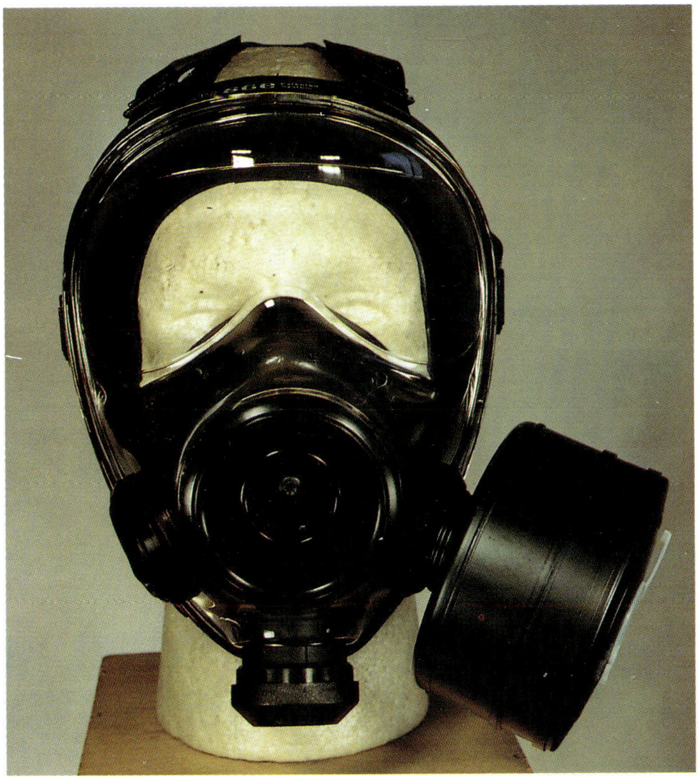

Italian SGE 1000 NBC Respirator, 1992. One of the most unusual designs in the "fourth generation respirator" group, the SGE design features a polycarbonate facepiece to which a component face-seal and harness assembly has been bonded. The mask provides a clear field of vision far in excess of most other masks of the conventional type and also provides a great degree of protection to the face.

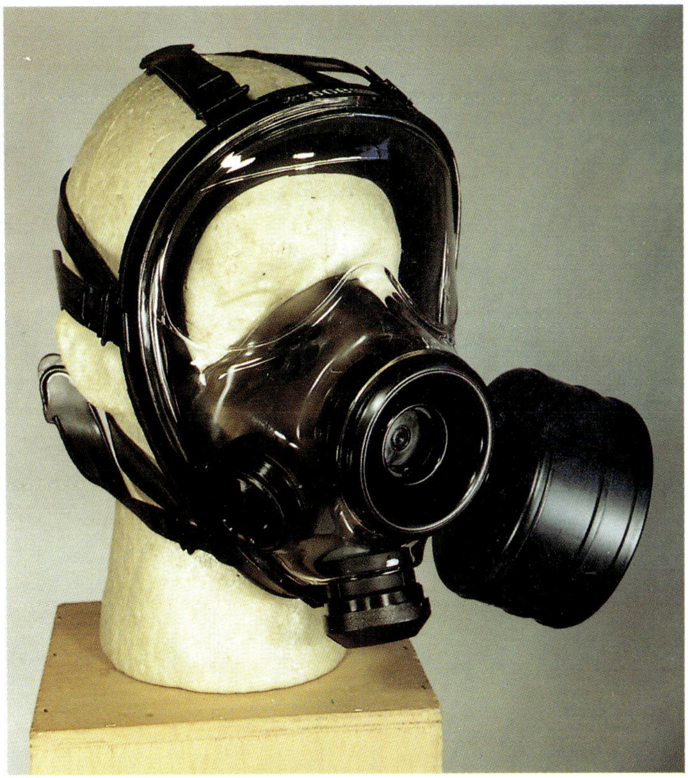

Italian SGE 1000 NBC Respirator, 1992. The internal oronasal cup is made of soft silicone rubber for excellent sealing and bilateral filter attachment ports. This mask is available in the U.S.A and has proven exceptionally useful for law enforcement applications involving crowd control and riot agents.

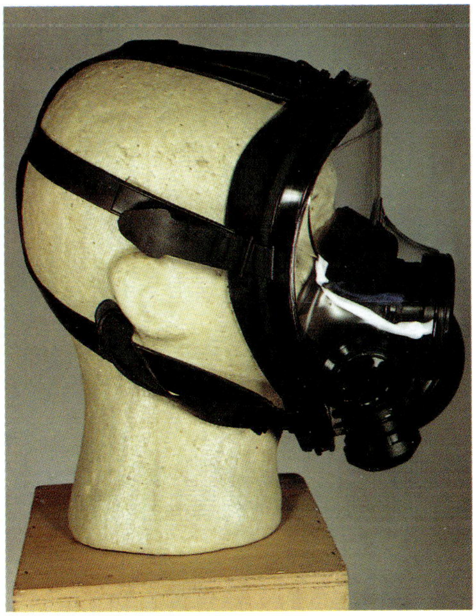

Italian SGE 1000 NBC Respirator, 1992. The drink port for this mask is located centrally in the voicemitter component and uses a bayonet type canteen adapter. The exhalation valve is located at the bottom of the facepiece, which promotes drainage of moisture.

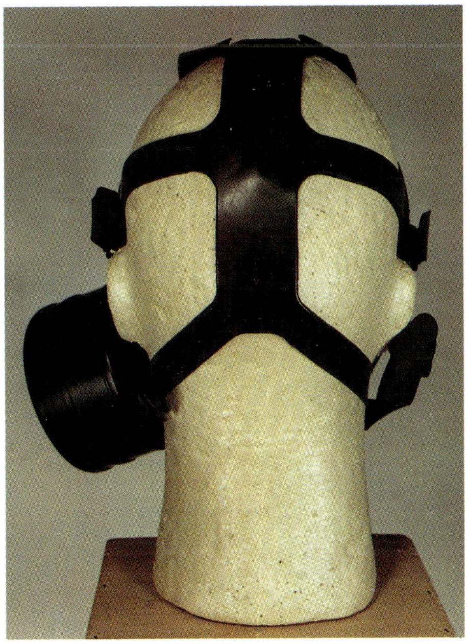

Italian SGE 1000 NBC Respirator, 1992. Rear view showing the rubber head harness strap assembly, which functions similarly to the UK S-10 type.

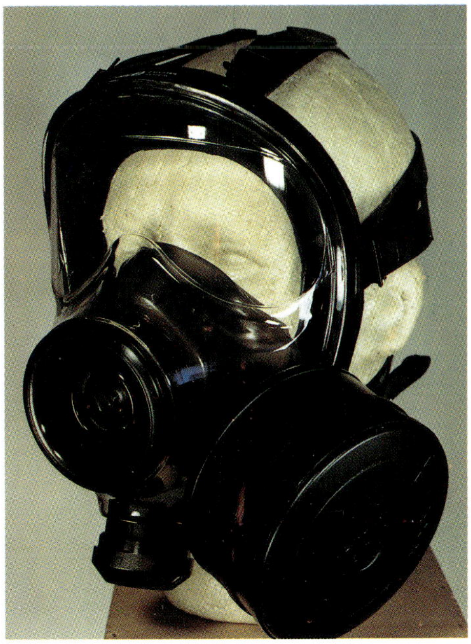

Italian SGE 1000 NBC Respirator, 1992. Left oblique view of the SGE mask shows detail of the facepiece and illustrates excellent field of vision.

MF-11 NBC Respirator, 1985

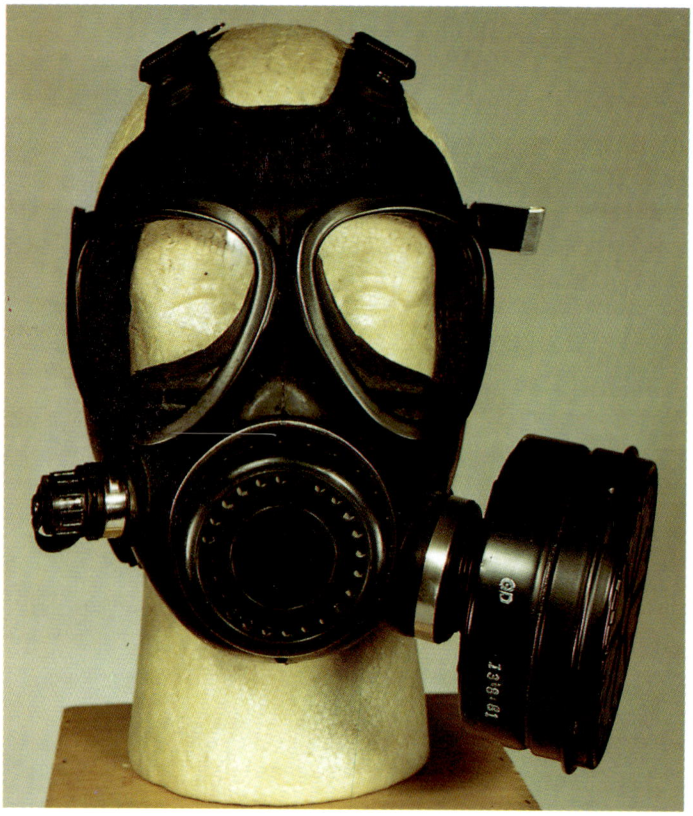

MF-11 NBC Respirator, 1985. This mask is a reworked version of the Chinese Peoples Republic M85 mask, marketed in the U.S.A by K.X. Industries. It is shown with a UK No. 2 Mark I filter fitted, and has a natural rubber facepiece. Drink tube is fitted to the right side of the mask and functions similarly to that found on Dräger (German) masks.

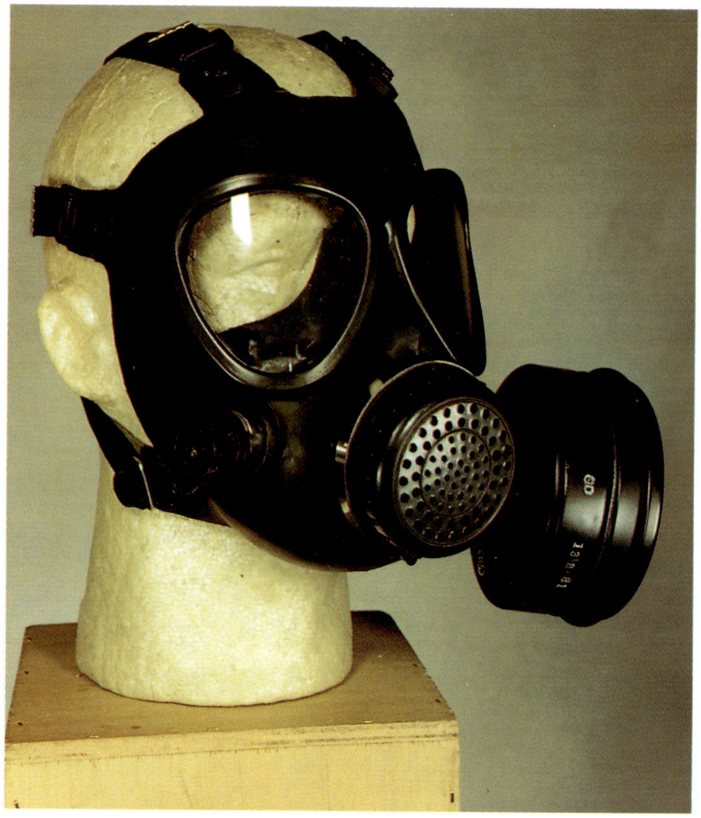

MF-11 NBC Respirator, 1985. Shown in right oblique view, the mask is simple, sturdy and functional. Design ergonometry was based upon Asian studies.

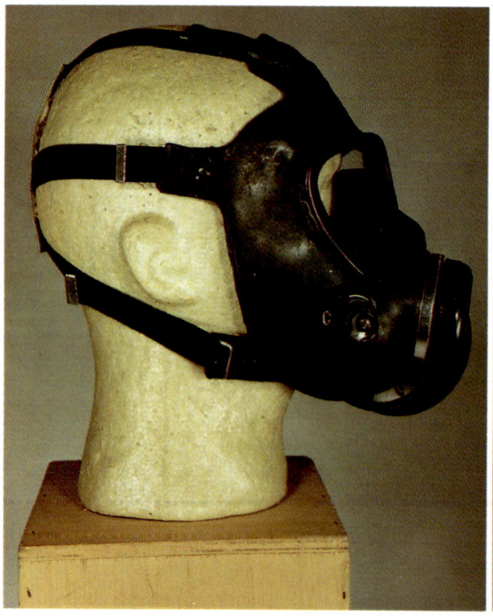

MF-11 NBC Respirator, 1985. Right profile of the M85/ MF-11 mask. Fittings and detailing are not of the highest quality but overall the mask is functionally adequate.

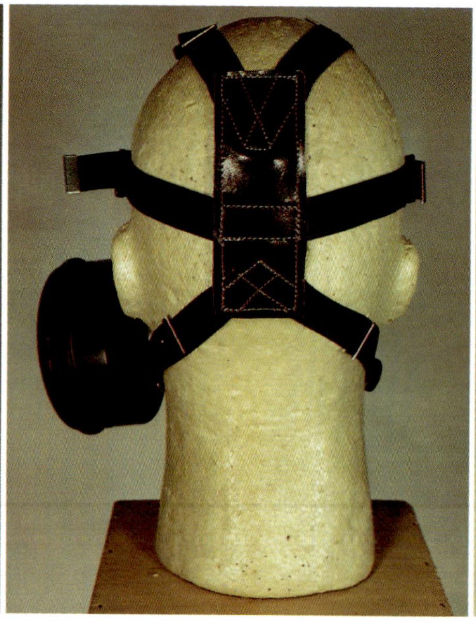

MF-11 NBC Respirator, 1985. Rear view shows head harness to be based upon U.S. elasticized type with synthetic central pad serving as juncture for 6 straps.

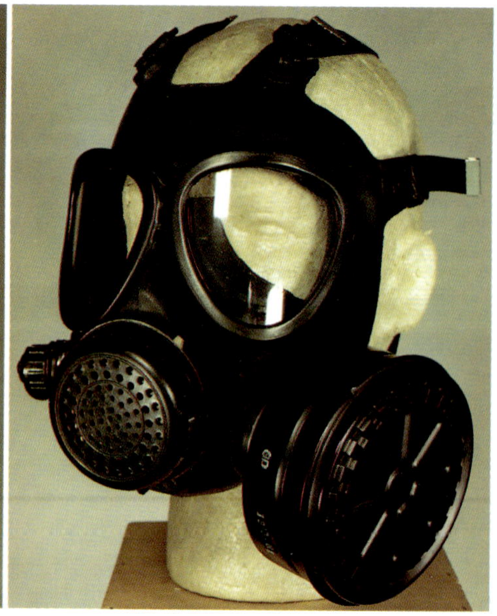

MF-11 NBC Respirator, 1985. Good left oblique view reveals detail of plastic voicemitter/exhalation valve housing and drink tube valve. Plastic molding detail is not particularly well done. British Type 2. Mark I filter is shown fitted.

Czech Republic M10M NBC Respirator, early 1980s

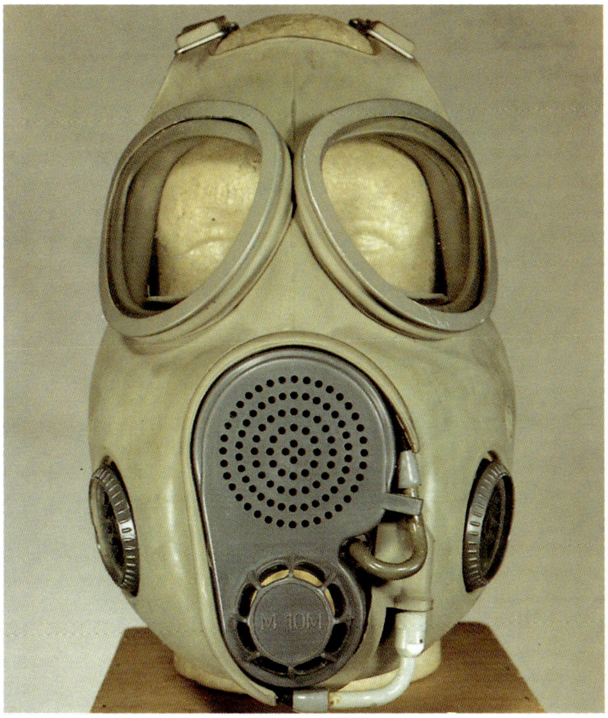

Czech Republic M10M NBC Respirator, early 1980s. Frontal view shows the M10M to be a carefully produced and engineered protective respirator. Overall similar to the M17 mask, the M10M version with drink tube is an updated modification of the M10, which first appeared several decades ago. Despite similarities to the U.S. M17, there are no interchangeable parts or components.

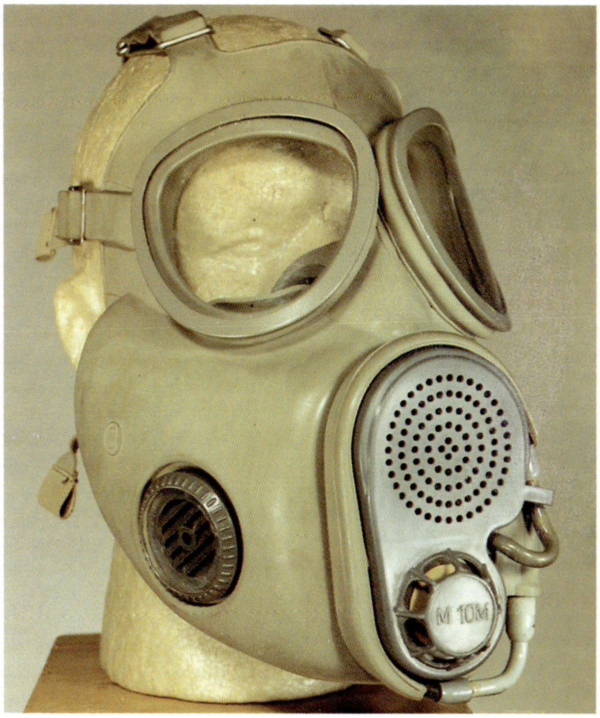

Czech Republic M10M NBC Respirator, early 1980s. Right oblique view highlights resemblance to U.S. M17 series, with bilateral cheek fitted filters inserted and removed from within the mask. Note mask model identification clearly molded into exhalation valve guard. This mask is still quite suitable for NBC protection, especially when used with the component hood that is similar to the U.S. M6A2 series.

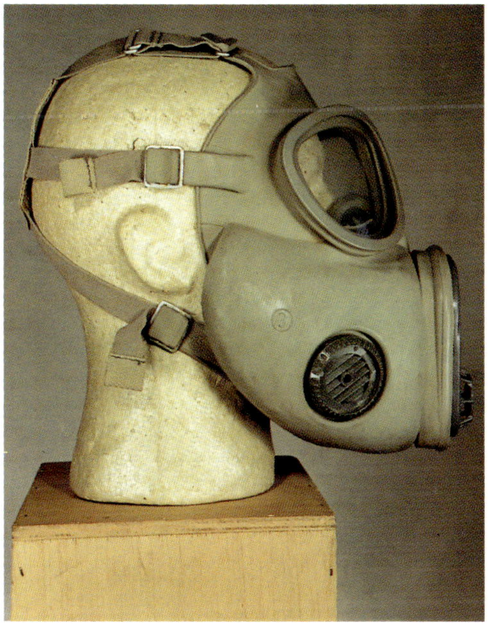

Czech Republic M10M NBC Respirator, early 1980s. Right profile shows inlet valve detail and size molded into facepiece (3). Many of these were acquired and issued to civilians by the Saudi government during the Gulf War, although a great number came from old Soviet Bloc war stockpiles and had missing or damaged components. In new, serviceable condition the M10 mask provides good CB protection.

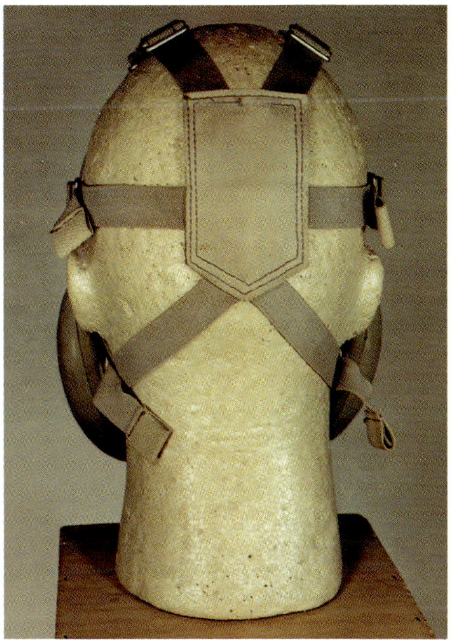

Czech Republic M10M NBC Respirator, early 1980s. Rear view show head harness to be based on U.S. M17 type harness, although elasticized strap material seems particularly strong and robust.

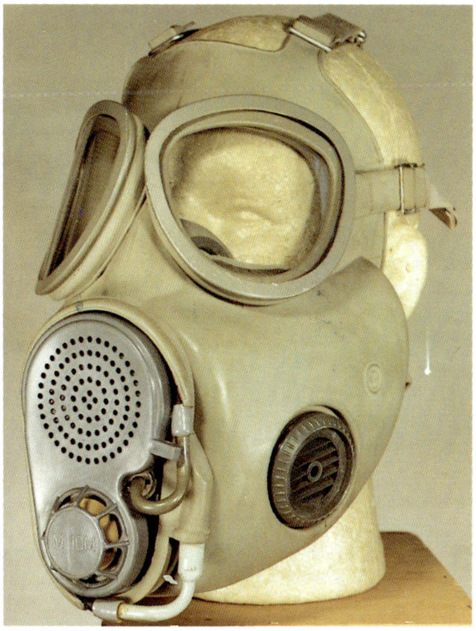

Czech Republic M10M NBC Respirator, early 1980s. Left oblique view shows off detail of drink tube and valve. Eye lens 'outserts' are fitted to the mask, which are usually used when the accessory hood is attached.

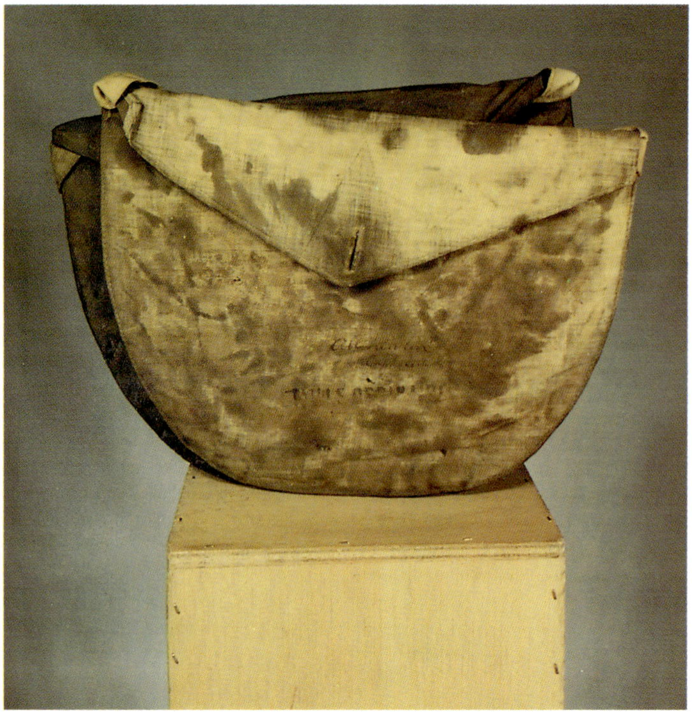

French M2 type mask carrier, WWI. Two are shown, one in front of the other. The material was of waxed cotton fabric with a buttoned flap. A carrying strap was provided.

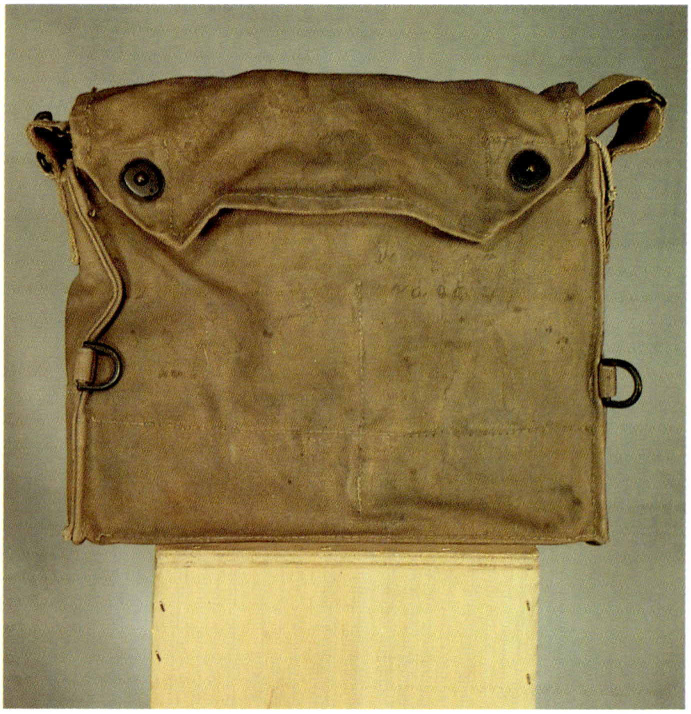

Carrying satchel, U.S. C.E.M. gas mask, WWI. Canvas duck material with snap closure; size is notably smaller than that used with ASBR types; carrying strap is stowed inside.

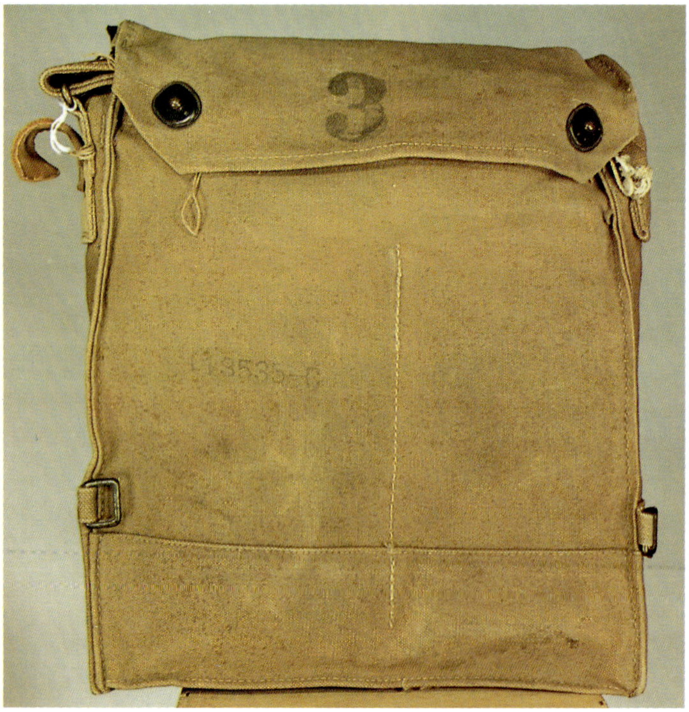

Carrier satchel, British Small Box Respirator (BSBR), WWI. Cotton duck material with snap closure flap. Size of mask carried is 3. Carrying strap is secured inside.

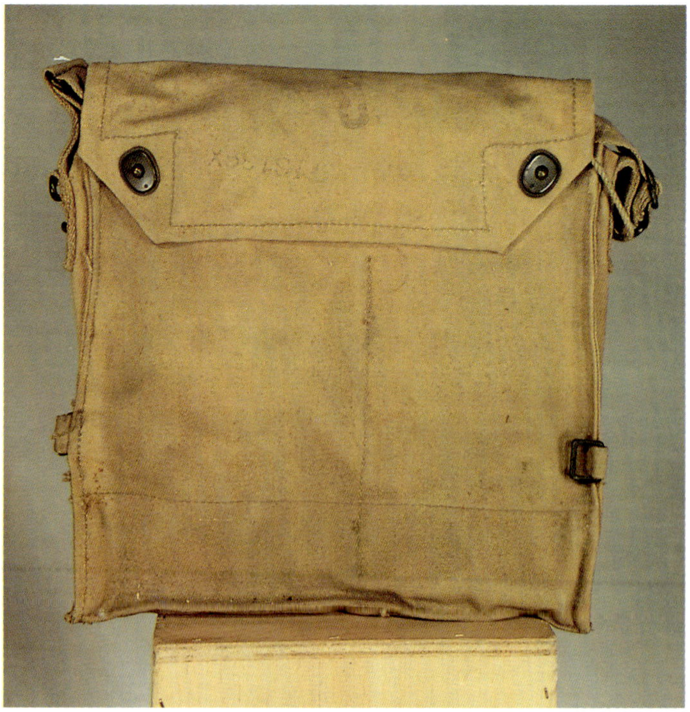

Carrying satchel, U.S. ASBR (Training Gas Mask), WWI. Canvas duck material. Size of mask carried within is indicated as 3. Carrying strap is stowed inside.

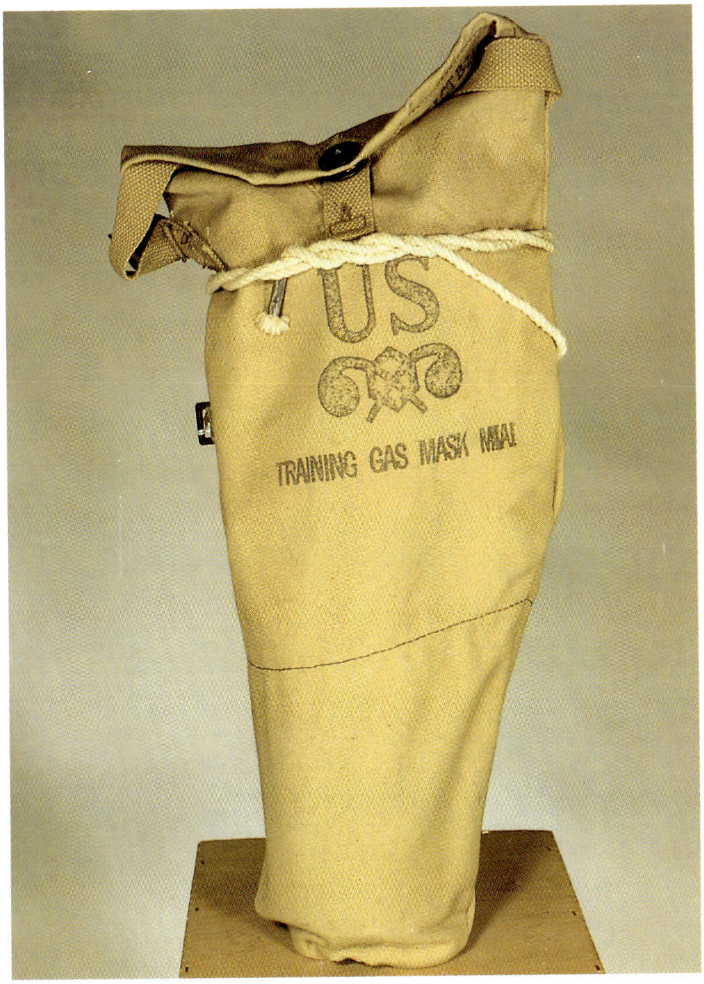

Carrying satchel, U.S. MIA1/M2A1 Training Gas Mask, 1940. Canvas duck with single snap flap and carrying strap.

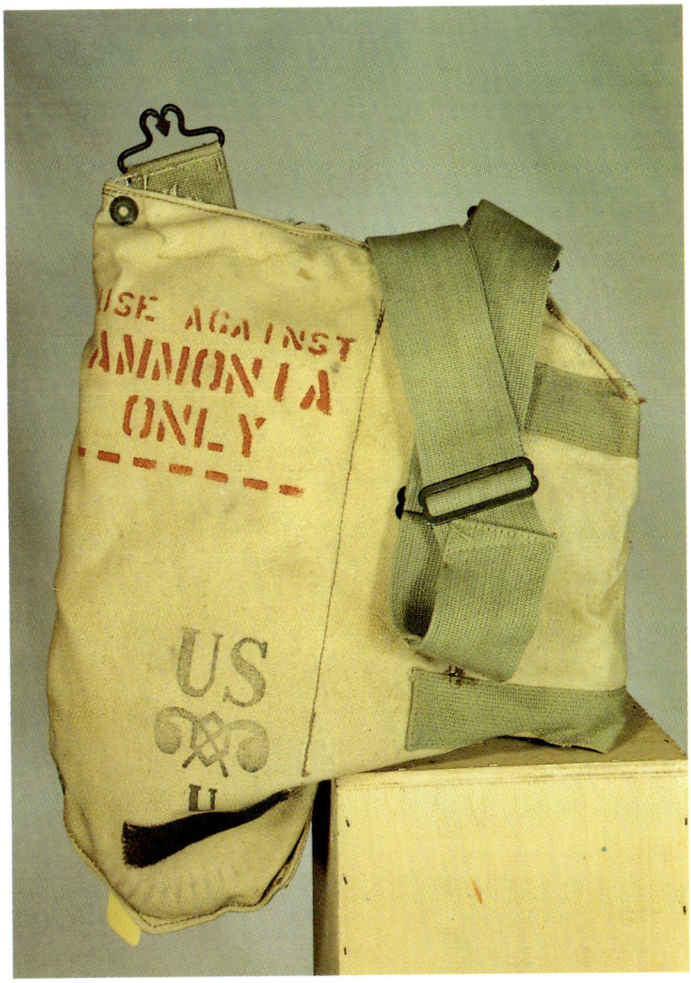

Carrying satchel, U.S. M2 type Ammonia Mask (Heavyweight), 1942.

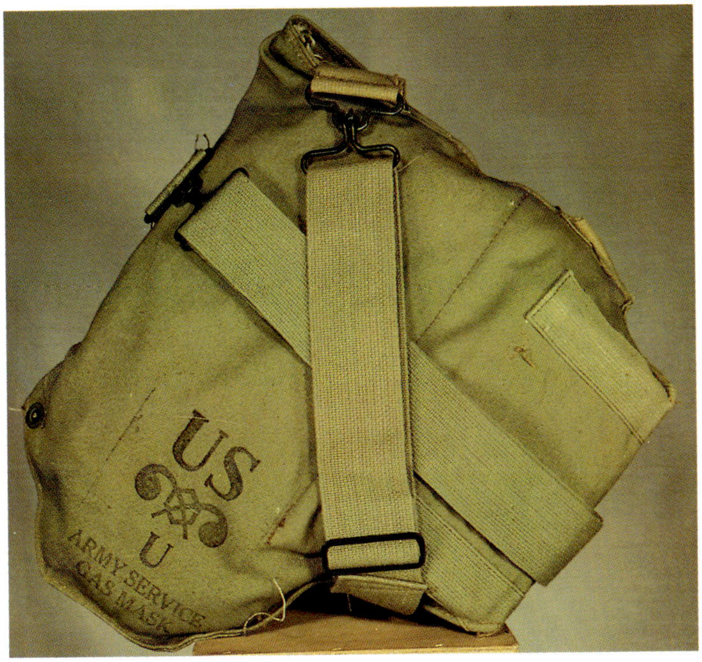

Carrying satchel, U.S. M2 type Army Service Gas Mask (Heavyweight), 1942.

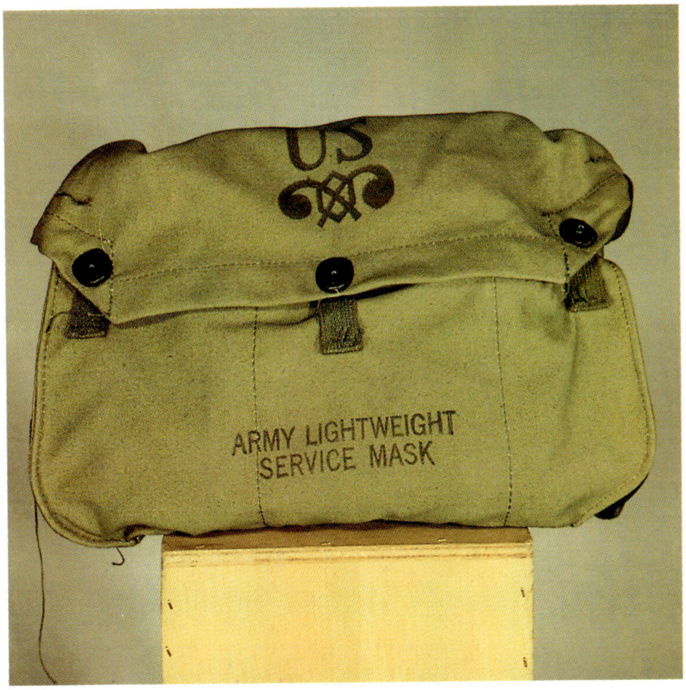

Carrying satchel, U.S. M3/M4 type Army Service Gas Mask (Lightweight), 1943/4.

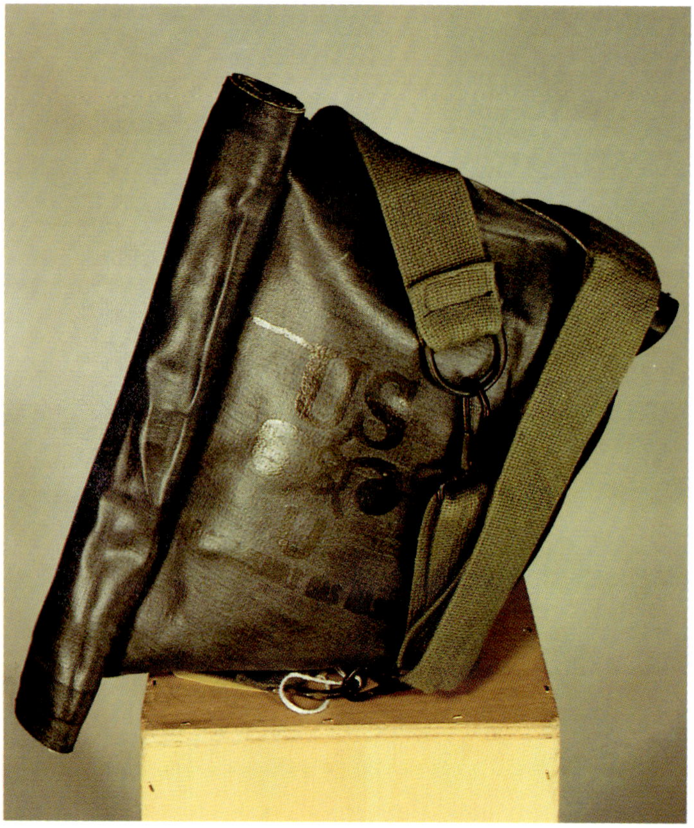

Carrying satchel, U.S. M5 Assault Gas Mask (Combat Service Mask), 1944. Rubber coated duck, which could be used as an emergency life preserver by assault landing troops.

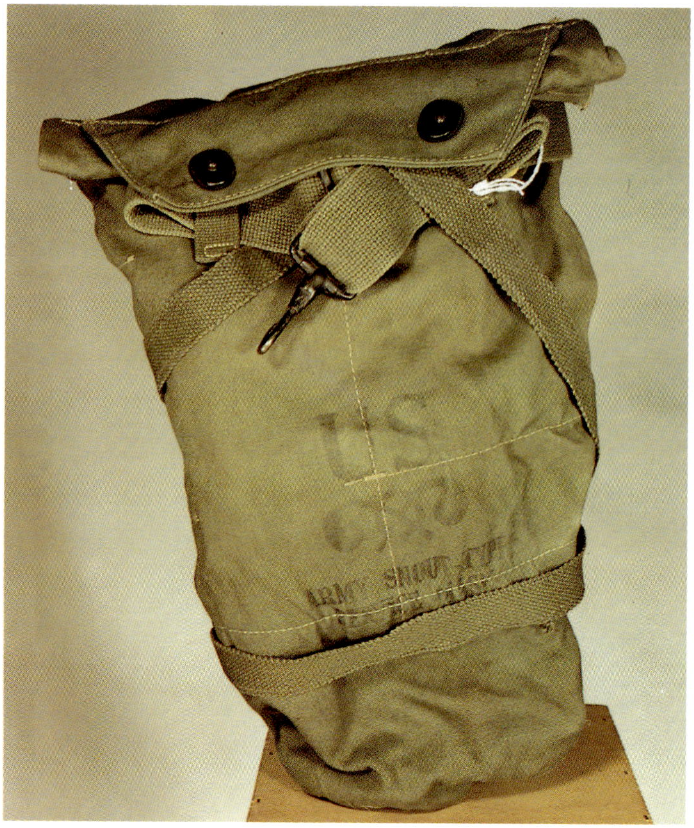

Carrying satchel, U.S. M8 Snout Type Gas Mask, 1945. OD colored fabric.

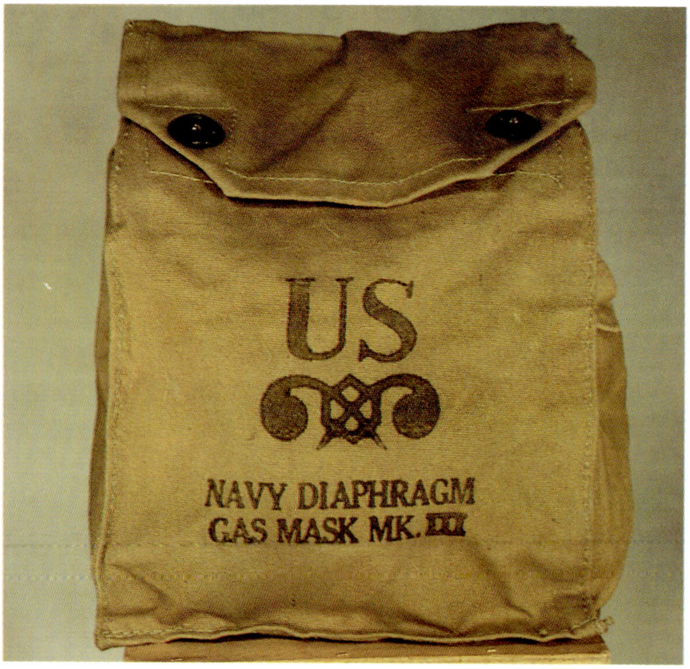

Carrying satchel, U.S. Navy Diaphragm Gas Mask Mk. III, 1943. Unusual in that the fabric of the U.S. Navy carriers was usually gray and the chemical corps 'crossed retorts' marking is usually seen on the U.S. Army version, and not on the Navy version.

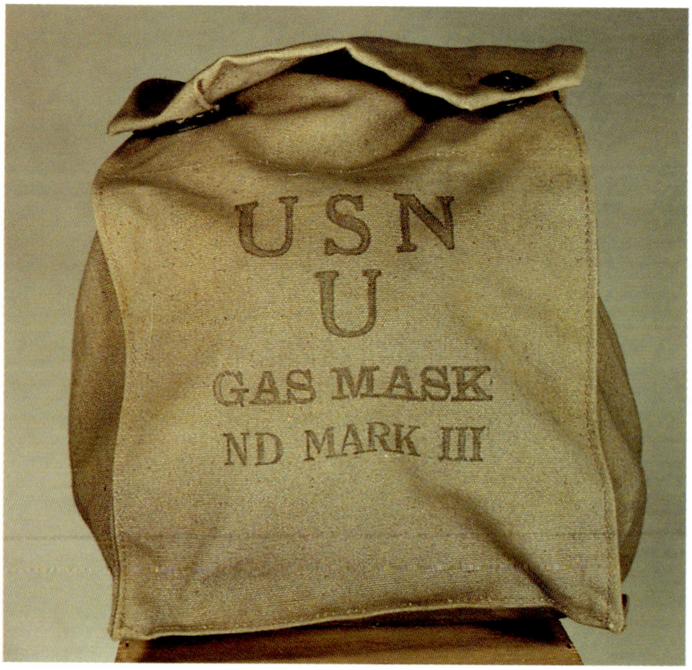

Carrying satchel, U.S. Navy Diaphragm Gas Mask Mk. III, 1943. This is the usual color and marking for the USN diaphragm and optical masks.

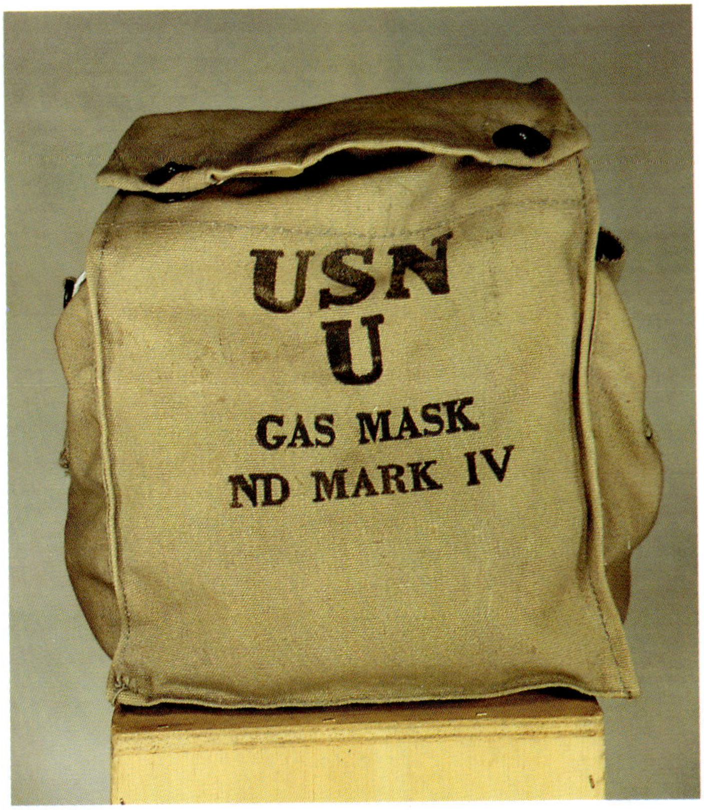

Carrying satchel, U.S. Navy Diaphragm Gas Mask Mk. IV, 1944. Typical USN gray duck fabric and markings.

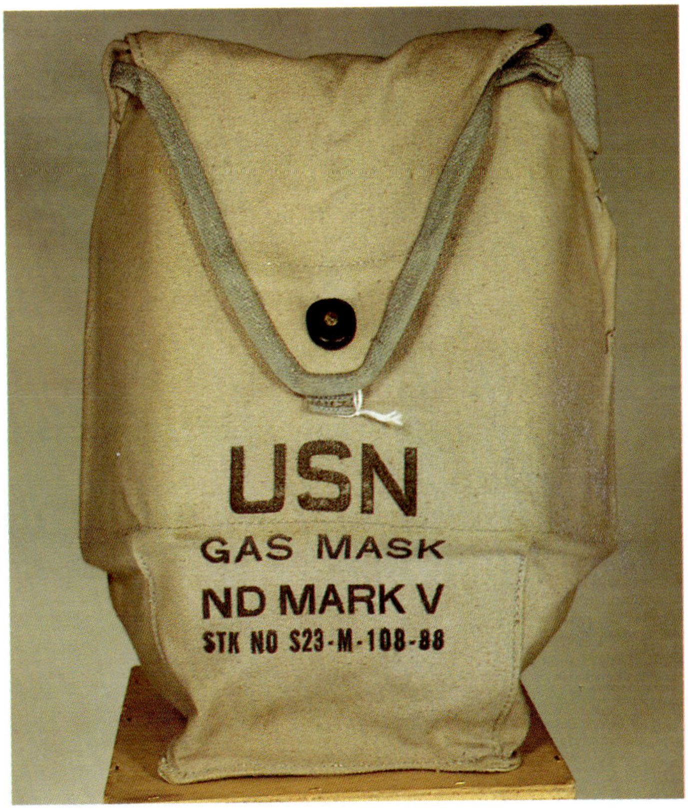

Carrying satchel, U.S. Navy Gas Mask Mk. V, 1955. Later versions of this carrier were marked "Mask, Chemical and Biological, ND Mk. V." Gray duck fabric.

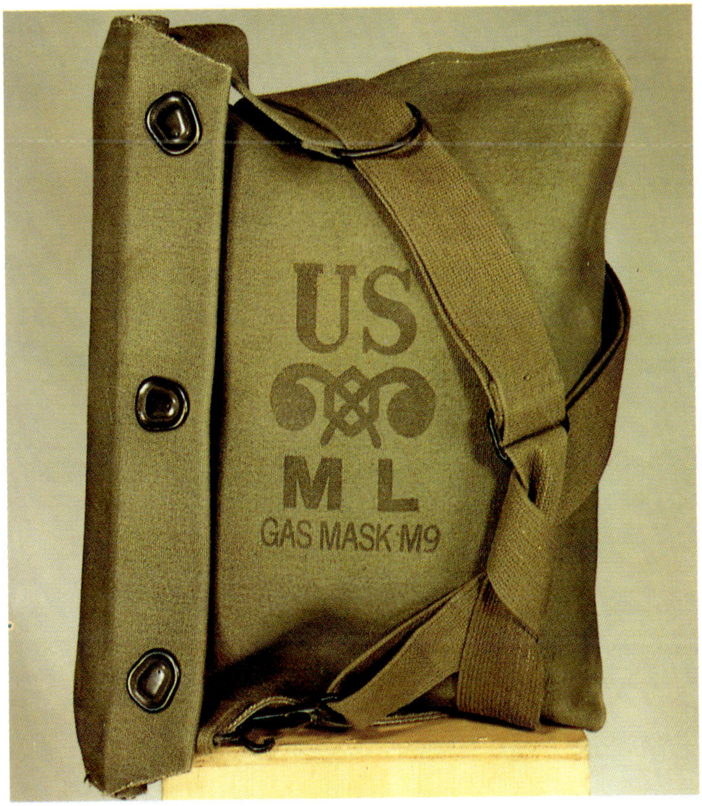

Carrying satchel, U.S. Army Field Protective Mask, M9 (C15R1 carrier), early 50s. OD fabric with three snap closure flap. Very similar in cut and shape to earlier M5 Assault Gas Mask carrier, but not proofed externally.

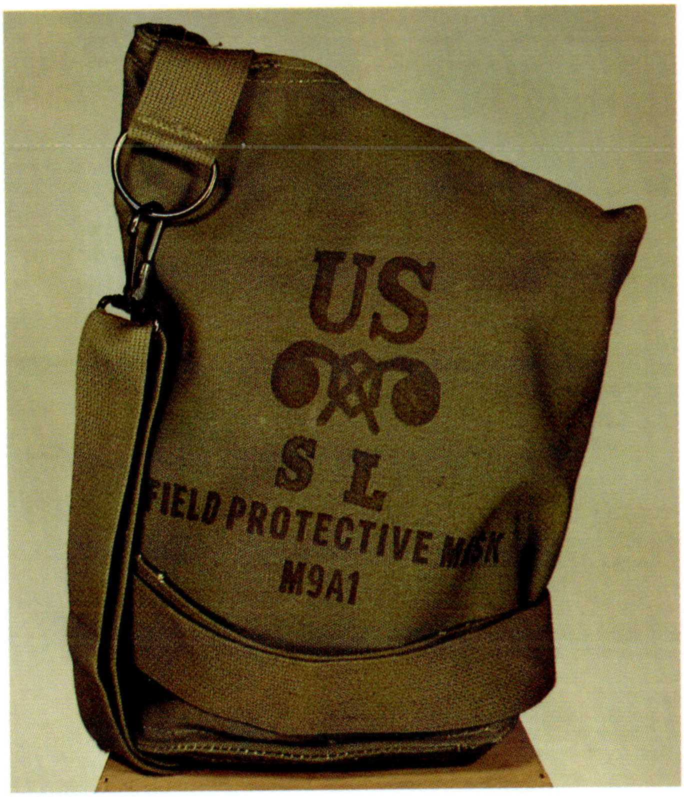

Carrying satchel, U.S. Army Field Protective Mask M9A1, mid-50s. Mask was identical to earlier model but carrier was new, resulting in mask nomenclature change (M11 carrier). OD cotton duck.

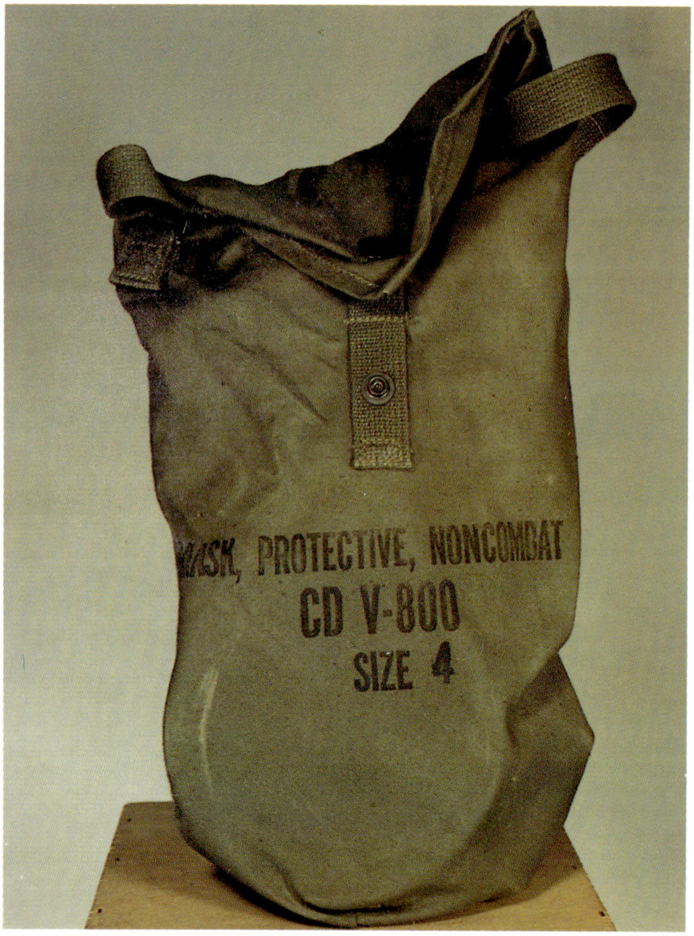

Carrying satchel, U.S. Civil Defense V-800 NBC Protective Mask, late 50s

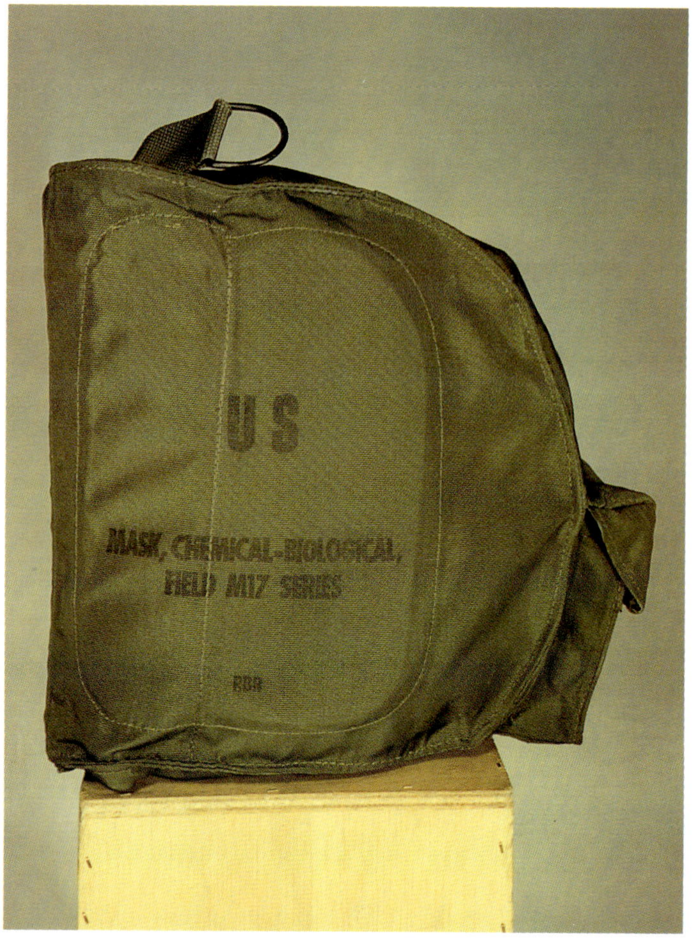

Carrying satchel, U.S. Army Field Protective Mask M17 Series, 1988. Relatively late model which was manufactured (cotton duck) as replacement/issue for all three M17 variants is shown. Final model was identical in all respects but made from OD nylon duck.

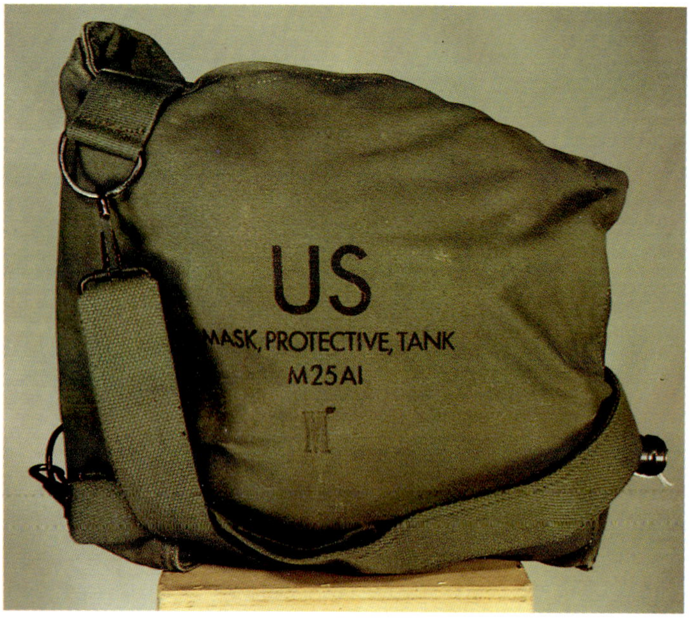

Carrying satchel, U.S. Army Mask, Protective, Tank, M25A1, mid-80s. OD cotton duck. Aircraft version (carrier for M24 mask) was identical, except mirror copy—worn on opposite side of body. Note protruding hose connector on distal end of filter (right side of photograph).

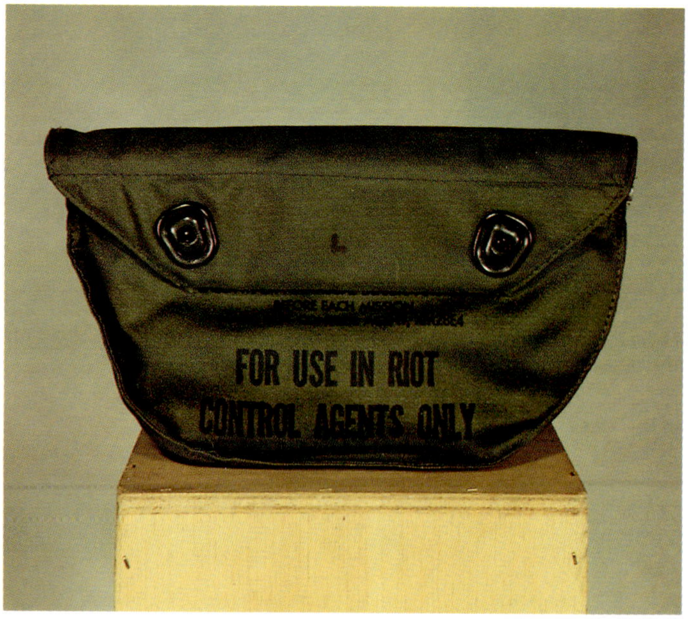

Carrying satchel, U.S. Army Protective Mask, Riot Control Agent, M28, 1960s. Small plastic lined carrier was half the size of the M28 mask, which had to be folded upon itself prior to stowing in carrier.

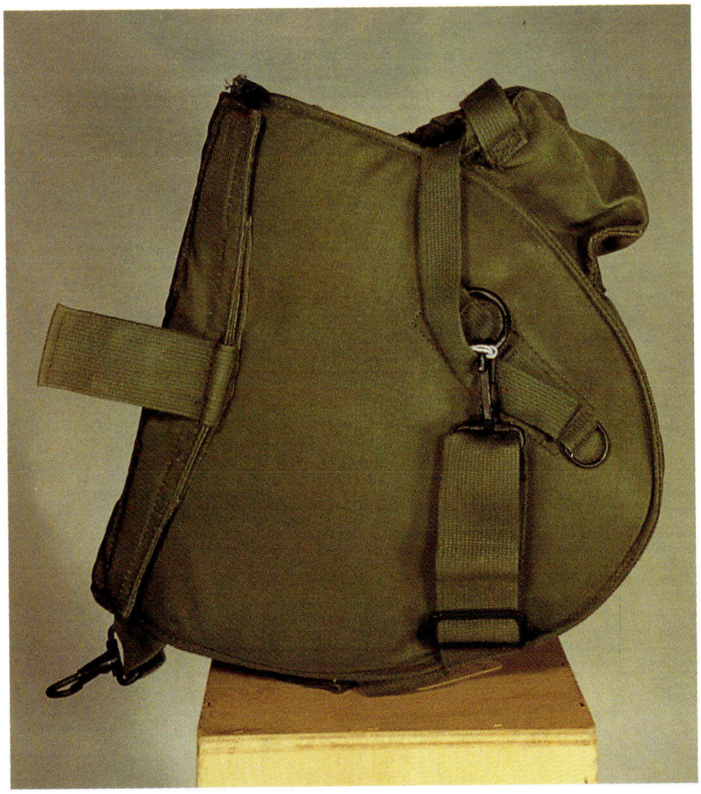

Carrying satchel, Mask, NBC Protective, MCU-2/P, late 80s. OD nylon duck, characteristic crescent shape, Velcro closure flap. External pocket for M258A1 or M291 individual decontamination kits.

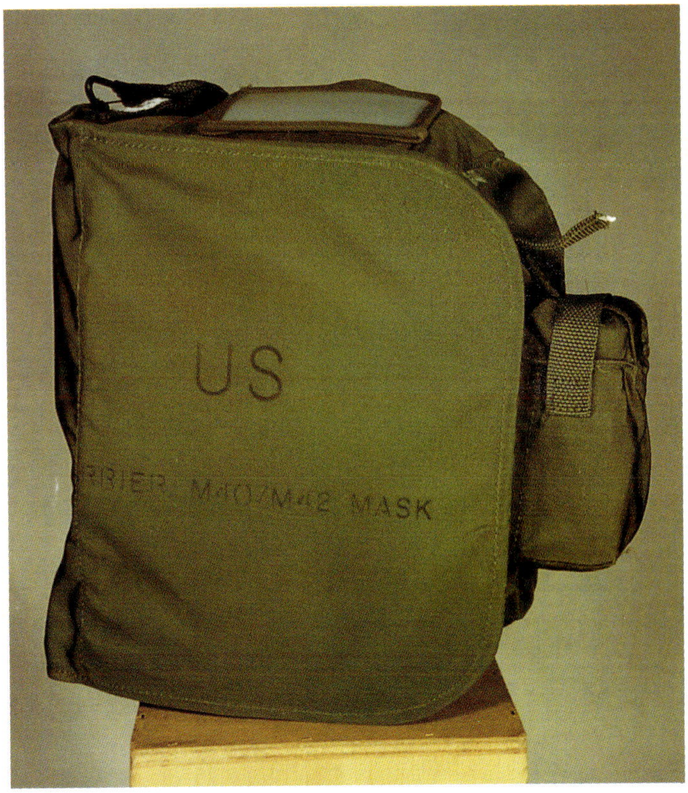

Carrying satchel, M40/M42 Series Masks, early 90s. OD nylon duck material, characteristic rounded rectangular shape, with external pocket for M258A1 or M291 personal decontamination kit. User identification pocket (white rectangle, uppermost side) is viewable.

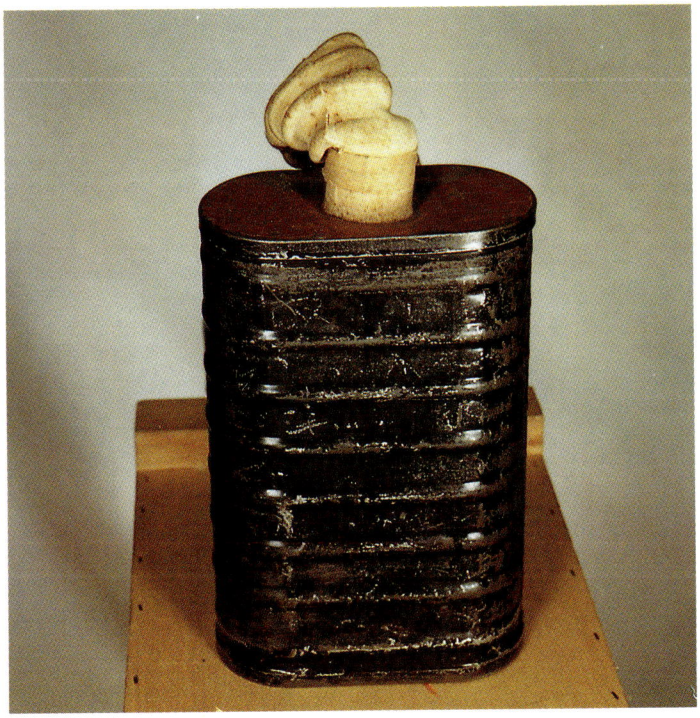

Filter, ASBR (Training Gas Mask) type, WWI. Characteristic black color on tin body, with red top to warn of training use only. This filter is taller by about an inch than the subsequent yellow J and green H Filters (C.E.M. and R.F.K. masks).

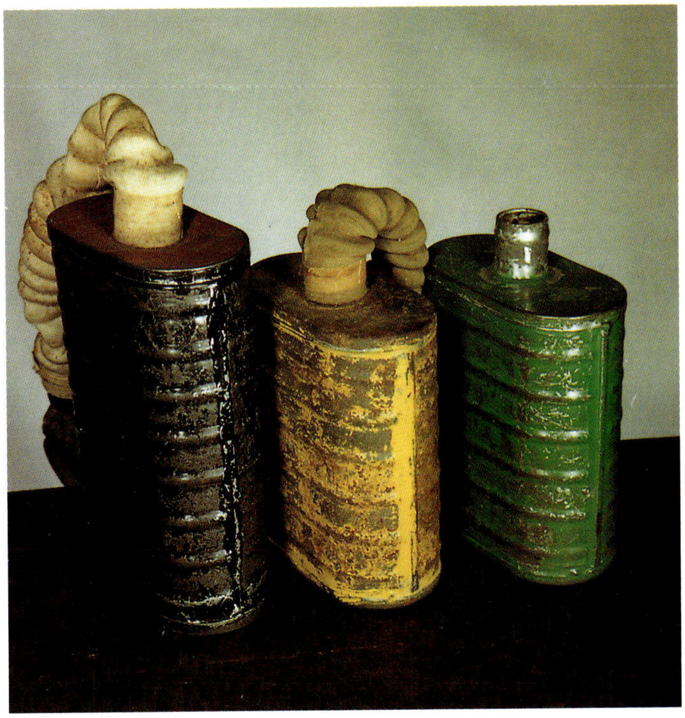

Filters, Black ASBR type next to yellow C.E.M and green R.F.K. types, WWI.

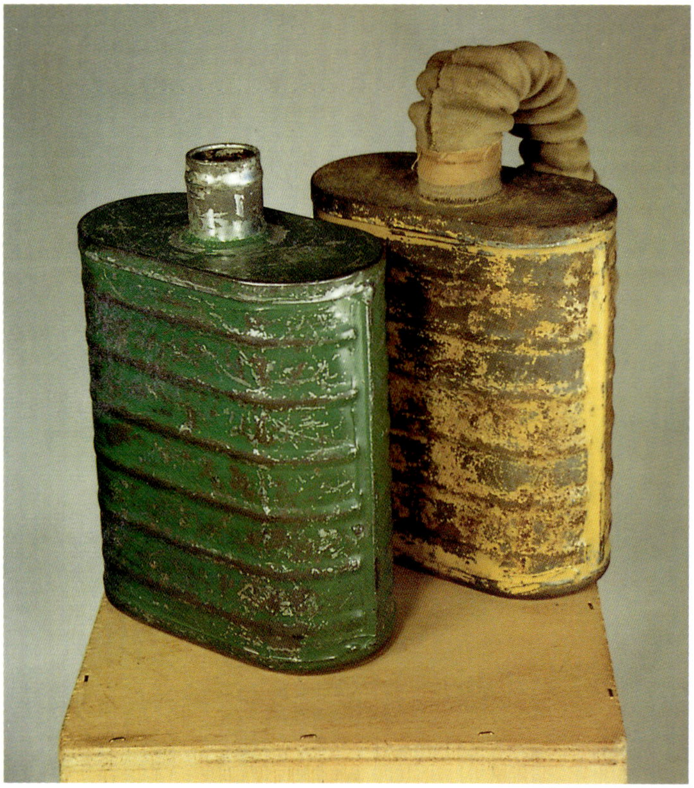

Filters, Type J (yellow), and Type H (Green), WWI. Last WWI type filters produced were the K and L types.

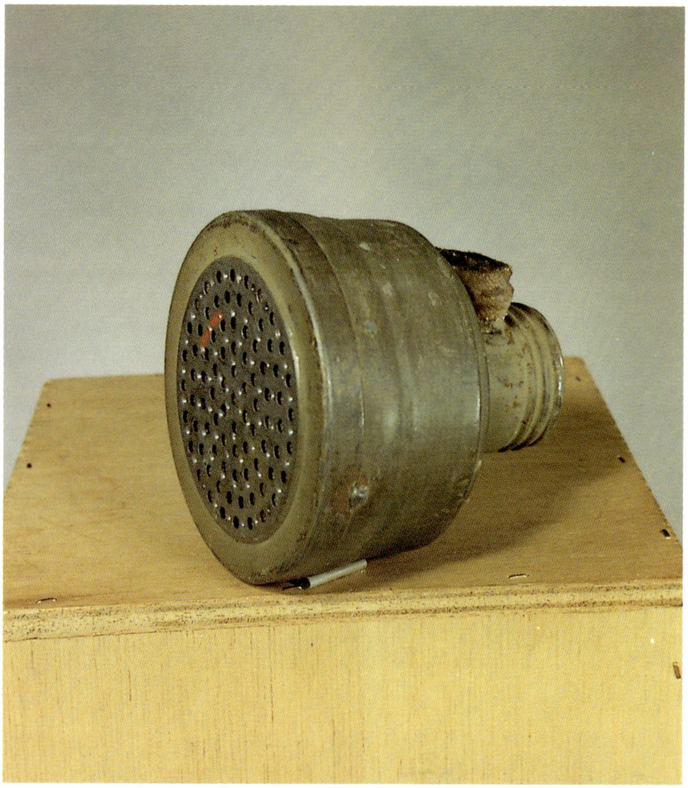

Filter, U.S. Navy Mouth Canister Gas Mask, (old) Mark I, 1918. Note exhalation valve outlet (rubber MI flapper valve missing) between main filter body and screw threaded connector.

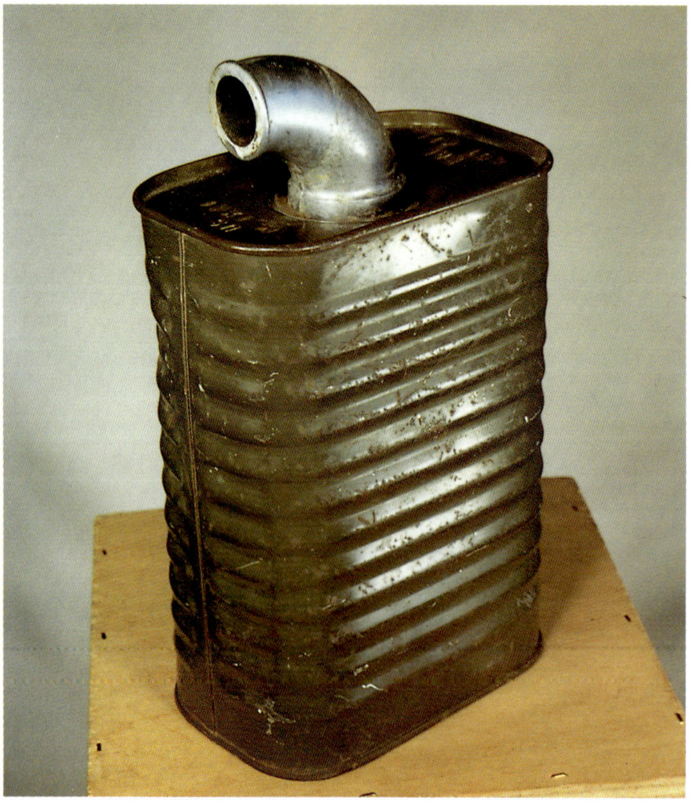

Filter, U.S. Army Type MIXA1, 1942. Most commonly used with all "heavyweight" type U.S. gas masks in Second World War.

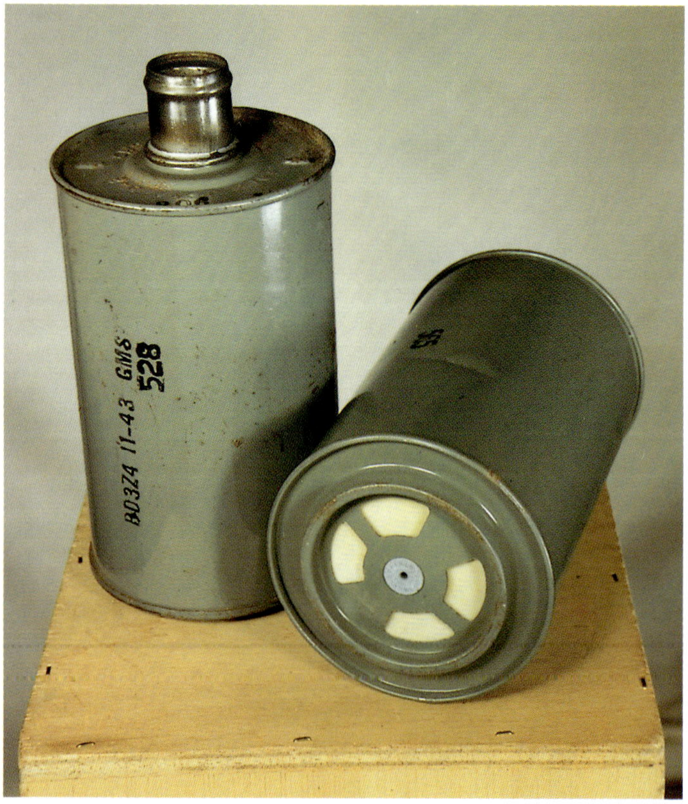

Filter, U.S. Army Type M10A1, 1943. Most commonly used with all U.S. "lightweight" type gas masks in WWII and still in use on M24/M25 type masks, although being phased out.

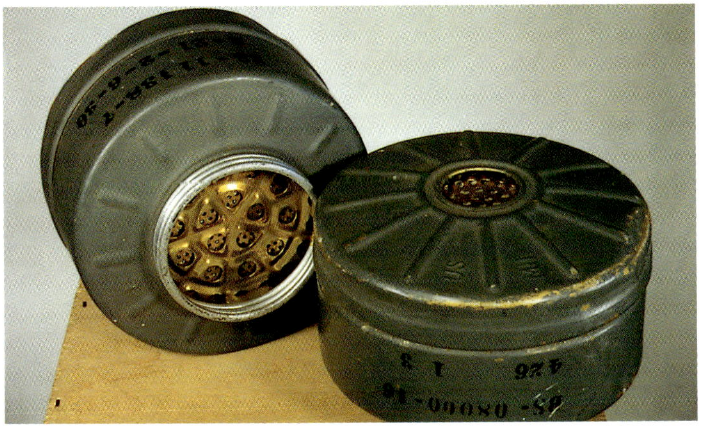

Filter, U.S. Army Type M11, first used in WWII, last used on M9A1 type masks. This filter was modeled after the German WWII Fe-42 axial flow filter.

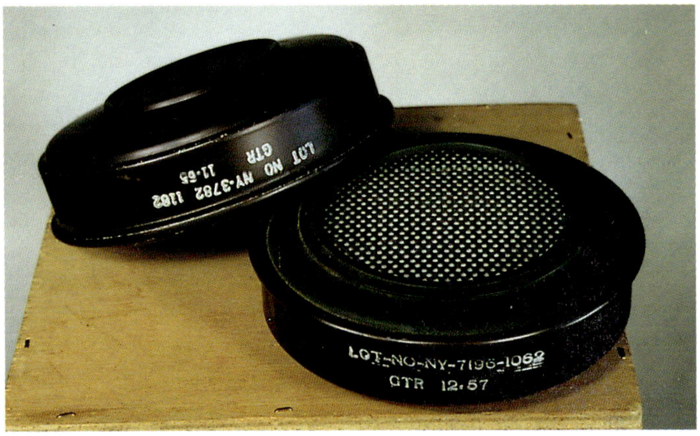

Filter, U.S. Navy C-1 filter, used with Mark V NBC mask, 1950s.

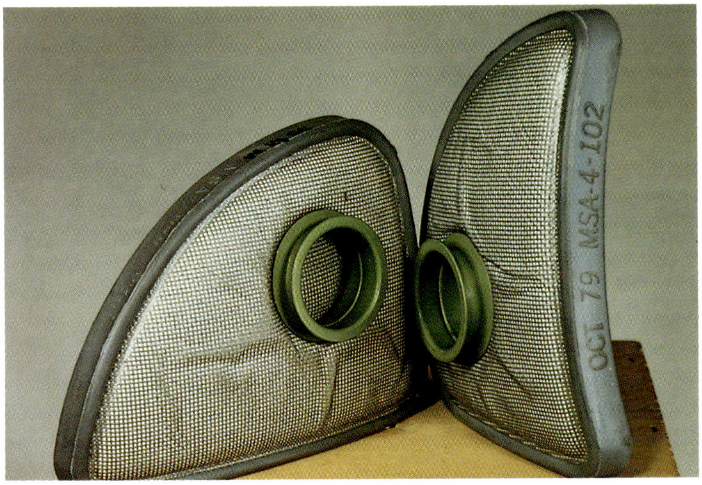

Filter, U.S. Army Type M13A2 ("pork-chop") filter set, 1960s. Four standard filter sets of this type were issued: M13 filter sets with black anodized inlet ring, M13A1 filter sets with either gold or black anodized inlet rings, and the M13A1 filter set with green anodized inlet ring. The green anodized inlet ring M13A1 was the authorized war filter for all M17 series masks, but the gold ring M13A1 was also in use against CB agents; all black ringed filter sets were relegated to training use only. Note date of manufacture and lot numbers on side of filter.

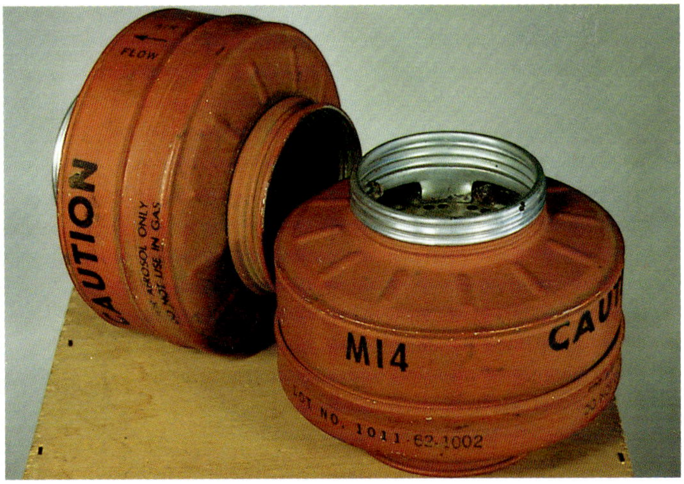

Filter, U.S. Army Type M14, 1950s/60s. These unusual filters were used in special laboratory situations and had 58 mm screw threaded ports on either end (one female and one male). They were intended to be used in pairs (joined together) and were for laboratory aerosol filtration only (not for field protective or gas filtration use).

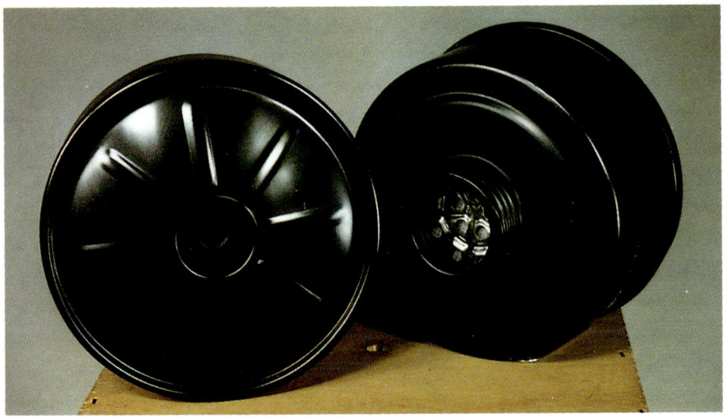

Filter, U.S. Army Type C2, 80s/90s. This is the standard U.S. military NBC filter and is distinctive, with its black anodized aluminum body, from the newest C2A1 filter (dark green metallic anodized aluminum body). Both the C2 and C2A1 filters are used with all modern U.S. Army NATO (STANAG 4155) filter compatible masks.

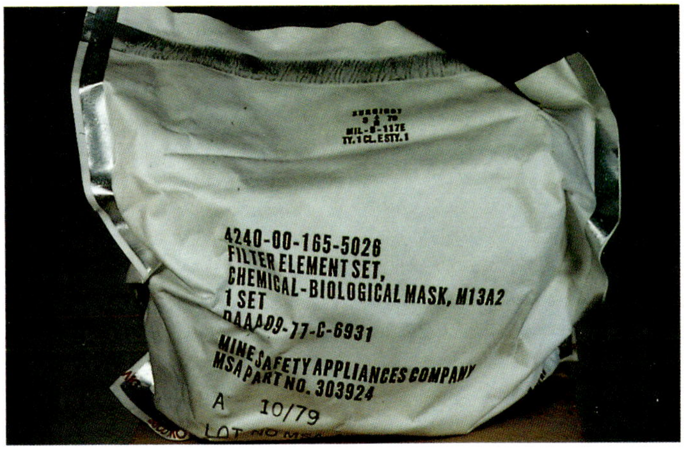

Packaging, M13A1 filter sets. This type of hermetically sealed, aluminized/plasticized composition packaging material is characteristic of the manner in which many U.S. NBC items were protected for storage in the 60s, 70s and 80s.

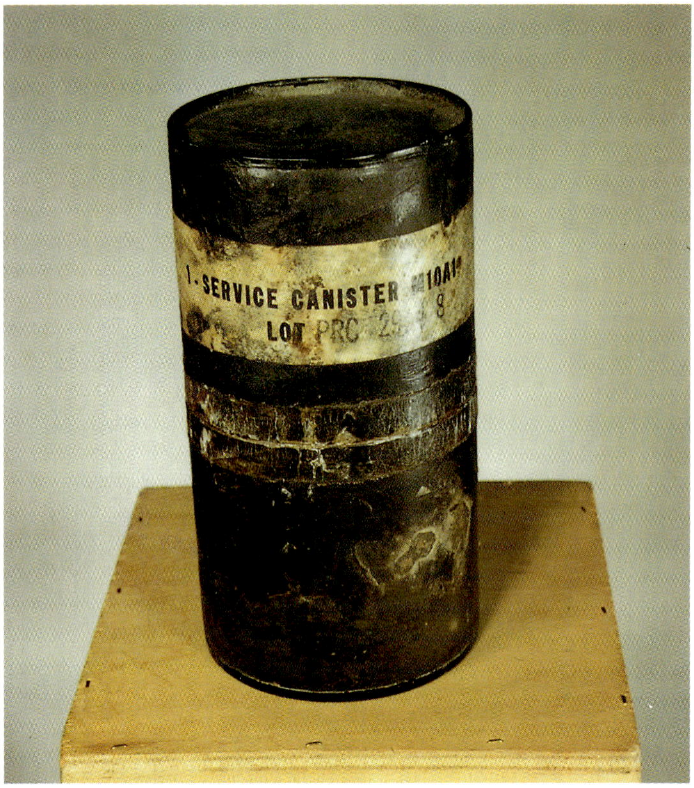

Packaging, M10A1 Filter, 1940s. Example of early M10A1 filter packaging for long term storage, which consisted of heavily waxed cardboard tube with metal caps.

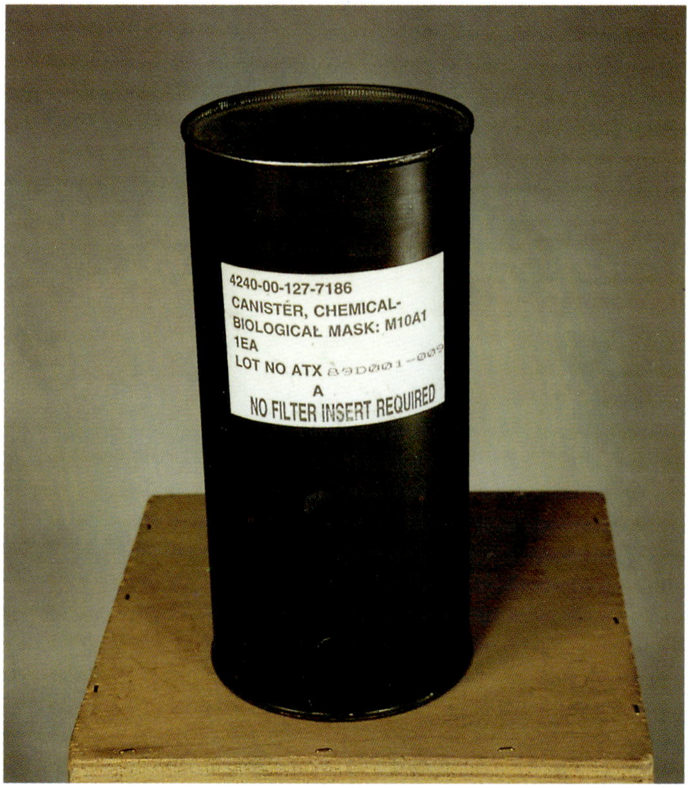

Packaging, M10A1 Filter, 1960s/70s. Example of later style M10A1 filter packaging, consisting of metal can with metal ends.

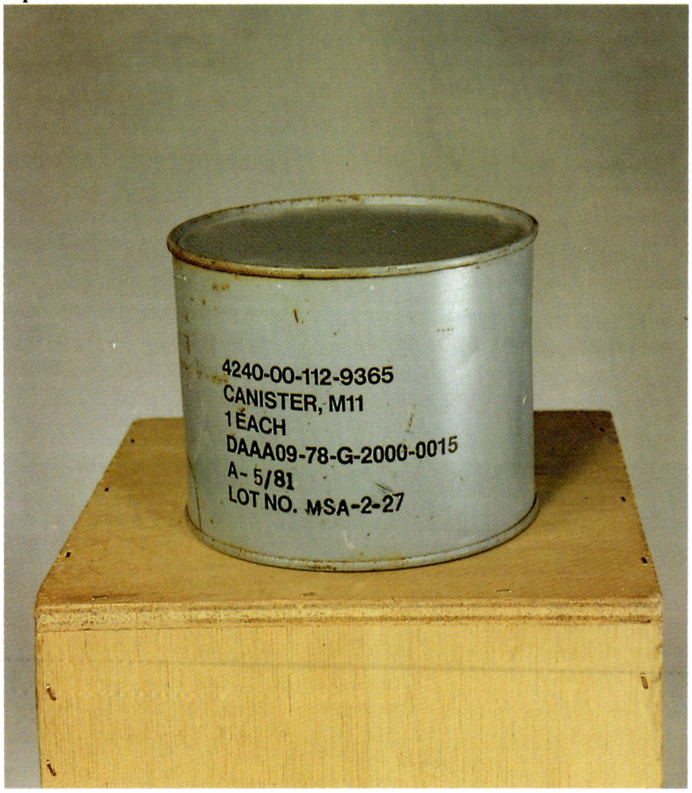

Packaging, M11 Filter, 1980s. Typical hermetically sealed can used for storage of M11 type filters in later years. Earlier versions, produced in the 40s and 50s, also used a similar type of can storage but the tins were of a darker black outer coloration.

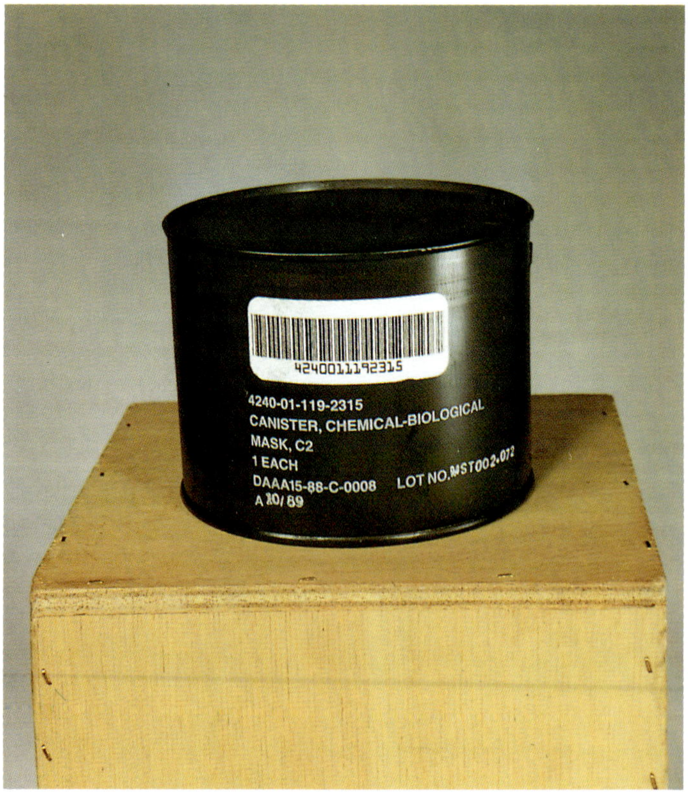

Packaging, C2 NBC Filter, 1980s/90s. Typical modern hermetically sealed filter storage can with identifications and bar coding, used for all current M40/M42 mask compatible filters.

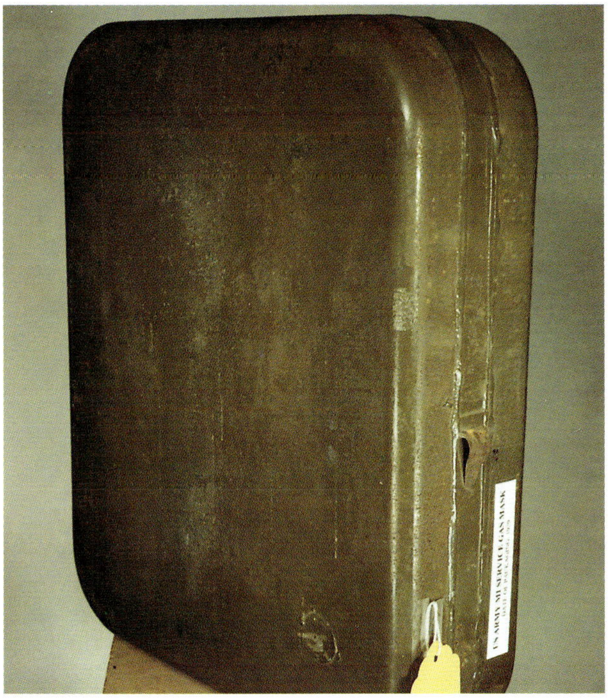

Packaging, U.S. Army Service Gas Masks, 1920s and 30s (early). Pictured is the Storage Container, Gas Mask, Type MI, which was used for long term storage of early MI type service gas masks. The container consists of two metal shells which were joined together with a soldered pull-strip. The air was replaced by Nitrogen gas, although oxidation and rust generally penetrates and releases the inert gas over a period of decades. This type was replaced by the Type II container.

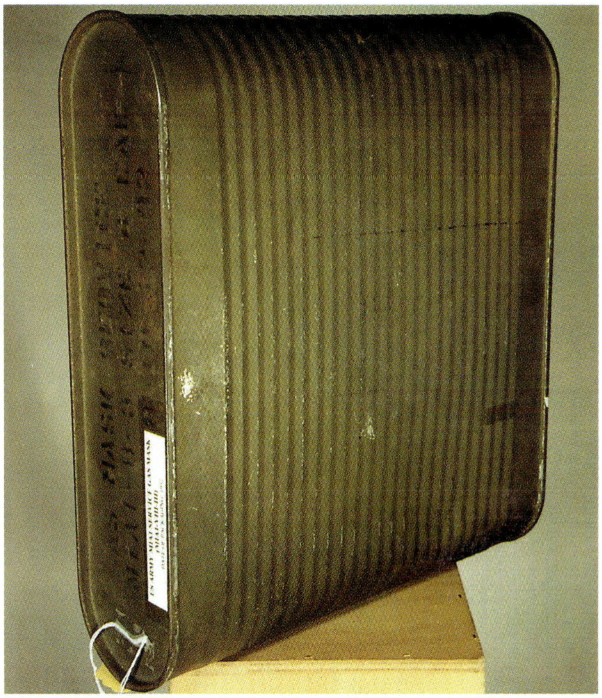

Packaging, U.S. Army Service Gas Masks, 1930s and 40s (late). Storage Container, Service Gas Mask, Type MII. This type of corrugated metal, flattened tube type can replaced the earlier Type MI storage container. It was also filled originally with inert Nitrogen gas, but penetration due to rust frequently results in release of the inert gas and contamination of contents with moisture carrying ambient air.

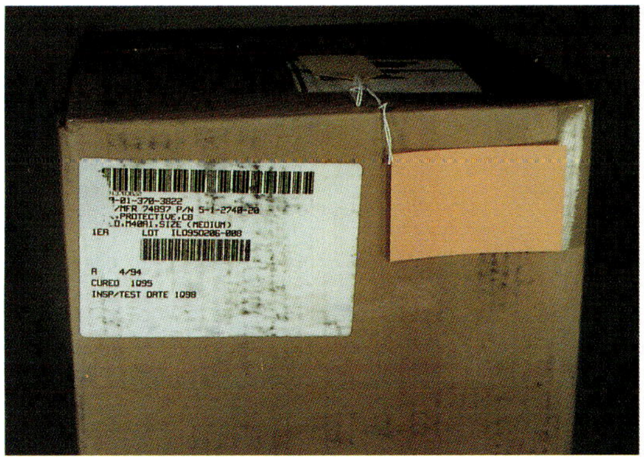

Packaging, U.S. Army M40/M42 Field Protective and Armored Vehicle NBC Masks, 1980s/90s. Shown specimen is an M40A1 Field Protective Mask which, along with its separate accessory and component items, is packed in a series of cardboard boxes and sealed plastic bags.

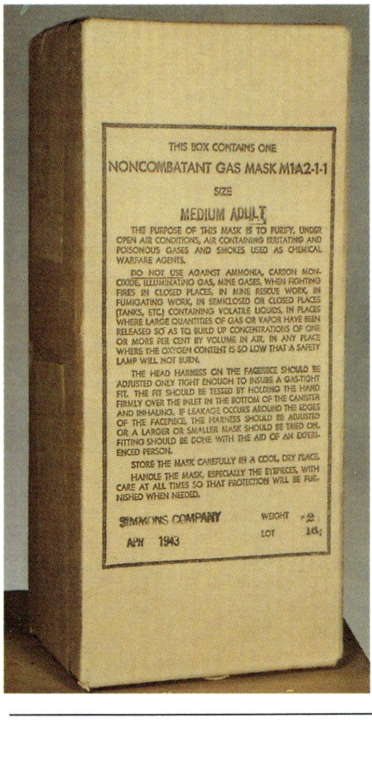

Packaging, U.S. Army Lightweight and Noncombatant type gas masks, WWII. Cardboard boxes (with the mask sealed in transparent cellophane, inside) were frequently used to protect and store masks during the Second World War. The specimen shown in an MIA1 Noncombatant Gas Mask (civilian), dated 1943.

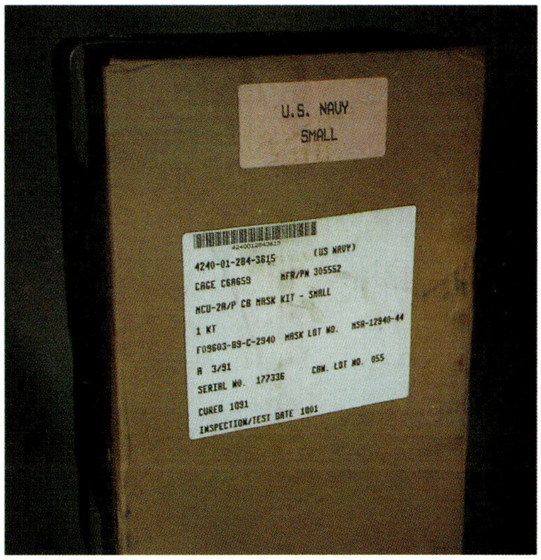

Packaging, USAF/USN MCU-2/P and MCU-2A/P NBC Protective Masks, 1980s/90s. Similar in style and content to the packaging illustrated in plate 467, the C2 and C2A1 filters (of which two are generally issued with each mask) are packed in standard hermetically sealed cans.

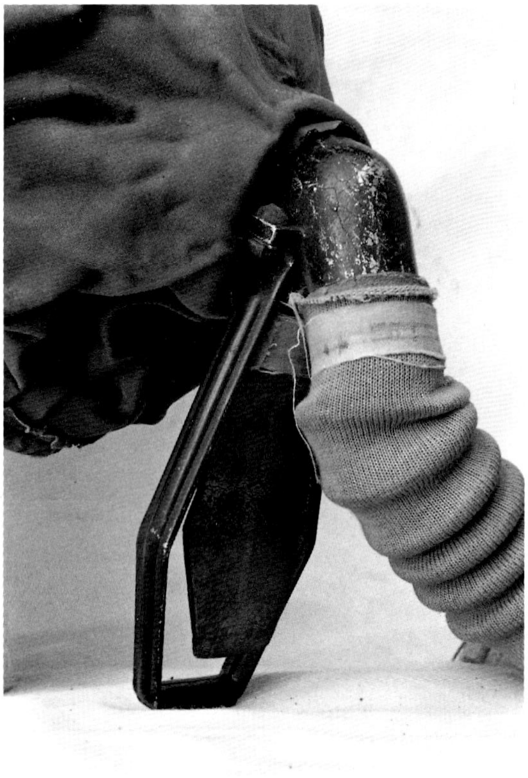

Detail of angle tube and exhalation valve (MI type, with metal guard assembly) on C.E.M. Mask, 1918.

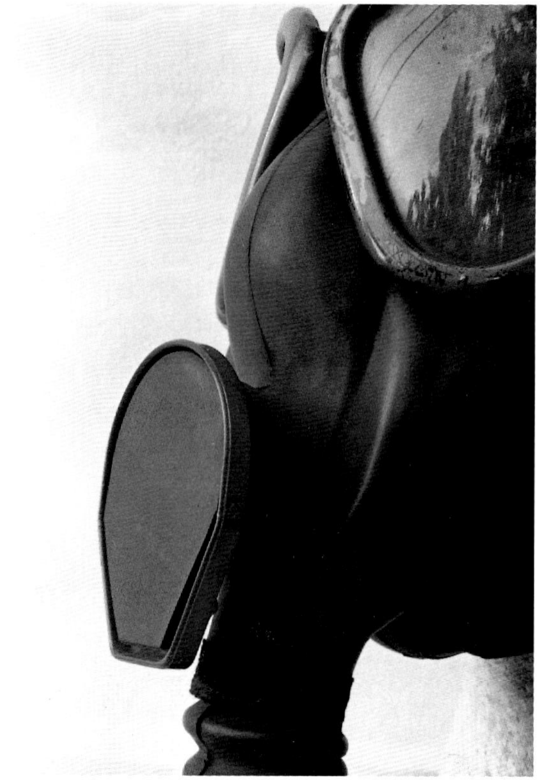

Detail of exhalation valve (Connell, type MV) on M2A1 Service Gas Mask (Heavyweight), 1941. Note plastic valve guard.

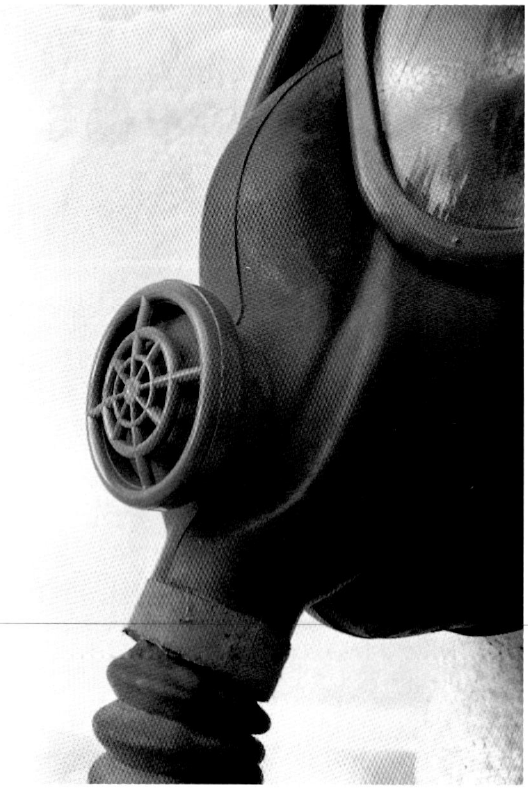

Detail of exhalation valve (Plastic cage, type M8) on M4A1 Service Gas Mask (Lightweight), 1944.

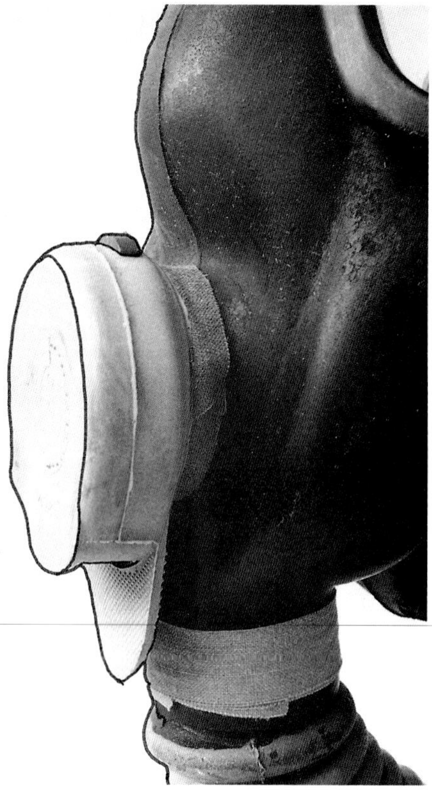

Detail of exhalation valve (rubber shrouded, type C15) on M3A2 Service Gas Mask (Lightweight), 1944.

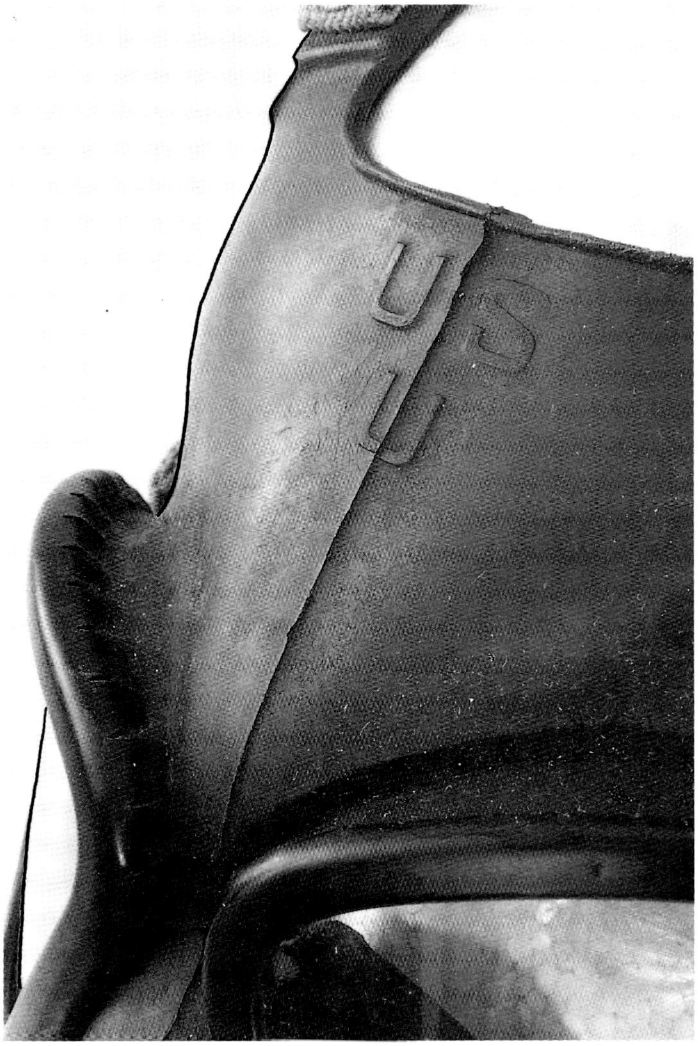

Detail of typical manufacturer ID and date mold marks on M17 exhalation valve shroud (60s) and later series mask (shown is an early M17, dated 64 and manufactured by MSA).

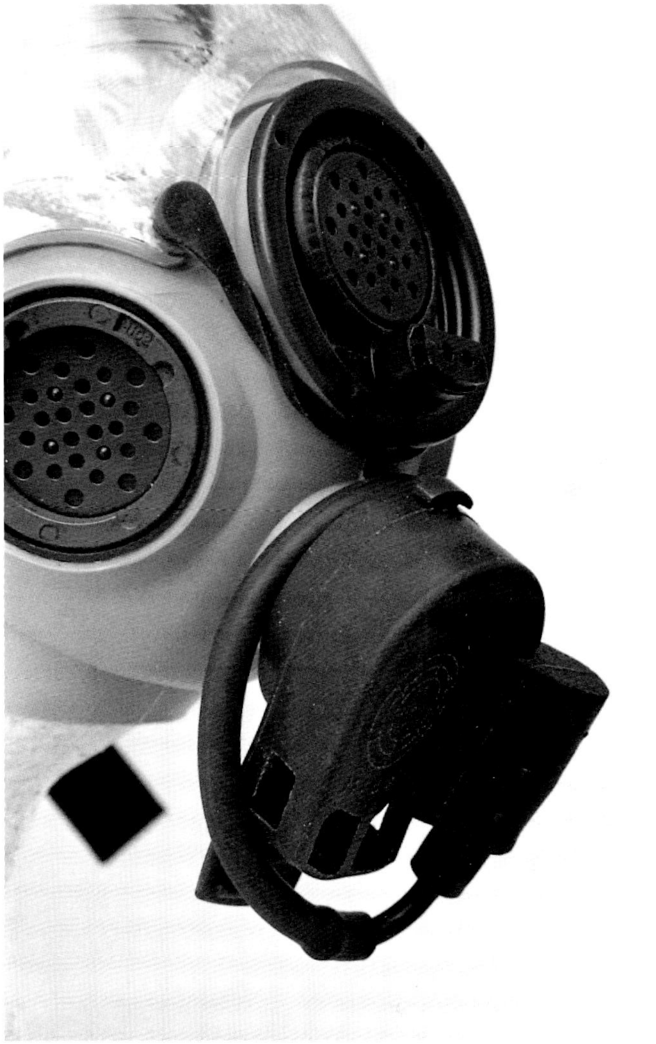

Detail of exhalation valve shroud and drink tube assembly (external) on MCU-2A/P type NBC mask (late 80s & 90s). Note ID/date mold mark on shroud.

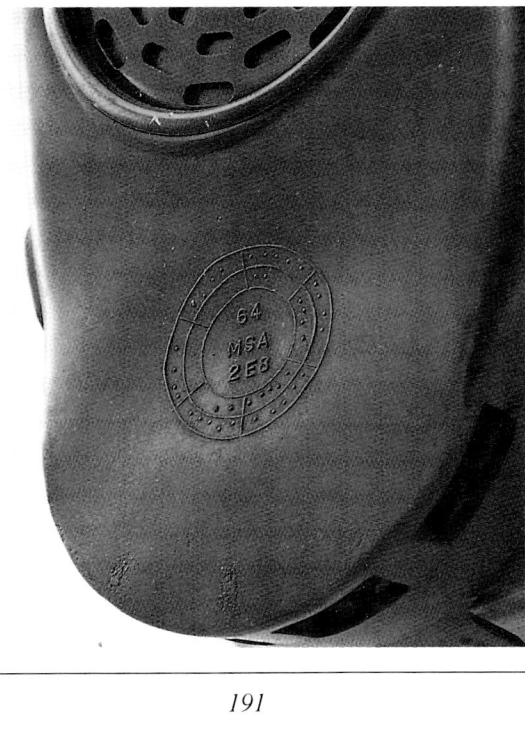

Detail of typical manufacturer ID and date mold marks on M17 exhalation valve shroud (60s) and later series mask (shown is an early M17, dated 64 and manufactured by MSA).

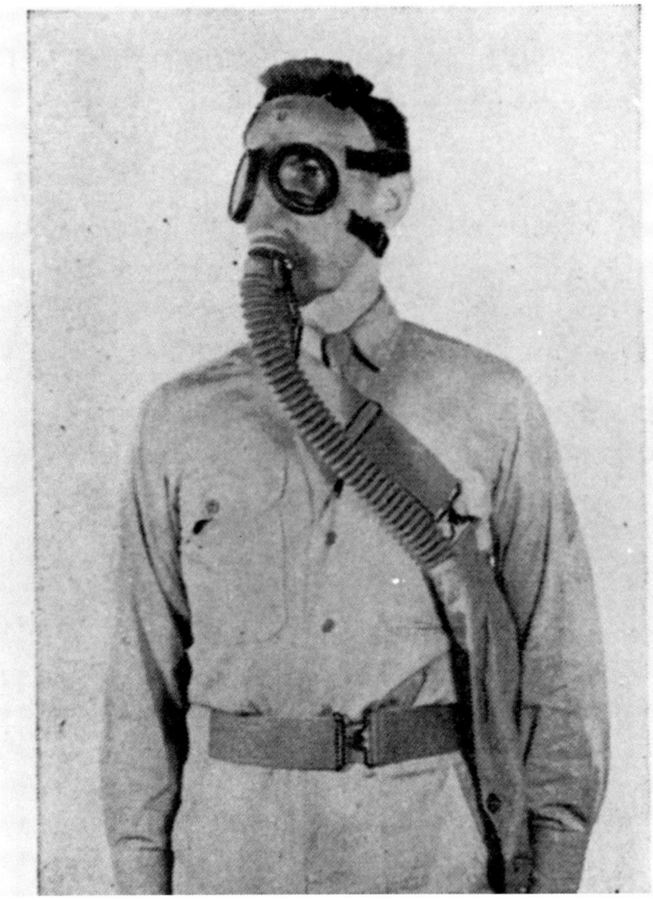

MIA2 Army Service Gas Mask (Heavyweight) as worn in actual use, 1936. (Courtesy of U.S. Army Chemical Warfare Museum, Ft. McClellan, Alabama).

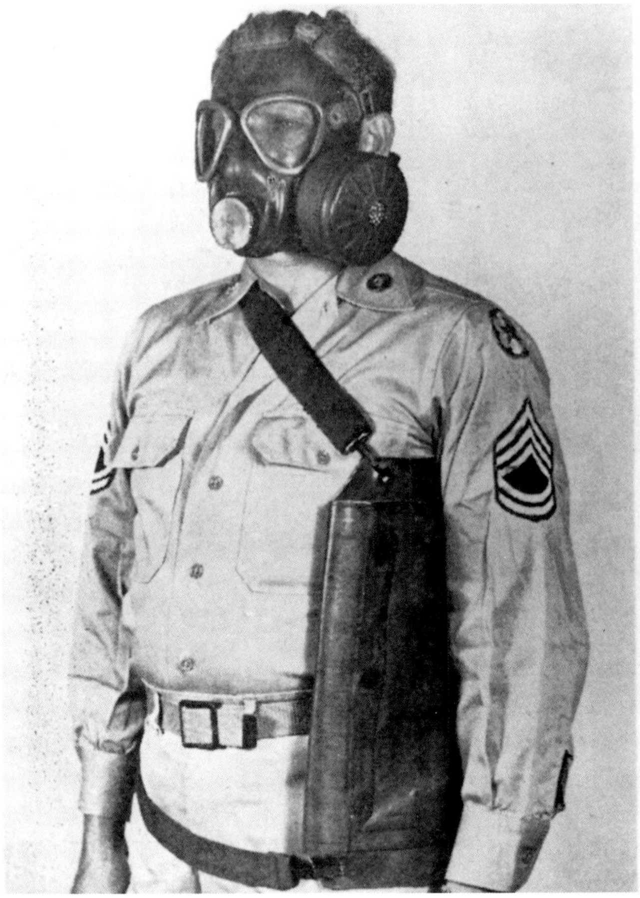

M5-11-7 Assault Gas Mask (Combat Service Mask), neoprene, as worn, 1944. Note watertight assault landing style carrier. (Courtesy of U.S. Army Chemical Warfare Museum, Ft. McClellan, Alabama).

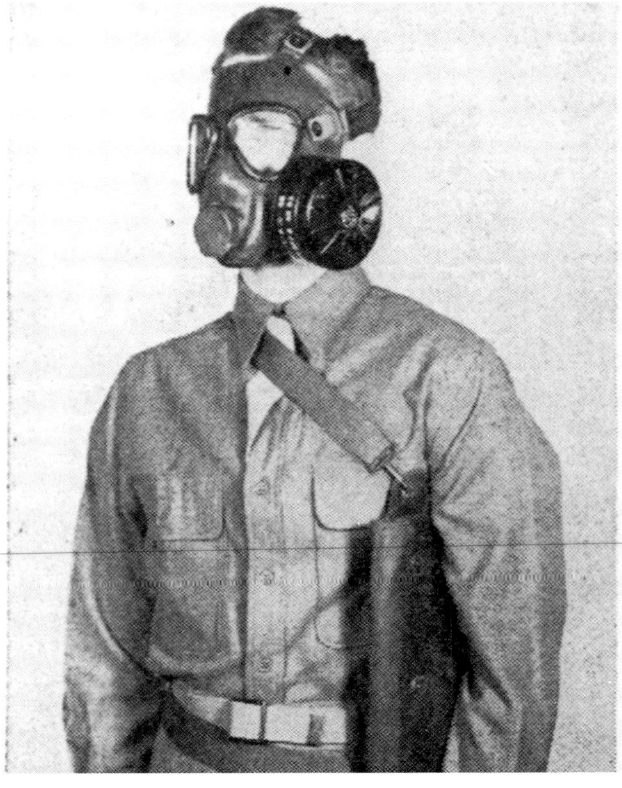

M5-11-7 Assault Gas Mask (Combat Service Mask), neoprene, as worn, 1944. A second example, showing the proofed, watertight carrier. (Courtesy of U.S. Army Chemical Warfare Museum, Ft. McClellan, Alabama).

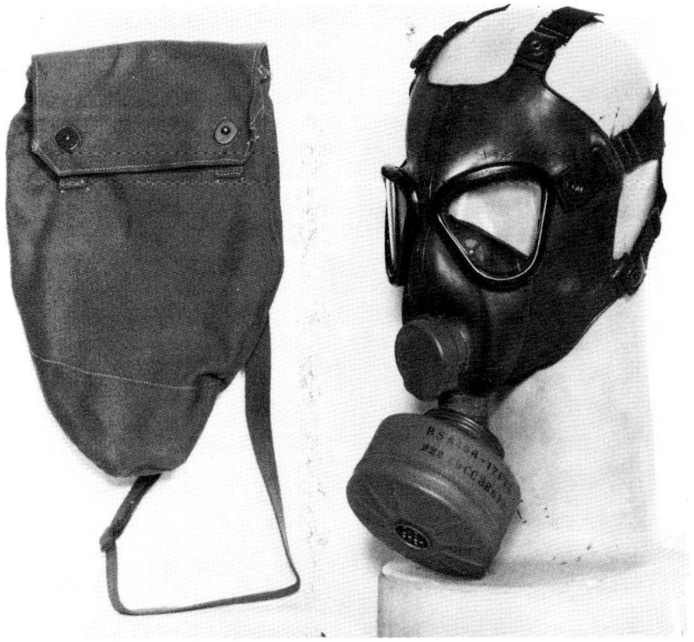

M8-11-10 Snout Type Gas Mask, neoprene facepiece, C15 exhalation valve, 1945. Shown with carrier and early M11 style filter. Note lack of 'rifle skids' on facepiece, indicative of later of two variants. (Courtesy of U.S. Army Chemical Warfare Museum, Ft. McClellan, Alabama).

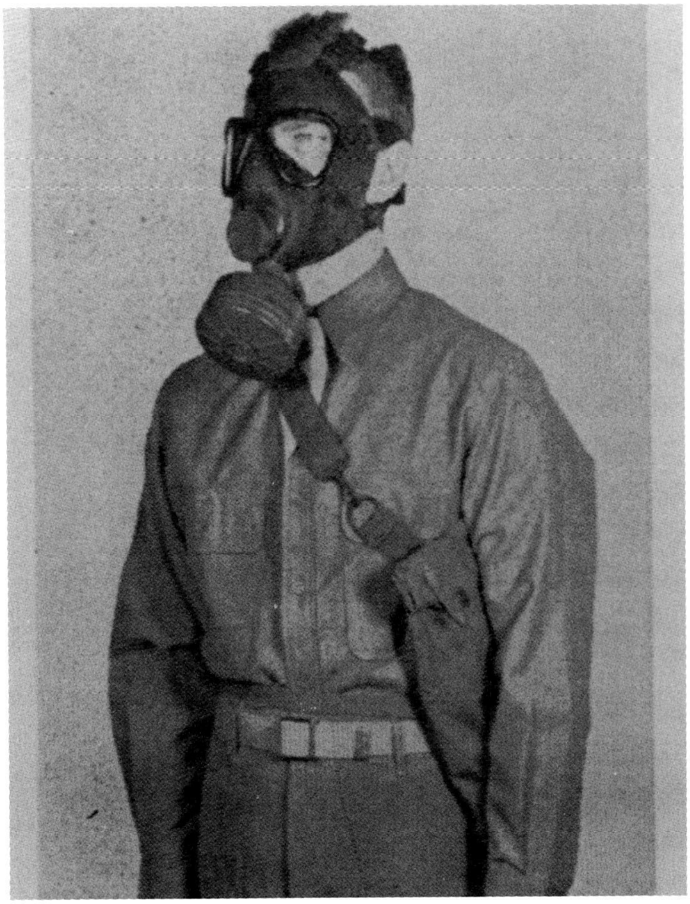

M8-11-10 Snout Type Gas Mask, as worn, showing M10 carrier, 1945. (Courtesy of U.S. Army Chemical Warfare Museum, Ft. McClellan, Alabama).

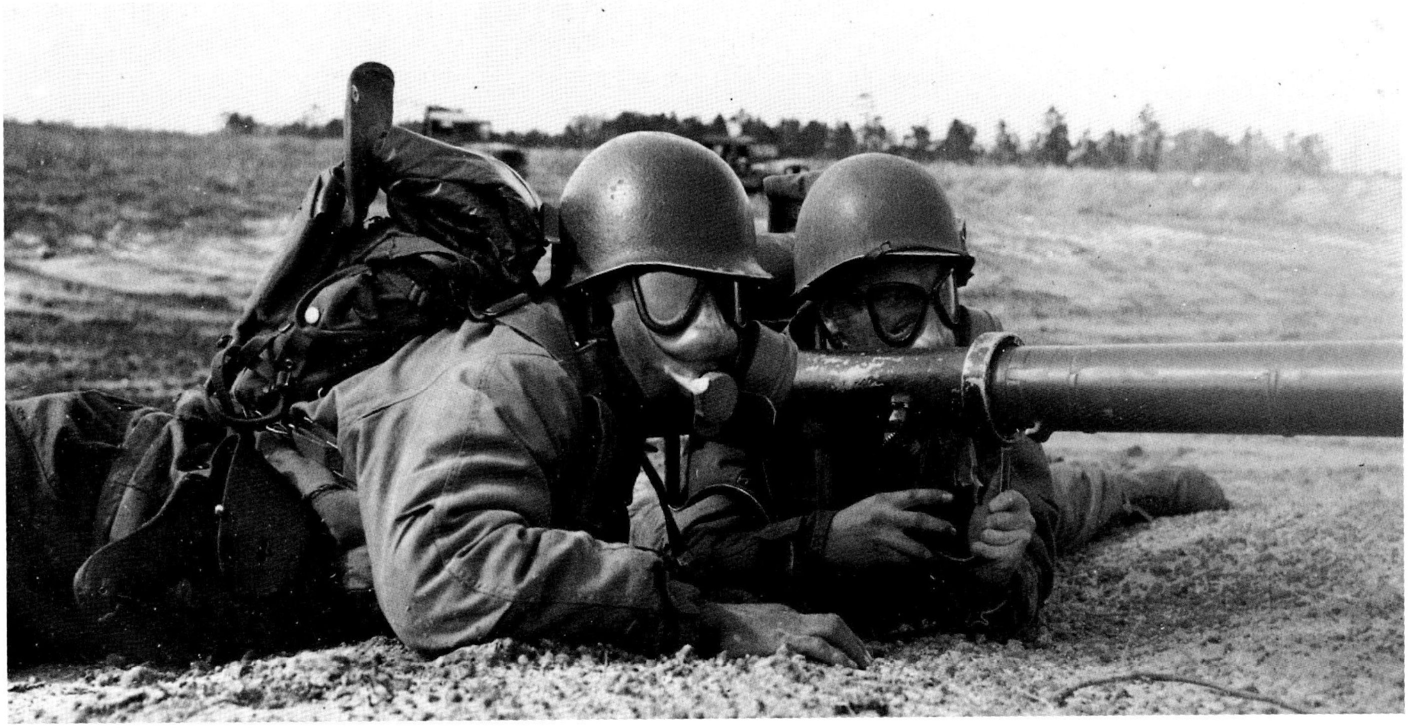

Action photograph showing two U.S. infantry soldiers wearing M9 Field Protective Masks while on field training exercises at Fort Benning, GA, 1950s. (Courtesy of U.S. Army Chemical Warfare Museum, Ft. McClellan, Alabama).

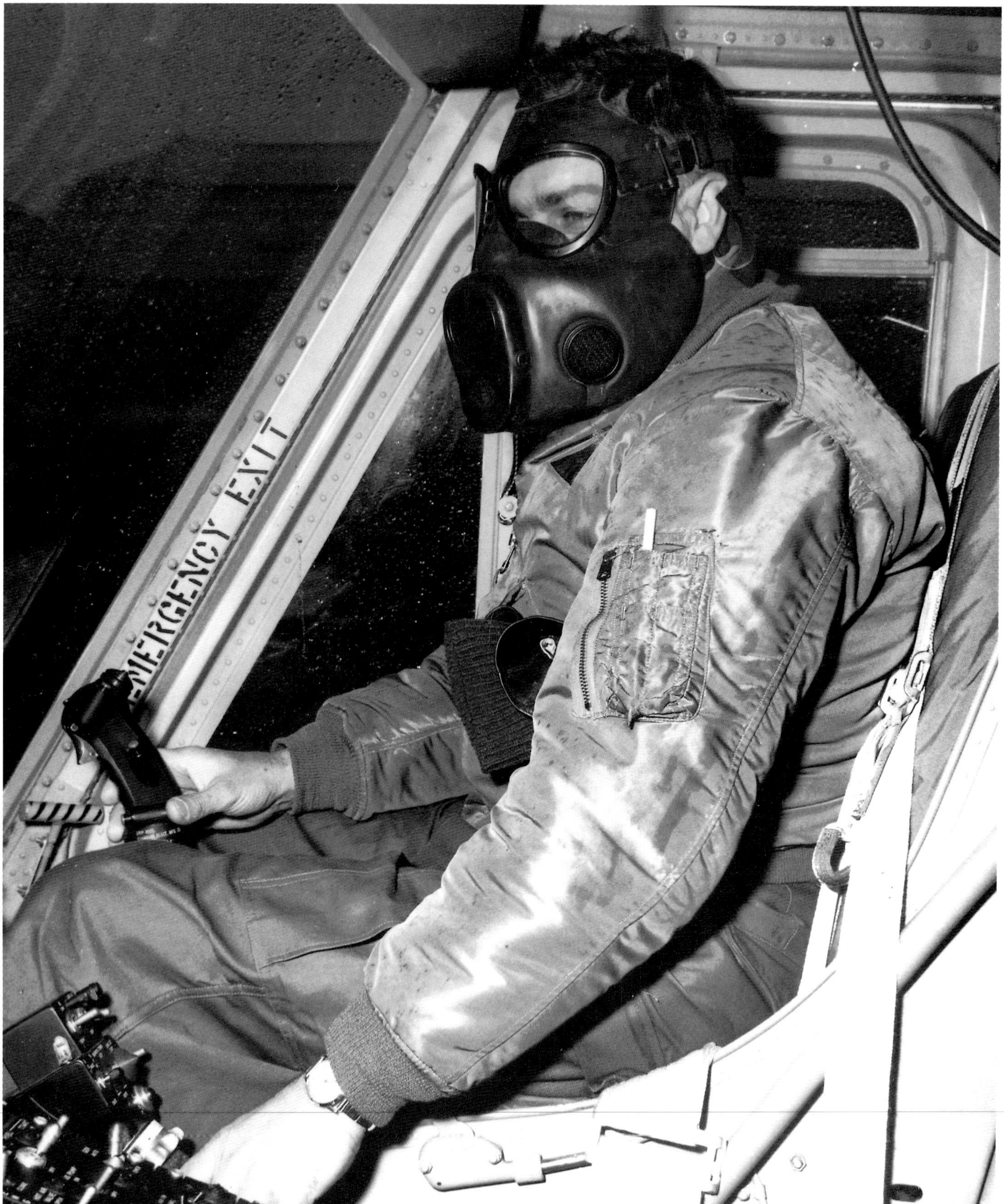

Photograph showing an Army helicopter pilot wearing an M17 mask on flight operations, 1963. (Courtesy of U.S. Army Chemical Warfare Museum, Ft. McClellan, Alabama).

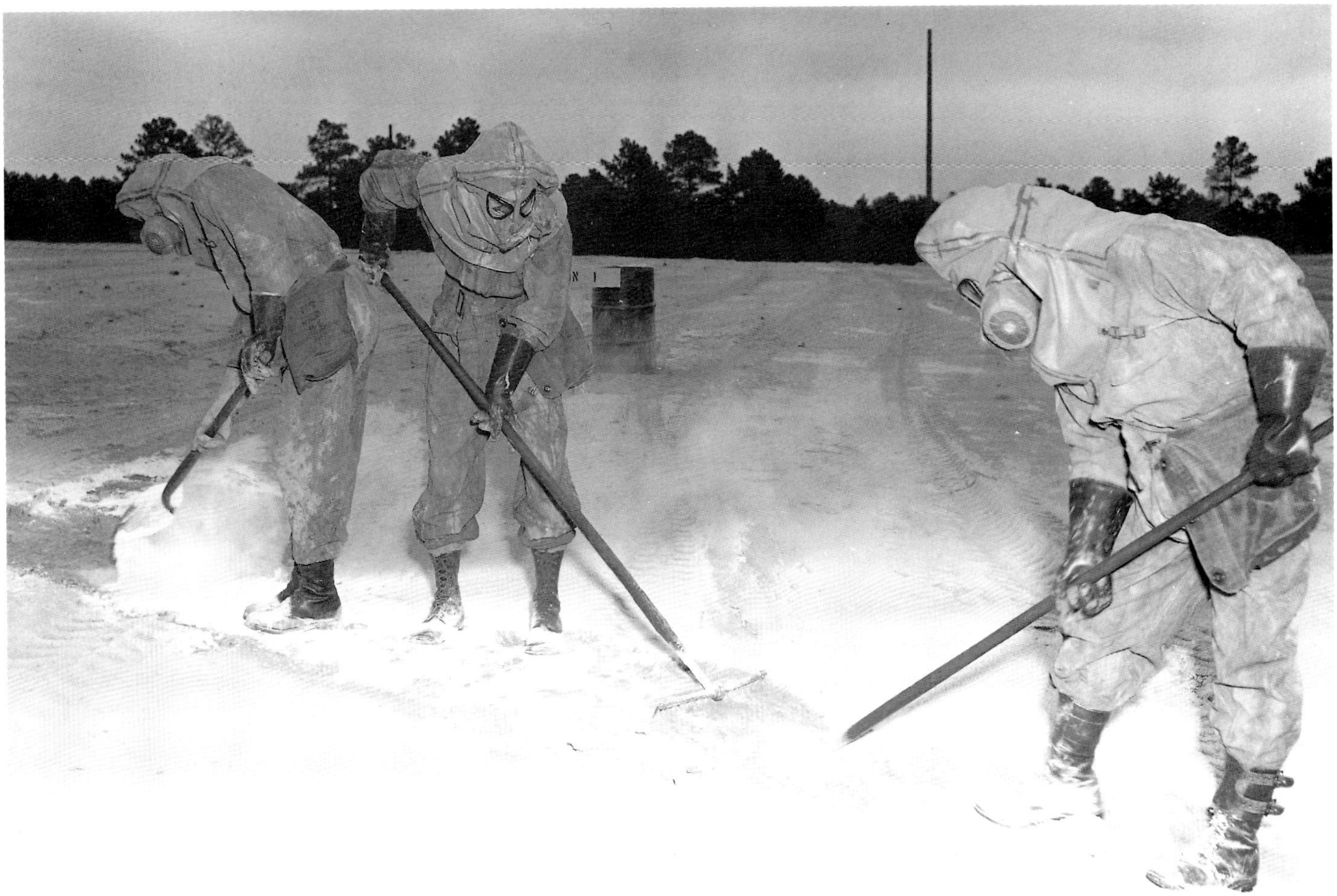

U.S. Army soldiers wearing full NBC protection, including M9 respirators, at Fort Bragg CBR School in 1957, while participating in a 5-day decontamination course. (Courtesy of U.S. Army Chemical Warfare Museum, Ft. McClellan, Alabama).

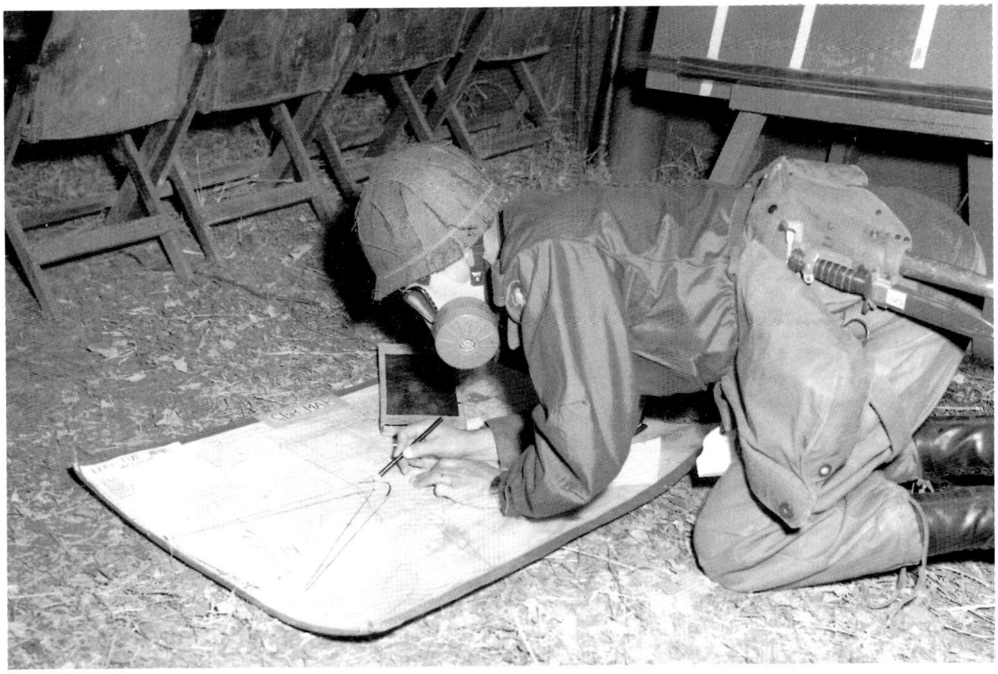

Member of 444th Transportation Company (Light Truck), plotting aggressor's location during simulated gas attack, 1962. (Courtesy of U.S. Army Chemical Warfare Museum, Ft. McClellan, Alabama).

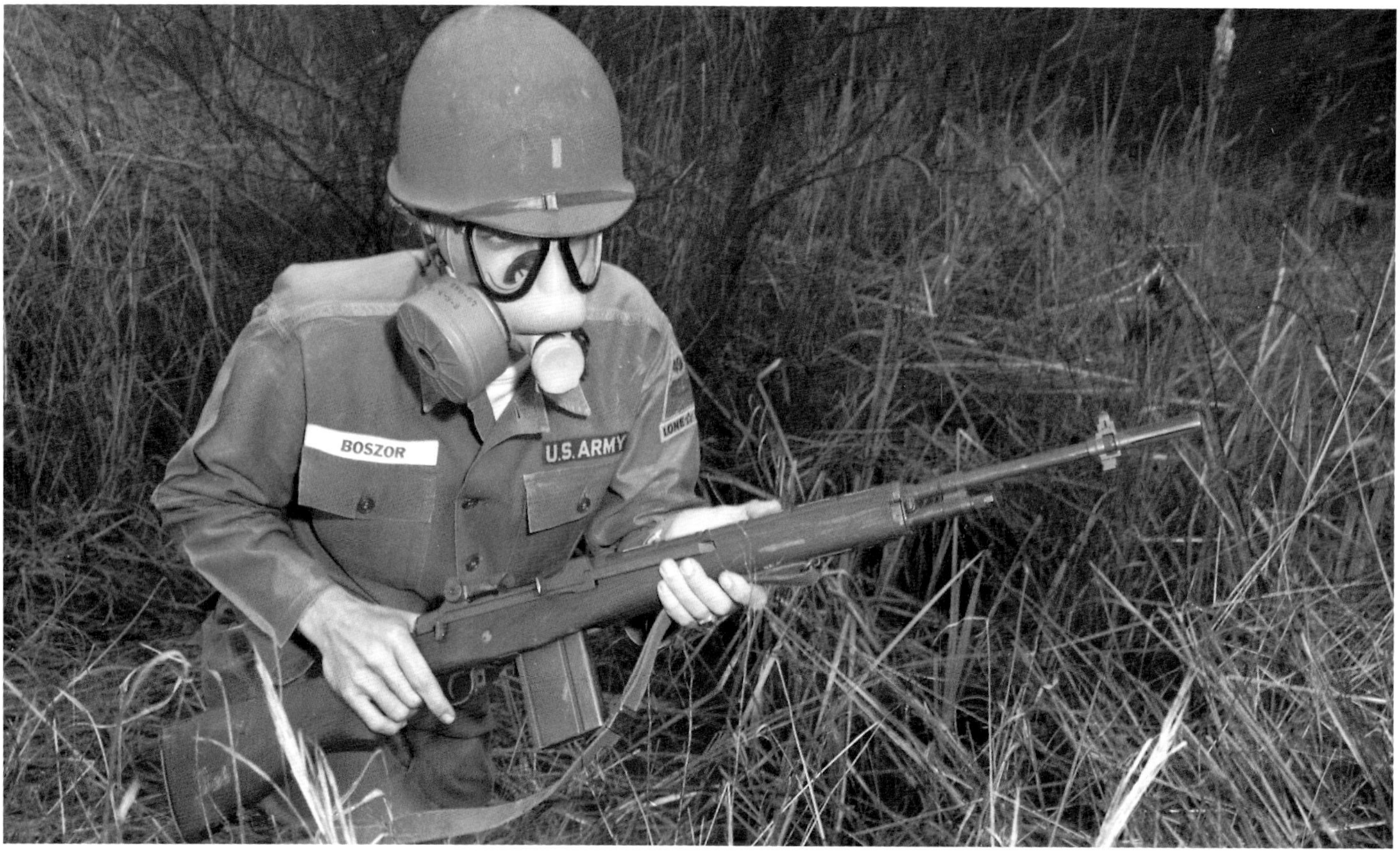

2Lt. Richard Boszor of 2nd Armored Battalion demonstrates use of M9A1 respirator during maneuvers at Fort Polk, LA, 1962. (Courtesy of U.S. Army Chemical Warfare Museum, Ft. McClellan, Alabama).

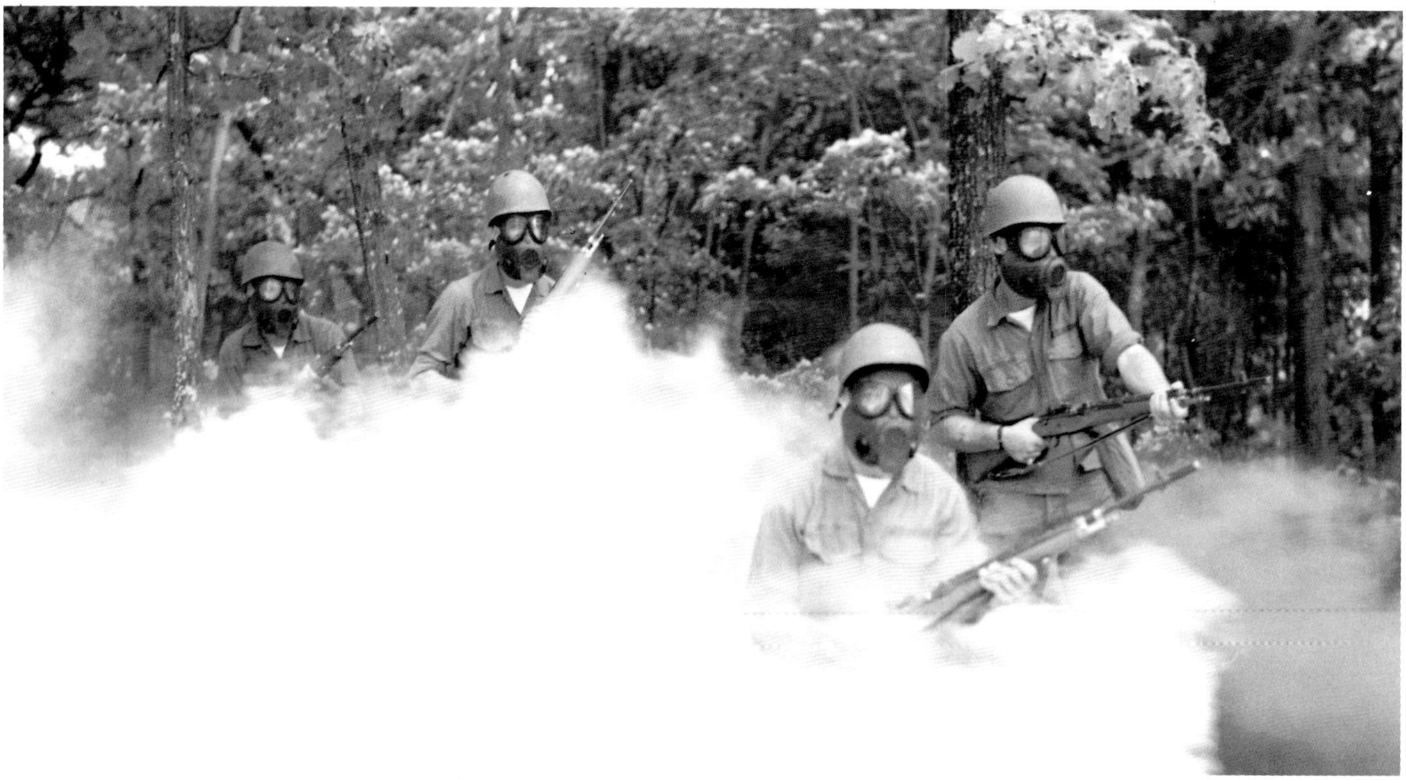

6th Infantry exercises conducted at Fort Campbell, KY, during 1968, included simulation of CBR attack scenarios. M17 respirator is being worn. (Courtesy of U.S. Army Chemical Warfare Museum, Ft. McClellan, Alabama).

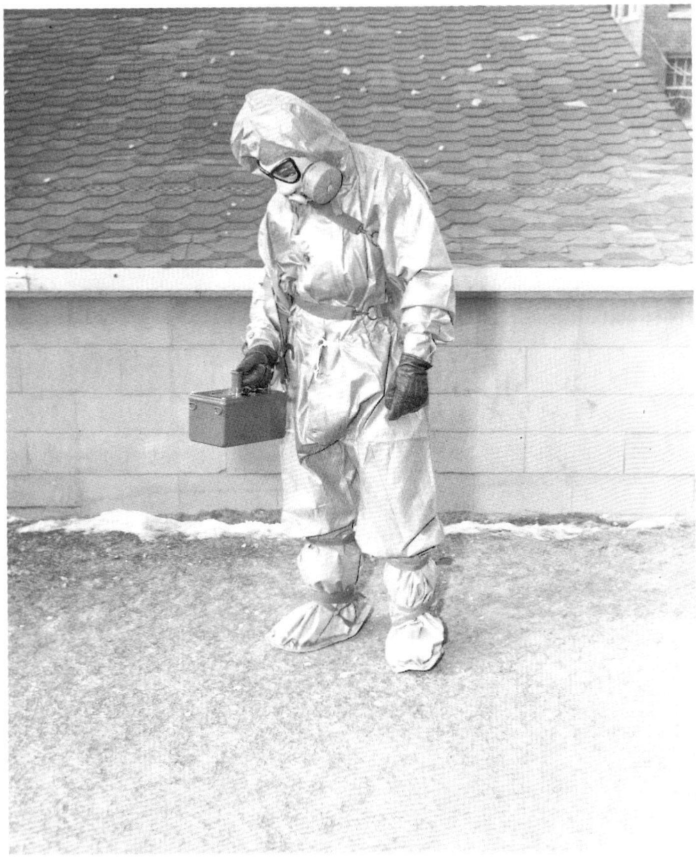

U.S. Army soldier demonstrates use of radiation detection equipment while wearing full CBR protective clothing (including M9A1 respirator), Fort Wayne, IN, 1960. (Courtesy of U.S. Army Chemical Warfare Museum, Ft. McClellan, Alabama).

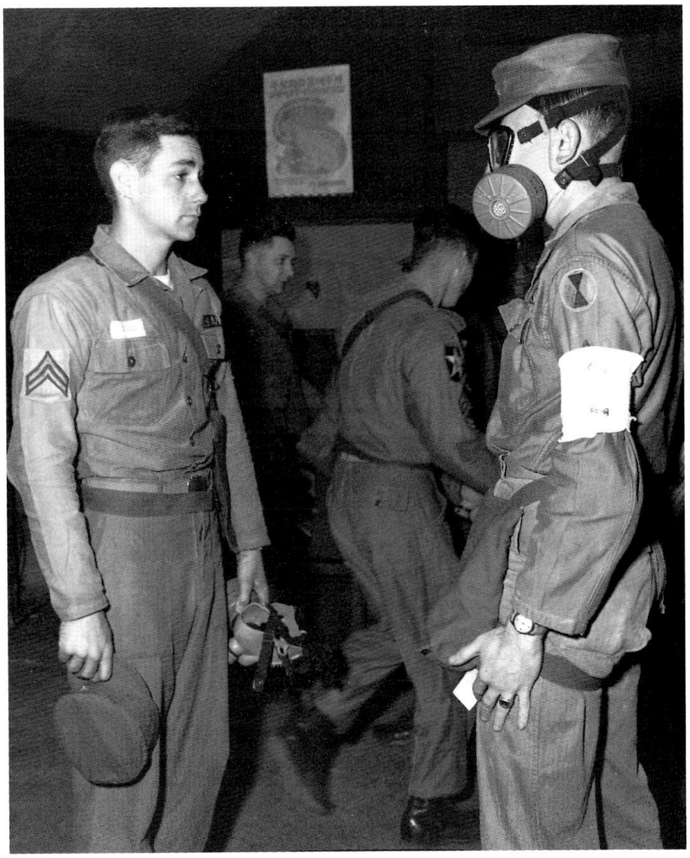

Members of the 7th U.S. Infantry Division, undergoing CBR training (use of agent CN), Korea 1955. (Courtesy of U.S. Army Chemical Warfare Museum, Ft. McClellan, Alabama).

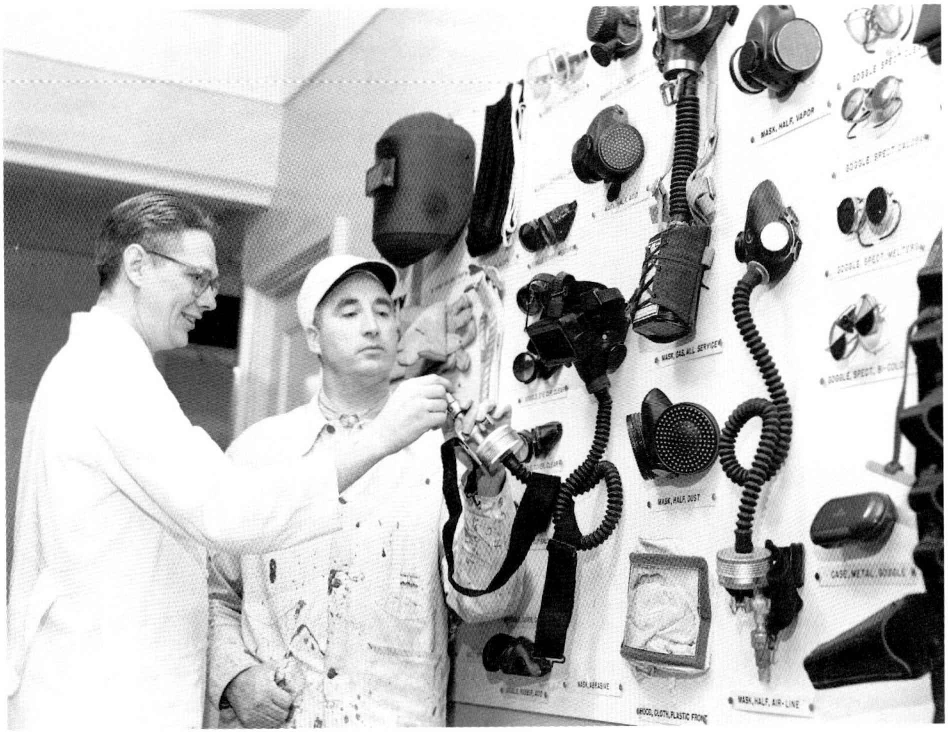

U.S. Navy civilian workers examine display of mid-50s respiratory protection equipment. Note M11/M12 type respirator at top of display board, circa 1956. (U.S. Navy photograph).

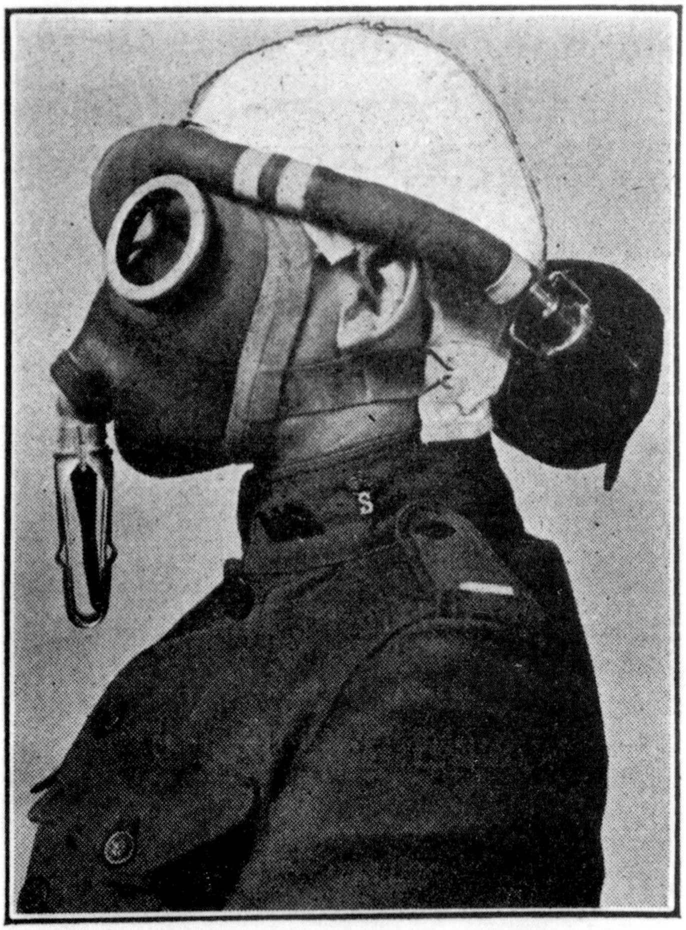

Photograph of early U.S. Navy "Head Mask and Canister" (1918), a predecessor of the later U.S. Navy Head Canister (old) Mark II respirator with which it is frequently confused. The design appears to have been put together using an A.T. type mask that has had its angle tube assembly modified (capped off) and bears some resemblance to the much later U.S. Army optical mask and U.S. Navy Diaphragm Gas Masks.

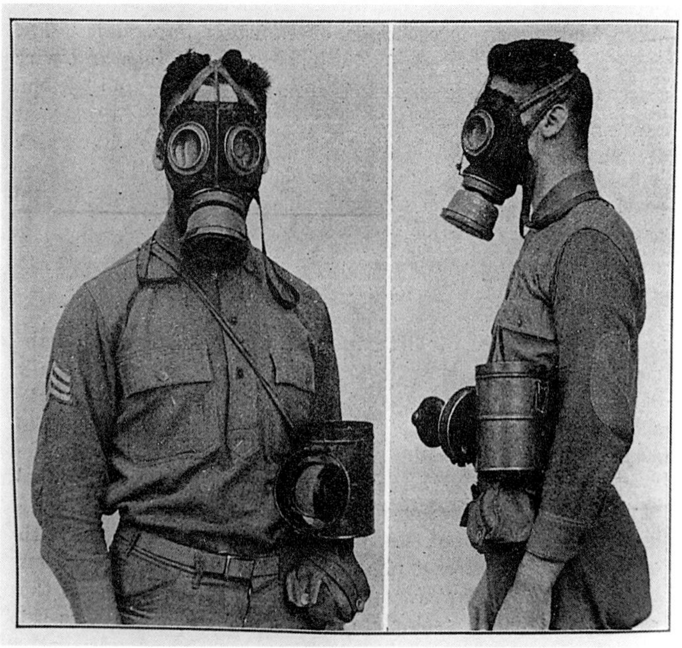

Photograph of the German World War One gas mask which was the inspiration for the U.S. Navy Mouth Canister (old) Mark I Gas Mask. The specimen shown was made with a leather facepiece, 1916.

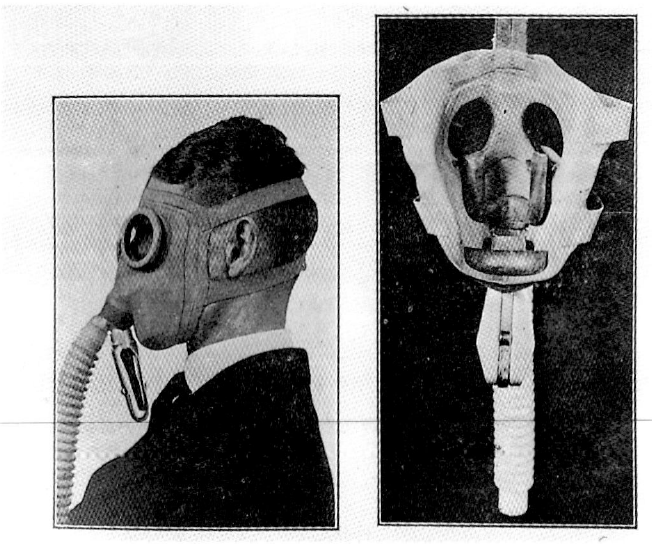

Photograph of an early American Tissot Mask (A.T. Mask), 1919. Along with the K.T. and final K.T.M masks, one of the important designs which yielded the Model 1919 (MI) mask.

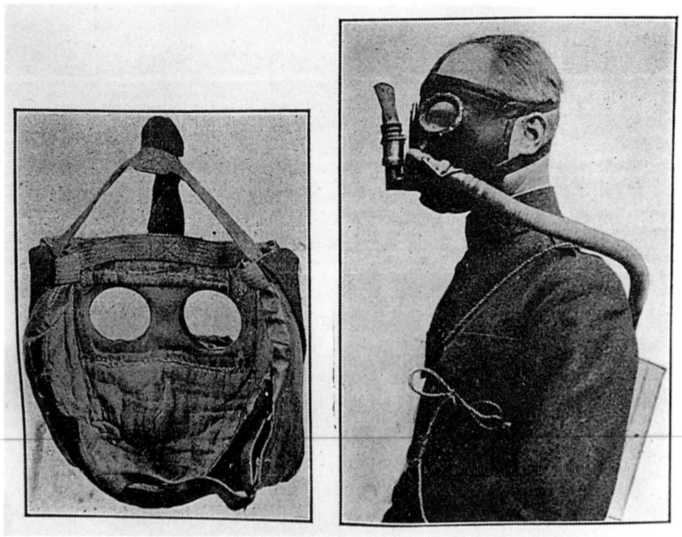

Photograph of the interior of the WWI French M-2 mask (left) and the exterior of the French Tissot-type Artillery Mask (right). The Tissot artillery mask's functional principles significantly influenced the development of U.S. gas mask design developments during and after the First World War.

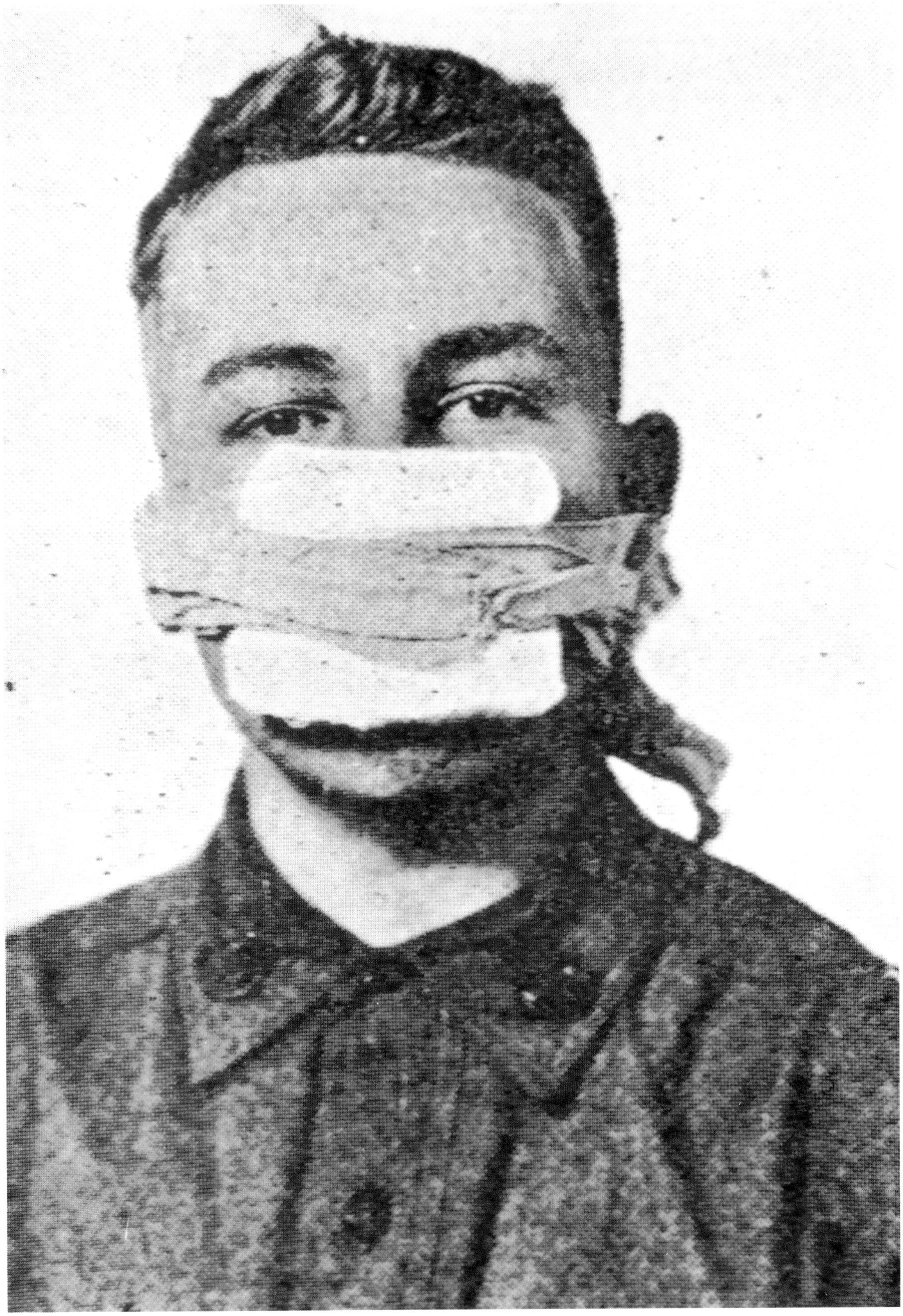

Photograph of very early British WWI anti-gas protection, known as the "Mouth Muff." Basically cotton pads wrapped in muslin gauze which were tied against the mouth and providing very poor protection when dry, their effect was enhanced if they were first soaked in water, urine or photographic 'Hypo.' (Photo from *Chemical Warfare*, by Fries and West).

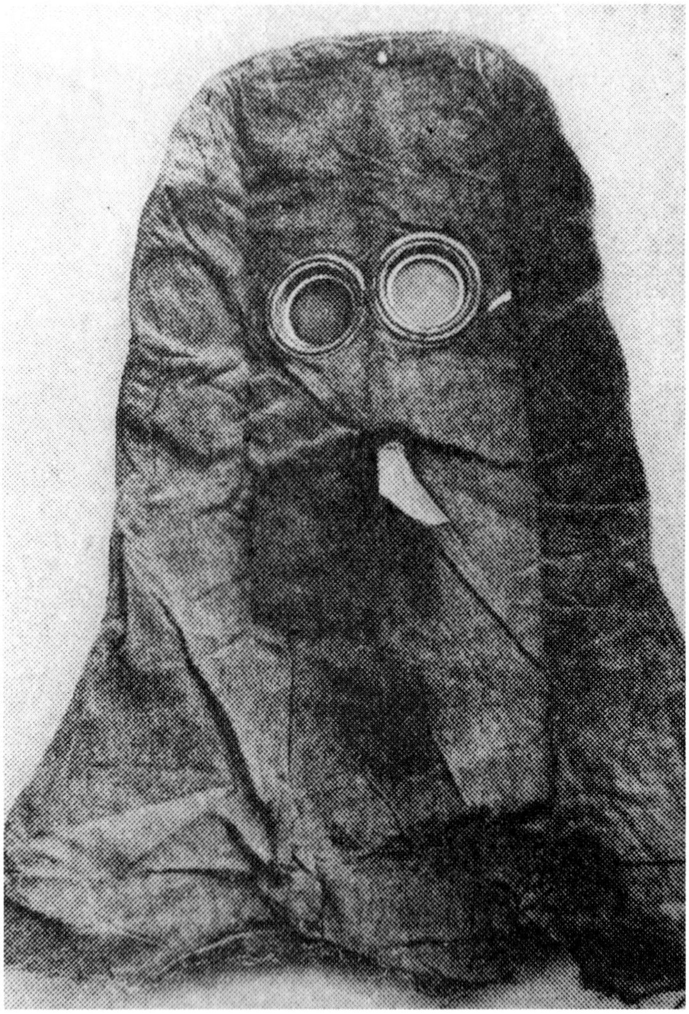

Photograph of the WWI British PH Helmet, which was made of 2 layers of flannelette material that had been pre-soaked in a solution of urotropin, caustic soda, phenol and glycerine. It offered no protection against lachrymals and goggles were issued to be worn under them. The PH Helmet was superseded by the Harrison Tower Box or 'Large Box Respirator' when it became obvious in 1916 that far more protection was needed. (Photo from *Chemical Warfare*, by Fries and West).

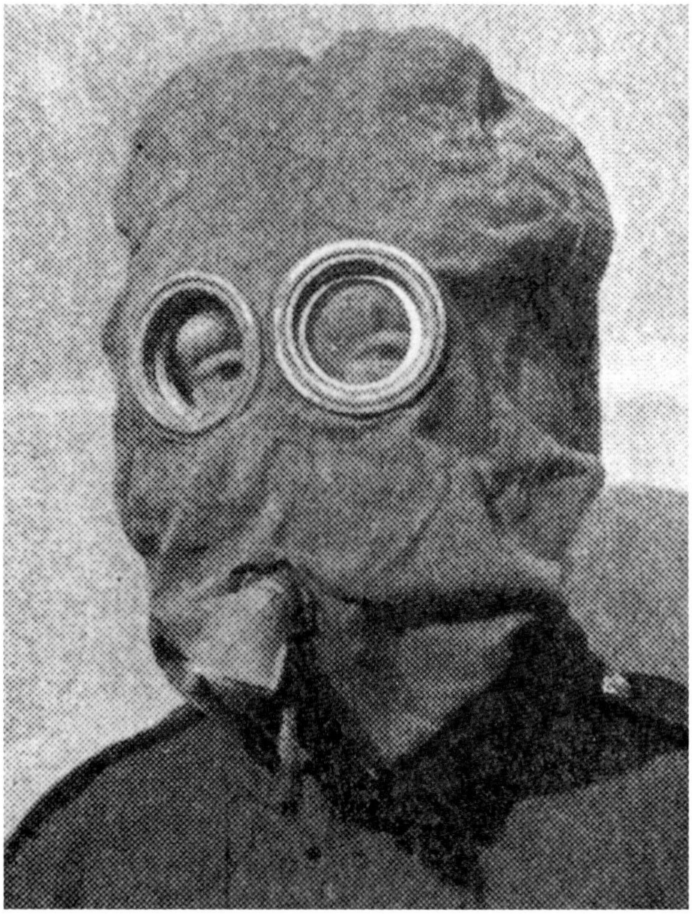

Another photograph of a WWI British PH Helmet being worn; note the rudimentary rubber 'flapper' valve and the lower skirt section of the helmet, which was normally worn tucked into the collar of the soldier's tunic. (Photo from *Chemical Warfare*, by Fries and West).

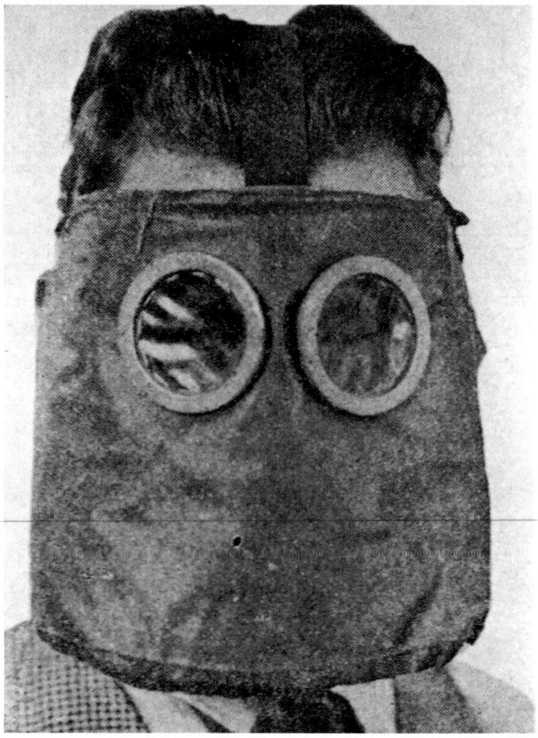

Photograph of the exterior of the WWI French M-2, which was carried by AEF soldiers as a spare or emergency back-up form of protection in the event their small box respirator failed. The M-2 used 40 layers of muslin gauze impregnated with two kinds of chemical preparation and had celluloid eyepieces. (Photo from *Chemical Warfare*, by Fries and West).

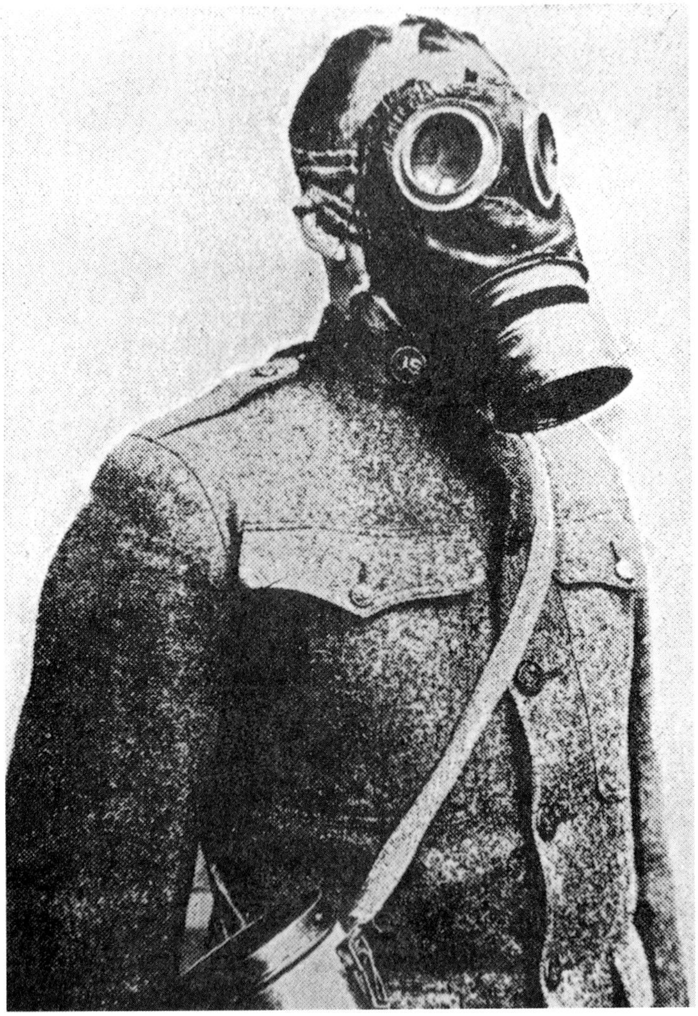

Photograph of an American soldier modeling WWI vintage 'The German Mask,' with its leather faceplece and snout-attached filter canister. The mask tended to 'bellow' with each respiratory cycle due its not having an expiration valve (air was taken in and exhaled through the filter). (Photo from *Chemical Warfare*, by Fries and West).

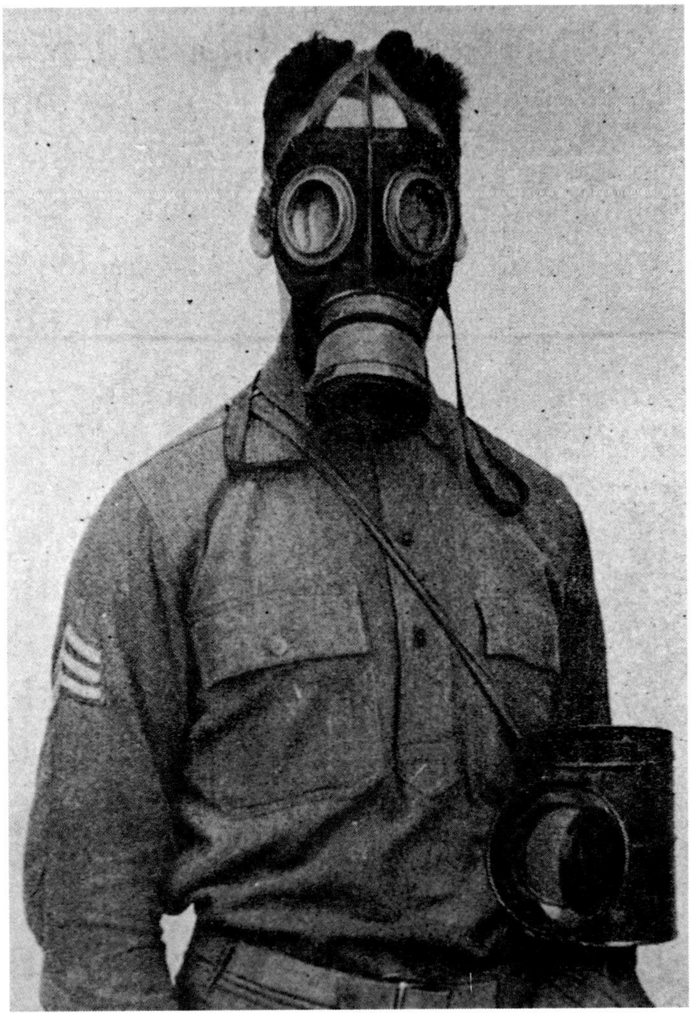

Another photograph of an American soldier wearing 'The German Mask.' Note the 'at the ready' neck strap and the enameled metal carrying container. The German mask influenced many other designs of the snout type and served as the direct inspiration for the US Navy's WWI vintage Mk. I Mouth Canister Mask, with which it shares a more than passing resemblance. (Photo from *Chemical Warfare*, by Fries and West).

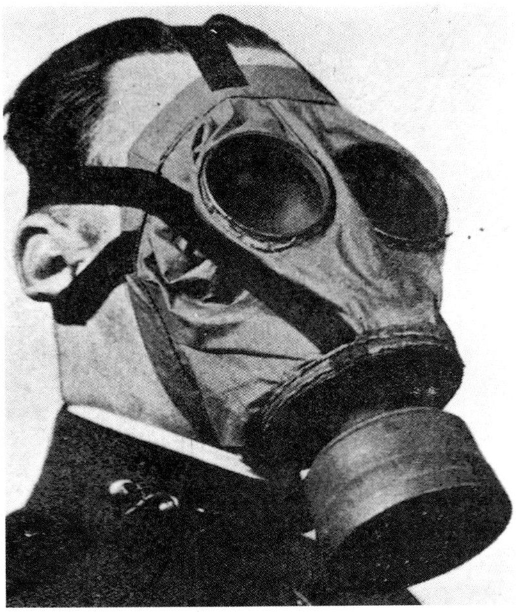

Photograph of the WWI US Navy Mk. I Mouth Canister mask, which was visually very similar to the Austrian (KuK) version of the German mask. Note external black canister weight bearing straps. Unlike the German and Austrian snout-type masks, the US Navy mask used a flapper type exhalation valve and did not bellow during the respiratory cycle. The US officer modeling the mask is wearing the crossed chemical retort insignia of the Chemical Service on his collar. (Photo from *Chemical Warfare*, by Fries and West).

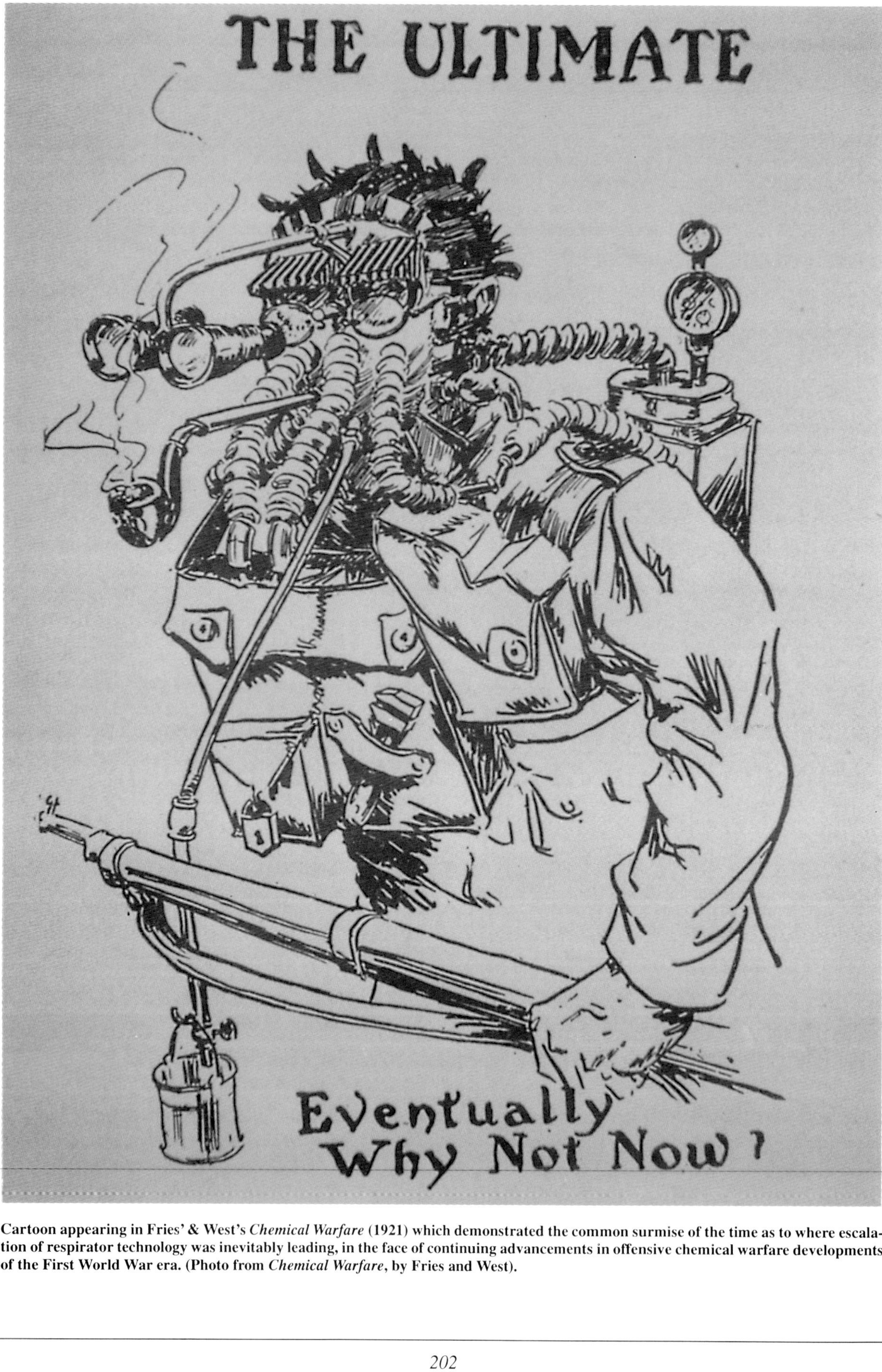

Cartoon appearing in Fries' & West's *Chemical Warfare* (1921) which demonstrated the common surmise of the time as to where escalation of respirator technology was inevitably leading, in the face of continuing advancements in offensive chemical warfare developments of the First World War era. (Photo from *Chemical Warfare*, by Fries and West).

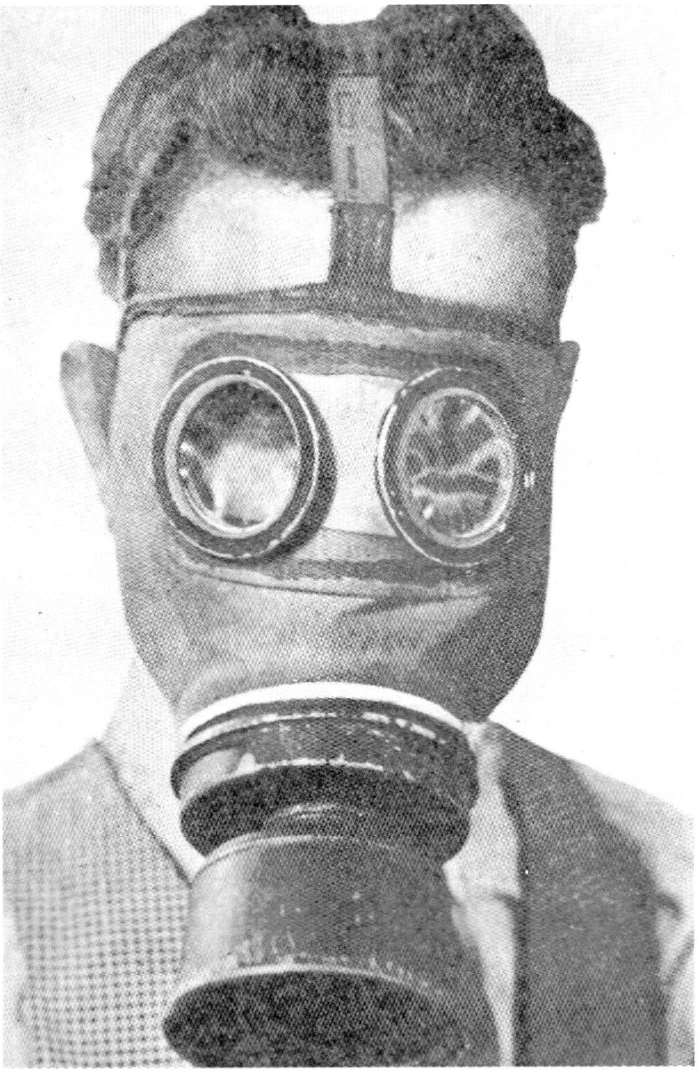

Photograph of a civilian wearing the post WWI vintage French A.R.S. Mask. Later versions used a slightly angled filter attachment plate, although the mask remained largely identical to its earlier form. Amazingly, this ancient mask has been seen worn by protesting French civilians a protection against police lachrymal agents as late as the early 90s. (Photo from *Chemical Warfare*, by Fries and West).

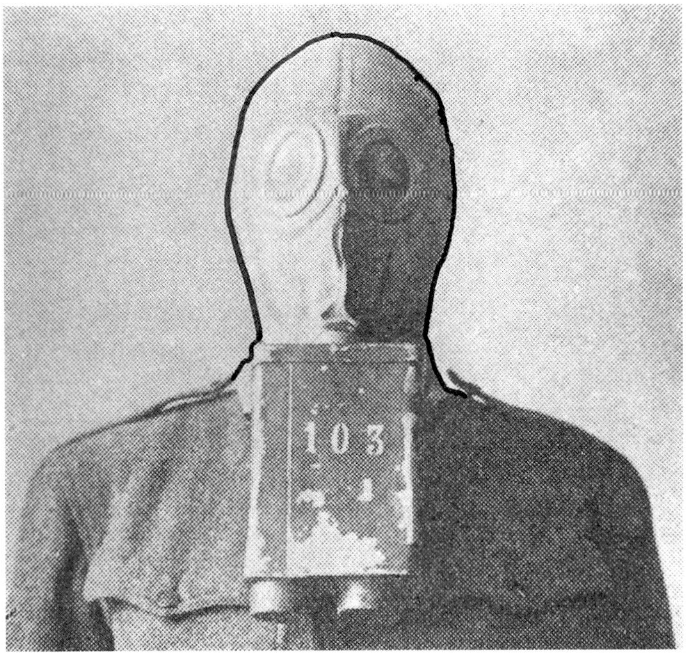

Poor quality photograph of the Russian Selinski-Kumandt protective respirator, which first used the rubber head-hood concept that would continue in use up through recent years, mostly in former Soviet Bloc nations and Russia. The rubber hood provided excellent overall protection but was hot and uncomfortable to wear for protracted periods. (Photo from *Chemical Warfare*, by Fries and West).

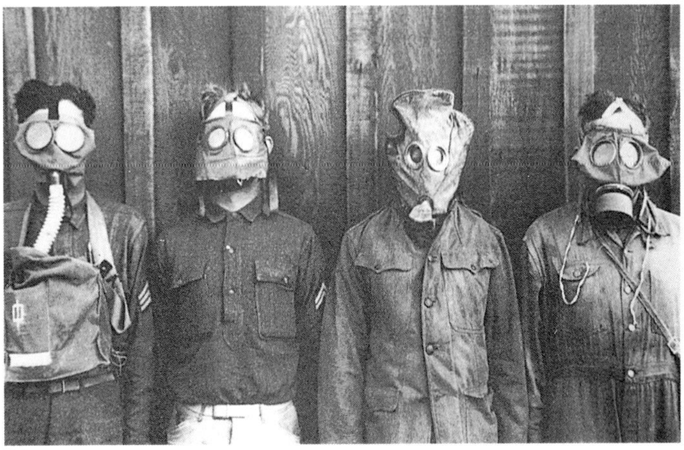

Photograph showing Allied (AEF) soldiers modeling 4 different WWI era chemical warfare respirators. From left to right are the American Small Box Respirator (ASBR), the French M-2, the British PH Helmet, and the Austrian (KuK) version of 'The German Mask.' (Photo from *Chemical Warfare*, by Fries and West).

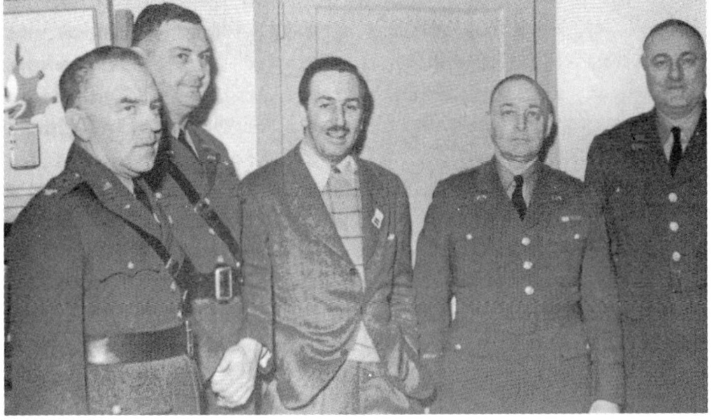

LEFT: Photograph showing senior officers of the WWII Chemical Warfare Service meeting with Walt Disney in a joint effort to investigate the possibility of producing a Mickey Mouse protective gasmask for children (January 1942). Note the illustration of the mask in reference on the wall of the office on far left. (Photograph from *US Army in WW II: The Techncal Services. The Chemical Service, Volume II: From Laboratory to Field*).

ENDNOTES

Chapter One

1 Although the Greeks originated the chemical solution known as 'Greek Fire,' knowledge of its use persisted for a considerable time after the end of the Greek civilization until Europe sank into the throes of the 'Dark Ages.' The secret was rediscovered again during the Renaissance and used to some effect in battle.

2 Conjecture continues to this day concerning the question of whether the spread of disease and contagion among Native Americans through distribution of infected blankets was deliberate or simply happenstance. It is *more likely* that the immune systems of Native Americans were so unable to cope with new diseases to which the white man was more resistant that contact between the races inevitably resulted in the epidemic smallpox which ravaged American Indian tribes; it is therefore reasonable to assume that the spread of smallpox was initially accidental, and not a contrived or deliberate use of 'biological weapons' at first. The devastating result of the smallpox epidemic among Indian populations was obviously recognized at some point, however, and may possibly have been exploited for genocidal purposes. There are several other accounts in the literature of instances in other eras and in different parts of the world where smallpox may have been deliberately spread to exterminate indigenous populations.

Chapter Two

1 This is a very difficult fact to prove positively and both sides were anxious to establish the fact that the other had used modern chemicals in war for the first time. The Germans used 105 mm howitzer shells filled with dianisidine chlorosulfonate in October of 1914, shortly after the French attack; however, these were relatively ineffectual offensive actions. The use of chlorine gas marked a radical escalation of the use of chemicals, in any event, and therefore the German action at Ypres is considered the originating date of the modern chemical warfare age.

2 These figures appears to be not only greatly exaggerated, but rather carelessly perpetuated in the face of substantial documentation to the contrary—as Dr. L.F. Haber of Bedford College (University of London) pointed out in his 1975 Stevenson Lecture (see bibliography) on gas warfare from 1915 to 1945.

3 Of interest is the reference to a pair of stockings, since an extra set of socks was frequently resorted to as an emergency filtering pad to cover the mouth during the first spate of gas attacks by the Germans against the Allied troops; therefore it was not really too unusual to find them carried in the respirator satchel. If they were anything, troops in the field were endlessly inventive and expedient—whatever worked!

Chapter Three

1 The very first German mask was actually made from rubber-backed fabric, and was very similar to the subsequent leather facepiece model; however, due to a shortage of rubber, the leather facepiece became the accepted type. Due to the close military associations between the German forces and those of Austro-Hungary, many early German and Austrian gas masks bore much similarity to each other from a design and fabrication standpoint.

2 This mistake is noted in none other than Dr. Augustin M. Prentiss' voluminous reference on early chemical warfare developments (which is otherwise an excellent reference) *Chemicals In War*, McGraw-Hill, 1937. Porton Down surely chuckles over this error, possibly due to a misunderstood English accent.

Chapter Four

1 So similar is the appearance of the R.F.K. mask to the C.E.M. that it is frequently difficult to distinguish one from the other. Although a few identifying marks were sometimes printed on the CEM (usually the letters "CE" under the chin, on the outside of the mask), there was very little else to serve as an aid in this task. One clue is the color of the canister: the CEM normally uses a yellow painted filter and the RFK mask's filter (while same physical dimensions as the CEM's filter can) is properly green. Another primary clue is the strap configuration of the harness (C.E.M. used 5 straps, R.F.K. used 6).

Chapter Five

1 Fries' excellent book, co-authored with West, remains one of the best available references for early chemical warfare developments (see bibliography).

2 It should be clarified that the MI/M2 Training Gas Mask preceded the M2 Service Gas Mask in that after the new M2 type facepiece was introduced first in the training mask, it became immediately clear that the new facemask would lend itself to adaptation for a very suitable new service mask design. This was accomplished simply by removing the cylindrical MI Training Filter and attaching a hose and a rectangular MIX type filter.

Chapter Six

1 This assumption was justified at war's end when it was determined that the excellent Allied emphasis on maintaining considerable chemical defensive capability was one of the primary factors which acted to deter Axis use of chemical agents during the Second World War.

2 It is interesting to reflect on the U.S. M5 neoprene mask's problem with 'cold-set' after noting that Germany used synthetic rubber to fabricate the facepiece of many of its GM-38 type masks. Did the Germans have a similar problem? The Dräger company molded thousands of their GM-38 type masks from a single, one-piece casting of black synthetic rubber, but the formulation of the material was probably very different from that of neoprene. This mask also featured an early form of reversed peripheral seal, although it is questionable whether or not the mask's designers *recognized* the true value of this feature—later German masks continued to use leather and fabric face-seal contact areas, suggesting that the *sweat-seal effect* was still not fully understood (from a conceptual standpoint) at that point in time. An examination of surviving German GM-38 masks today reveals *some* cold-set tendency, but not as much as that exhibited by the neoprene U.S. M3 and M5 facepieces.

3 The aluminum bodied U.S. M11 filter canister has become one of the most common, best known filter types in the world. It was used on several 'third-generation' respirators, including the interesting early 1950s Netherlands K Model, most of the M9 mask copies, and a few others, as well. Its resemblance to the German, DIN threaded FE type filters of the late war years (FE-42) is more than coincidental, as the M11 was modeled after that design (another example of the 'borrowing concept,' which is still very much a strong tradition in respirator design today).

4 Curious is the fact that although the U.S. war-time defense requirement which mandated substitution of neoprene synthetics for natural rubber remained in effect in 1943 and 1944 (while the M5 and some M3 respirators were being manufactured), a civilian restriction on use of rubber products in the shoe industry was reversed and rescinded in the same period!

Chapter Seven

1 A very interesting summary of naval CBW concerns for this early period may be found in Edward B. Vedder's book, *The Medical Aspects of Chemical Warfare* (1925). In that book, a section written by LCmdr. Duncan C. Walton (USN Medical Corps) provides insights into the navy's operations, based upon WWI experience and expertise. From a historical perspective, the chapter is informative.

2 Several early experimental models of the 'head-canister type' gas mask were developed and evaluated, prior to acceptance of the early Mk. II head-canister gas mask. These earlier models were quite similar to but substantially different in appearance from the final U.S. Navy Head Canister Mask, Mk II.

Chapter Eight

1 These should not be confused with the later 'Mk. I and Mk. II' gas masks, which were U.S. Navy versions of the Army MIA1 and MII Diaphragm gas masks.

Chapter Nine

1 What is not generally known about the 38 million or so 'perfect' British civilian respirators which were distributed on the eve of the new European war was that they were not completely effective against certain chemical agents possessed by the Germans. This fact, discovered to the chagrin of the British government, was kept rather hushed-up and unpublicized, although both Germany and the British were aware of the fact. The principle effect achieved by the respirator distribution program was one of providing a tremendous *morale boost* to the British civilian population, rather a distinctive parallel to the effect achieved by the Saudi Arabian government in distributing respirators to the civilians in that country during the 1991 Gulf War to allay similar anxieties among expatriates.

2 The anxiety potential posed to a small child by the ordinary chemical protective mask or hood was recognized astutely by one Col. George F. Unmacht, Territorial Coordinator for Civilian Gas Defense in Hawaii, who in 1941 masterminded a program there to fabricate some 50,000 infant gas protecting bags which had a resemblance to a bunny with floppy ears. The bags were hand made, through donated labor, and used old X-ray film for clear visor sections. The bag consisted of two layers, the outermost of which had been impregnated with a gas-resistant substance, and the inner layer consisted of paraffin treated lighter fabric. Completely separate (one contained within the other), the sacks were connected only by a small, porous section which was occasionally saturated with a 5% solution of sodium phenolate (to purify air). The children appeared to be considerably less frightened by the design than conventional infant-enclosing protection sacks (MI Infant Protector).

3 A modern example of the importance of providing satisfactory training (along with CBW protective equipment) for civilians is found in the 1991 Gulf War. Extensive difficulties presented themselves in both Israel and Saudi Arabia, having to do with a lack of adequate training, communication and understanding, during the course of developing and coordinating a comprehensive civilian CBW defense. At least one or more deaths occurred from the incorrect use of civilian respirators (failure to remove filter plug before fitting the mask) and misunderstanding of how to correctly store, maintain and use the basic respirator was rife.

Chapter Ten

1 This was generally true in the early stages of the war, but since the German advances had gone so well using the 'conventional' weapons of the blitzkrieg, there was no great incentive to pursue this idea. Later in the war, with Germany's industrial resources severely taxed by the existing war effort, it is questionable whether or not Germany possessed the capability to wage a strong offensive chemical war. In fact, a captured German general stated during interrogation that the OKW's impression was that the Allies were far better prepared with protective chemical clothing and other defensive materiel than was the German army.

2 Before the war had ended, an unusual artillery shell taken from a captured German ammunition dump was delivered to specialists in England's Porton Down. A hitherto unknown type, it was found to contain organophosphate chemicals (Tabun); this was the first *proof* that Germany had prepared a new type of chemical weapon. Britain had already determined that this type of chemical had war potential through prior research with organophosphates. Of special significance was a complete lack of any extant detection capability to protect against its use, although if some sort of warning system could have been devised, existing protective equipment *might* have been marginally adequate.

3 Remaining a current expression of the respirator art, little else appears to offer advantages over the cheek-mount configuration—at least as regards conventional face-only type masks. A possible exception is the new Belgian BEM-4GP, which features a unique 'swivel-mount' block on its lower frontal surface that enables a filter canister to be attached and then positioned either to the right, to the left, or downwards. In service right now, it remains to be seen how serviceable this complexly articulated component will remain in withstanding the rigors of actual service, since simplicity remains an important practical advantage in NBC protective equipment design.

4 The M9 design remains so well conceived, through the test of years, that it was used by Sweden's FOA (Defense Research Establishment) as a standard of respirator protection against which to measure the capabilities of new and existing military respirator models from several nations. Of course, the previous Swedish mask, the Skyddsmask 51, was virtually a direct copy of the American M9.

5 The M14A2 was in fact almost identical to the subsequent M25 tank respirator.

Chapter Eleven

1 This had to do with a defect resulting during manufacture and the fact that the original M13 filters were discovered to be subsequently unsuited for combat protection against toxic war agents was underscored in conversations with a prominent civilian expert in CBW defense matters.

2 The Slovensk, Locobnè, Zavodny company (in Hnùsta, Slovak Republic) apparently sold considerable numbers of these to Arab nations in the Southwest Asian area. Saudi Arabia issued the M10M version (with drink tube) in great numbers to civilian employees (through its Ministry of the Interior administered civil defense agency) along with the Czech CM-4 respirator (without drink tube), during the 1991 Gulf War crisis. They are comfortable to wear and provided a high degree of civilian protection, if and when proper training in their use accompanied issuance. Beards, such as those affected by religiously conservative Islamic individuals, proved to be a major problem in this context.

3 The M18 Headwound Protective Mask consisted of a large, hood-shaped helmet of gas-aerosol filtering fabric. Fitted with two vertically positioned transparent viewing panels, it presented a somewhat unusual appearance when secured as intended on the shoulders. Using straps under the arms to hold the sack in position on the head, a draw-cord is used to tighten an integrated inner collar which maintains gas-tight integrity. The lower area of the garment is joined to a butyl-proofed nylon cape, which forms the shoulder segment. Inhaled and exhaled air are both passed through the filter fabric of the hood itself, and there is no appreciable resistance to breathing. It is carried in a vinyl plastic bag (issued with it) after being folded flat.

Chapter Twelve

1 The 'memorandum of understanding' was signed in 1975.

2 The XM-30 (later MCU-2A/P) mask was rejected by the Army in 1983, after over 8 years of developmental 'teething.'

3 The Canadians disassociated themselves from the U.S./Canadian cooperation in early 1984. Their new C-2 filter canister (now in use by both the U.S. and Canada) was successfully completed by 1982.

4 Another excellent feature of silicone rubber is its resistance to ultraviolet light, ozone and other deteriorating environmental elements, all qualities desirable for a CBW protective facepiece. This is a major reason, along with its inherent softness and compliant nature, for its success as a basic material from which high-quality aviation masks and hoses were manufactured.

5 The Air Force accepted the XM-30 design as its MCU-2/P CBW respirator and placed an initial order for 10,000 of the masks, which were to be produced and delivered during late 1983 and 1984. These were the production masks produced (by Scott Aviation) with the translucent silicone faceblanks.

6 Due to a need for rapid resolution of the respirator development program, the XM-40 design drew heavily on the existing XM-30 development, hence the new XM-40 was substantially configured and initial prototypes produced by the end of 1983—not long after the Army had rejected the XM-30 proposal for its own needs.

7 Several contractors had initially submitted design proposals for the M40 respirator. These included Scott Aviation (a division of Figgie International), ILC, and Avon (UK). Their respective designs were designated XM-40 (Scott), XM-41 (ILC) and XM-42 (Avon). Avon had submitted a version of their S-10 development, altered to meet U.S. Army requirements, while the Scott and ILC designs approximated each other, hewing more closely to the proposed U.S. Army modification of the XM-30 mask. Other companies, including the MSA Company (long associated with the production of protective chemical respirators, both military and civilian) became involved, and testing of the prototype XM-40 design began in 1984. The original plan intended that production should allow delivery of the first M40

masks in July of 1985. However, by late 1986 the advanced phase of the prototype testing was severely behind schedule and a request for production proposals had not yet been issued. By 1987, testing was completed, and Scott Aviation was the successful bidder for a primary production run of 115,750 masks (contract was for 22+ million dollars). The contract called for two increments of production, of which that was the first, due to be fulfilled by December of 1989; the second increment would follow, as planned, for a total run of 300,000 of the new masks (total contract award: 51+ million dollars). In April of 1988, it was announced that the contract with Scott would expire after only one year, and the contract was reopened for bidding, which resulted in new awards to the ILC and MSA companies for 300,000 masks to be delivered by late 1992.

8 Not related to the XM-42 Avon proposal based on the S-10 (known as the "US-10").

9 With recent revelation of the somewhat shocking secret testing of nuclear materials on unknowing civilians conducted by official U.S. Government agencies throughout the 50s, and a previous history of deliberate 'stonewalling' on the part of the Pentagon to protect activities considered sensitive, an obvious question is raised as to whether information in this matter is being deliberately withheld by official (military) agencies from public disclosure.

10 A series of tests of the serviceability of the MCU-2A/P type mask in use in the U.S. Navy and Air Force determined an unusually high rate of failures both before and after corrective maintenance had been undertaken. These tests were conducted by the Army and Air Force in cooperation with a commercial organization which produces advanced face-fit testing equipment. One of the results of the tests was renewed concern over the importance of not just correctly fitting man to mask, but of maintaining face-seal and component functional capability through periodic testing. Debris contamination of exhalation valve in field use situations was also cited as a potentially serious failure area in masks lacking the 6th valve former spoke and the corrective metallic grid retrofit.

Chapter Thirteen

1 "Fourth generation" respirator is a term of reference originated by Swedish National Defense Research Establishment (FOA) scientist Per-Gunnar Jönsson, in association with comparative tests his NBC division of the FOA conducted of the current leading international respirator designs. The term relates to the four generations as being 1) WWI, 2) WWII, 3) Post WWII, and 4) Modern period. Actually, we are on the verge of a succeeding development phase as the 90s promote new scientific breakthroughs in polymeric chemistry, and methodologies (CAD is one of these 'new' elements).

2 The use of silicone rubber in the facepiece of the new M45 mask again raises concern over possible susceptibility to penetrating vessicant agents, for although Sulfa Mustard is one of the earliest and oldest of the 'modern era' chemical weapons, it is still one of the most dangerous and widespread CW agents in use around the world at this time.

3 Canada's DREO (Defense Research Establishment Ottawa), their equivalent of our U.S. Edgewood/Aberdeen facility in Maryland, invested in a McDonnell-Douglas CAD system which figured significantly in the very successful C-4 respirator development program. The CAD system not only allowed for rapid design development, modification and prototype production, it also allowed for a rapid transfer of the design and technical specifications and parameters to the production contractor, SNC Corporation of Ontario, so that production of the C-4 could commence with a minimum of delay. Canada's early use of a CAD type system for respirator development has served as an example to other international NBC defense groups engaged in similar work, and such systems are now being incorporated into the current "state-of-the-art." Canada's C-4 program benefited so much from their use of CAD that their C-4 prototype, which existed as an engineering model in 1986, was produced in a limited run of 1500 masks for extensive field testing in Europe and Canada (this was completed in two years). An interim production run of the final, fully refined mask design allowed the Canadian troops deployed in the 1991 Gulf War to be equipped with the new C-4. One final aspect of the Canadian program was a rigidly enforced cost-benefit review and analysis of every phase of the program, which enabled the very best possible respirator to be produced for the least possible outlay—something which American efforts ought to take serious note of, in view of typically costly (and frequently severely wasteful) U.S. research, development and production efforts in similar areas.

BIBLIOGRAPHY

Books

Auld, S.J.M., Maj., RE, *Gas and Flame in Modern Warfare*, Geo. H. Doran & Company, New York, NY, USA, 1918.

Battelle Memorial Institute, *Worldwide NBC Mask Handbook,* Battelle Edgewood Operations/CBIAC, Edgewood, Maryland, USA, 1993.

Cole, Leonard A., *The Eleventh Plague: The Politics of Biological and Chemical Warfare,* W.H.Freeman & Company, 1996

Dando, Malcolm, *Biological Warfare in the 21st Century,* Macmillen & Company, 1994.

Douglass, Jr., Joseph D., (co-author), *America the Vulnerable: The Threat of Chemical and Biological Warfare*, Lexington Books, New York, NY, USA, 1987.

Doull, John, Klassen, Curtis D., and Amdur, Mary O., (Editors), *Casarett & Doull's Toxicology: The Basic Science of Poisons,* Macmillen & Company, NYC, NY, USA, 1980.

Elo, Mikko, *Suojeluvarikko: 1944-1994*, Gummerus Kirjapaino Oy, Jyväskylä 1994, {ISBN 951-25-0719-6].

Farrow, Edward S., *Gas Warfare,* E.P.Dutton & Company, New York, New York, USA, 1920.

Fries, Amos A., and West, Clarence J., *Chemical Warfare,* McGraw-Hill Book Company, New York, New York, USA and London, UK, 1921.

Gander, Terry J., *Nuclear, Biological and Chemical Warfare,* Ian Allen Limited. Publishers, London, UK, 1987 [ISBN: 0 7110 1722 0].

Gander, Terry J., *Jane's NBC Protection Equipment (Annual, 92/93),* Jane's Information Group, London, UK, 1992.

Gripstad, Birger, *FOA Briefing Book on Biological Warfare Agents,* Swedish National Defense Research Establishment, Sweden, 1986.

Harris, Sheldon, *Factories of Death,* Routledge, London & New York, 1994 [ISBN: 0-415-09105-5].

Hersh, Seymour M., *Chemical and Biological Warfare: America's Hidden Arsenal,* Bobbs-Merrill Co., Indianapolis, IN., 1968.

Hessel, F.A., *Chemistry in Warfare: Its Strategic Importance,* Hastings House, NYC, NY, 1940

Ivarsson, Nilsson, & Santesson, *A FOA Briefing Book on Chemical Weapons,* Swedish National Defense Research Establishment, Umeå, Sweden, 1992.

Prentiss, Augustin M., PhD, LTCol, USA, *Chemicals in War: A Treatise on Chemical Warfare,* McGraw-Hill Book Company, New York, New York, USA, 1937.

Richter, Donald, *Chemical Soldiers: British Gas Warfare in World War One,* University of Kansas Press, Lawrence, Kansas, USA, 1992 [ISBN 0 7006 0544 4].

Somani, Satu M., PhD, *Chemical Warfare Agents,* Academic Press, Incorporated, San Diego, California, USA, 1992 [ISBN 0 12 654620 7].

Spiers, Edward M., PhD, *Chemical Warfare,* Macmillan Publishers, London, UK, 1986.

Spiers, Edward M., PhD, *Chemical Weaponry: A Continuing Challenge,* St. Martin's Press, New York, New York, USA, 1989.

Spiers, Edward M., PhD, *Chemical and Biological Weapons: A Study of Proliferation,* Macmillan Publishers, London, 1994 [ISBN 0 333 56420 0].

Stanton, Shelby, Capt., USA, *US Army Uniforms in World War Two,* Greenhill Books, London, UK, 1991.

Vedder, Edward B., LTCol, USA, *The Medical Aspects of Chemical Warfare,* Williams & Wilkins Company, Baltimore, Maryland, 1925.

Williams, Peter, and Wallace, David, *Unit 731: Japan's Secret Biological Warfare in World War Two,* The Free Press (Div. of Macmillen), NYC, NY, USA, 1989, ISBN 0-02-935301-7.

Manuals, Reports and Technical Publications

FM 21-40, *Defense Against Chemical Attack,* War Department, US Army, 1 May 40.
FM 21-40, *Defense Against Chemical Attack,* War Department, US Army, 11 Jun 46.
FM 21-40, *Chemical, Biological, Radiological & Nuclear Defense,* Department of the Army, 17 May 71.
FM 8-9, *Nato Handbook on the Medical Aspects of NBC Defense Operations,* AMedP-6, Departments of the Army, Navy & Air Force, 1 May 83.
FM 100-2-3, *The Soviet Army, Troops, Organisation & Equipment,* Department of the Army, 16 Jul 84.
TM 3-205, *The Gas Mask,* Department of the Army, Chemical Warfare Service, 9 Oct 41.
TM 3-4240-269-12, *Operator & Organisational Maintenance Manual, Including Repair Parts & Special Tools Lists: Mask, Riot Control Agent, XM28E4,* Department of the Army, 8 Apr 68.
TM 3-42-40-279-10, *Operator's Manual, Mask, Chemical & Biological, Field, ABC-M17/M17A1 and Accessories,* Department of the Army, 29 Aug 75.
TM 3-42-40-279-20 & P, *Organisational Maintenance Manual, Including Repair Parts and Special Tools List, Mask, Chemical and Biological, Field, ABC-M17/M17A1 and Accessories,* Department of the Army, 29 Aug 75.
TM 3-4240-280-10, *Operator's Manual, Mask, Chemical & Biological, Aircraft, ABC M24 and Accessories, and Mask, Chemical & Biological, Tank, M15/M25A1 and Accessories,* Department of the Army, 22 Mar 76.
TM 3-4240-280-23 & P, *Organisational & Direct Support Maintenance Manual, Including Parts & Special Tools Lists, Mask, Chemical & Biological, Aircraft ABC M24 and Accessories, and Mask, Chemical & Biological, Tank M25/M25A1 and Accessories,* Department of the Army, 22 Mar 76.
TM 3-4240-300-10-1, *Operator's Manual for Chemical & Biological Mask, Field, M40,* Department of the Army, 15 May 91.

Pamphlets and Small Booklets

Chemical Defense Experimental Establishment, Porton Down, *A Brief History of the Chemical Defense Experimental Establishment, Porton,* March 1961 (declassified).
Gimingham, C.T., Captain, Royal Engineers (Royal Army), *The Evolution of the Small Box Respirator,* 20 Jan 19, privately printed, PRO Nr: WO 142/254.
War Office (Great Britain), *Medical Manual of Chemical Warfare, 1943,* His Majesty's Stationery Office (HMSO), February 1943, 26 Pubs.5112.

Other Publications

CGSC, (US Army Command & General Staff College), RB3-1, *Selected Readings in Nuclear & Chemical Operations,* 8 Jul 82.
K.u.K., Armeeoberkommando, Österreichisher Chef des Generalstabs, *Vorbeitungen für Gasangriff,* Juli 1918.
K.u.K., Armeeoberkommando, Österreichisher Chef des Generalstabs, *Instruktion für dem Gasschutz und Frontwetterdienst,* Jänner 1917.
Saddique, Abdulaziz, MD, and Seraj, Mohammed, PhD, *Brief Notes & Guidelines on Toxic Chemicals and Their Effects,* Saffir Press, Riyadh, Kingdom of Saudi Arabia, 1991.
Steadman, Major S.J., et al, British Intelligence Objectives Subcommittee, *Drägerwerk Factories at Lübeck, Hamburg, and Uetersen,* London, UK, 24 May 45 through 1 Jun 45 (declassified).

Papers and Articles

Azizi, F., Elyasi, H., Sohrab-pour, H., Jalali, N., & Nafarabadi, M., "Serum Concentrations of Various Hormones Following Exposure to Chemical Weapons Containing Sulfar Mustard," (oral presentation & paper), 1st Int. Med. Congress on Chem. Warfare Agents, Mashad, Iran, 1988
Barry, John, and Watson, Russell, "A Gulf Cover-up?", *Newsweek* Magazine, 11 Nov 1996.
Cardwell, A/SLt. Mark, "Masked Marvel," *Sentinel* (Canadian Armed Forces Magazine), Feb 91.
Carey, Christopher T., "Desert CBW: Renewed Attention to Future Protection Requirements," *ASA Newsletter,* Issue 93-2, 10 Jun 93.
Carey, Christopher T., "Focus on Respirators: The Canadian (SNC) C4," *ASA Newsletter,* Issue 93-2, 8 Apr 93.
Carey, Christopher T., "Focus on Respirators: The M9 Family," *ASA Newsletter,* Issue 93-1, 10 Feb 93.
Carey, Christopher T., "The Strange Case of the Orphaned S-10s," *ASA Newsletter,* Issue 94-3, 10 Aug 94.

Carey, Christopher T., "Focus on Respirators: The Forsheda NBC Type F2," *ASA Newsletter,* Issue 94-2, 10 Jun 94.
Carey, Christopher T., "Focus on Respirators: The Finnish M95," *ASA Newsletter*, Issue 96-4, 10 Oct 96.
Carey, Christopher T., "NBC Protection: Substance, Reality, Fantasy," *American Survival Guide,* Vol. 19, No. 1, February 1997.
Carey, Christopher T., "Focus on Respirators: The French ARFA Series," *ASA Newsletter*, Issue 97-3, 10 Jun 97.
Carey, Christopher T., "CBW Self Defense: Individual Respiratory NBC Protection," *American Survival Guide,* Vol. 19, No. 6, June 1997.
Carey, Christopher T. Carey, "Defense Against the Poor Man's Nuclear Bomb: A Three Part Exploration of the Modern Biological Threat," *American Survival Guide,* Vol. 19, Nos. 8,9, 10 (Aug-Sept-Oct 1997).
Cole, Leonard A., "The Specter of Biological Weapons," *Scientific American*, December 1996, pp 60-65.
Green, Brian, "Battling Gulf War Syndrome," *Air Force Magazine*, 'Capital Hill', December 1994.
Harrison, Dr. B.H., and Main, L.A., "Mask Marvel: Canada's New NBC Respirator," *Forum,* July/August 1987.
Hirsch, Dr. Walter, "Soviet Biological Warfare and Chemical Warfare Preparations and Capabilities", (prepared for) Intelligence Branch, Plans, Training and Intelligence Division, Office of the Chief, Chemical Corps, (translated by Zaven Nalbandian), 671 pages, 1951 (unclassified 1974).
Jönsson, Per-Gunnar, "A Cooperative Study of Fourth Generation Military Respirators," (oral presentation and report), *Proceedings Supplement:: 4th International Symposium on Protection Against Chemical Warfare Agents,* (FOA), Stockholm, Sweden, 1992.
McCall, Sherman, "A Higher Form of Killing," *Proceedings* (US Naval Institute Journal), February 1995.
Mai, Jochen, "Giftgas im Märchenland," *Münchner Zeitung*, 9 Dec 1994, München, Deutschland.
Mäkinen, Markku, "Animal Gas Protection: A Short Historical Review," (oral presentation & paper), *Chemical Protection '92: Proceedings of Symposium on NBC Protection,* Finland, 1992.
Mäkinen, Markku, "The Finnish Military Gas Masks, 1930-1939," (oral presentation & paper), *Chemical Protection '92: Proceedings of Symposium on NBC Protection*, Finland, 1992.
Nash, Colleen A., "Cooler Wear for Desert Warriors," *Air Force Magazine,* December 1990.
Osterman, Maj. Joseph, USMC, "Who Will Answer the Chem/Bio Call?", US Naval Institute *Proceedings,* December 1996.
Riley, Maj. Victor J., USMC, "We Need to Learn the ABCs of NBC," *US Naval Institute Proceedings,* August 1993.
Rivera, Matthew, "Chemical Agents: Identification, Detection and First Aid," *American Survival Guide,* October 1996.
Sheldon, Jim, "The Scourge of 1915 and Modern Warfare," *Antiques and Collectibles Magazine,* July/August 1982.
Sheldon, Jim, "The Development of Gas Masks in Defending Against Chemical Warfare," *Antiques and Collectibles Magazine,* September/October 1982.
Sohrab-Pour, H., Masjedi, M., *et al*, "Late Complications of Sulfur Mustard in Respiratory System," Medical Journal of the Islamic Republic of Iran, Vol. 2, No. 3, 171-174, 1988.
Sohrab-Pour, H., MD, FCCP, "Observation and Clinical Manifestation of Patients Injured with Mustard Gas," *Medical Journal of the Islamic Republic of Iran*, Volume I, Rabiolaval 1408 (Nov. 1987), pp 32-37.
Thornton, LTCol. John, USA, "Iraqi Chemical Preparedness in the Gulf War," *ASA Newsletter,* Issue 93-4, pp 1/14-15, 12 Aug 93.

Memoranda, Communications and Correspondence

Letter, "Establishment of Project 4-80-02-12, Gas Mask, Noncombatant," to Chairman of Chemical Corps Technical Committee, dated 11 Oct 48, Chemical Corps Technical Committee, US Army Chemical Center, Maryland, USA (unclassified/obtained through FOIA).
Letter, "Classification of Mask, Protective, Noncombatant, M16 (E51R15-11-22R1) as a Standard Type," to Chairman of Chemical Corps Technical Committee, dated 19 Jul 57, Chemical Corps Technical Committee, US Army Chemical Center, Maryland, USA (unclassified/obtained through FOIA).
Letter, "Materièl Status Record Submission," to Commander, US Army Materièl Command, from LTCol C.E. Rose, Executive Officer, Development, Research & Engineering Division, dated 13 Mar 75, Department of the Army, HQ, US Army Armament Command.
Letter, "Civil Preparedness Requirements for NBC Defense Materièl," to Commander, US Army Materièl Command, from J.E. Davis, Defense Civil Preparedness Agency (DCPA), dated 31 Aug 73 (unclassified/obtained through FOIA).
Letter, "Classification of the Mask, Protective, Civilian, M22 (E52R27 / CD V-805) as a Standard-A-OCDM Type," to Chairman, Chemical Corps Technical Committee, dated 15 Jul 60 (unclassified—obtained through FOIA).
Letter, "Materièl Status Record Submission," to Commander, US Army Materièl Command, from R.A. Chandler, Chief, Engineering Support Office, dated 22 Sep 87 (unclassified—obtained through FOIA).
Telephone communications (series) with Derek Griffiths, late of CBDE, Porton Down, UK, 1991-92.
Telephone communications (series) with CSM George Murray of the US Army Chemical Corps Museum, Fort McClellan, Alabama, 1992-94.

Special References

Brophy, Dr. Leo P., and Fisher, Col George B., *US Army in World War Two: The Technical Services Series, The Chemical Warfare Service, Volume I: Organizing for War,* Office of the Chief of Military History, US Government Printing Office, 498 pages with illustrations, Washington DC, 1959.

Brophy, Dr. Leo P., Miles, Dr. Wyndham D., and Cochrane, Dr. Rexmond C., *US Army in World War Two: The Technical Services Series, The Chemical Warfare Service, Volume II: From Laboratory to Field,* Office of the Chief of Military History, US Government Printing Office, 498 pages with illustrations, Washington DC, 1959 (reprinted 1970).

Kleber, Dr. Brooks E., and Birdsell, Dr. Dale., *US Army in World War Two: The Technical Services Series, The Chemical Warfare Service, Volume III: Chemicals in Combat,* Office of the Chief of Military History, US Government Printing Office, 697 pages with illustrations, Washington DC, 1966.

U.S. War Department, Office of Military Intelligence, *Enemy Capabilities for Chemical Warfare*, GPO, Washington, DC, 156 pp, illustrated, classified intelligence study, 1943 (declassified, 1960s).

APPENDIX I: CBW Respirators Marketed but Not Manufactured in the USA

In addition to CBW defense respirators of entirely U.S. design and manufacture, there are several masks, originating overseas, which are marketed in this country. Some of the designs are moderately reworked or slightly modified before sale, while others are imported directly and offered for sale in their original configuration.

Two which fall into these categories are the KX Industries Model MF-11, and the KX Model MF-10. The first is the U.S. modified Chinese Peoples Republic NBC respirator type M-85, and the second is an extremely well made copy of the highly regarded British S-10 mask, manufactured under license in Pakistan. Both are available as general purpose NBC respirators for military or civilian application, and both feature voicemitters and drinking devices (a valved canteen cap comes with the mask to facilitate fluid uptake).

No one needs an introduction to the well-known British S-10 respirator, due to its preeminence in the world as an NBC trendsetter design. The Pakistani copy, marketed by KX Industries as the MF-10 (also known as the PK-10), appears to be an exceptionally well-made and carefully manufactured clone of the original. There are no apparent differences between the British version and the foreign-made copy with the exception of the head-harness (the British S-10 uses a polymer-rubber strap assembly and the MF-10 copy has an elasticized fabric strap harness). The foreign S-10 model will take any STANAG 4155 (40 x 3.63 mm) threaded filter canister, which ensures a wide range of possible choices. It is capable of providing excellent protection against CBW agents, just like the original AVON model.

The KX modified Chinese M-85 (KX Industries Model MF-11) uses the Chinese-manufactured facepiece to which a few upgraded components have been substituted for the originals, to assure enhanced serviceability. Low per-unit cost and high level respiratory protection are attractive features of the MF-11 (M-85). As with the SGE mask, the MF-11 has been marketed favorably to law enforcement agencies. Like the S-10 copy, the MF-11 (M-85) also uses any STANAG 4155 threaded filter canister.

In addition to these respirators, the most recent years following the 1991 Gulf War have seen a broad-range importation of foreign military surplus NBC respirators. Commonly found in this category are the German Dräger-type masks (Dräger M-65, Kareta-M and earlier precursors) and the Czech M10 and M10M model copies of the U.S. M17 mask. Both types of mask were issued extensively to Gulf Cooperative Council (Saudi Arabia, Kuwait and UA Emirates) civilians and are very good NBC protective respirators when properly fitted and maintained. The Czech M10M has apparently also been license-manufactured in former East Germany by the Sturm Company, and is now being imported to the U.S. in unissued condition in substantial quantities. More rarely seen are the Czech CM-4 and CM-5 NBC type respirators, which provide excellent NBC protection for civilians (the CM-4 has twin eye lenses and the CM-5 features a single panoramic eye lens). The latest models of the CM-4(M) and CM-5(M) feature drink tube attachments.

Another commonly found NBC respirator in the U.S. is the Shalon Chemical Company (Israel) civilian defense mask; both it and the Israeli M15A1 military mask (also imported) trace their lineage to the German (Dräger/Auer) post war masks (which trace *their* origin to the GM-38 of WWII). The Israeli filter used with the Shalon mask is a license-made copy of the standard mid-60s German *Zivilschutzfilter (ZF-68,* RM 7970*),* manufactured by Auer and Dräger.

Finally, small quantities of the excellent British S-10 respirator are now finding their way into the U.S. civilian and militaria collector market. Stories abound of the near legendary S-10, highly regarded during the Gulf War by those who were knowledgeable in NBC protection, which was worth as much as $1000 on the Saudi Arabian black market prior to the immediate outbreak of the Gulf War hostilities (filter now made by Sabre Ind., UK).

APPENDIX II:
U.S. Army Respirator Identification Nomenclature

Standard nomenclature for designating and identifying U.S. Army NBC defense respirators is described in U.S. Army TM 3-205, *The Gas Mask*, dated 9 Oct 41, and in U.S. Army TM 3-205, *The Gas Mask*, dated 2 March 1951.

Gas masks and their components are identified as to item by nomenclature which consists of a model number and a name (i.e. M9 gas mask, C15 expiration valve, E49 facepiece, etc.). Experimental mask designs feature an X before the model designation (example: XM-45); developmental items use E and a number (example: E1); standardized items have an M and a number (example: M9), or a C and a number, depending on whether item in question is an end item or a component.

Developmental Items:

E-numbers are used to identify items during experimental stages, starting with E1 for the first model of any item (or group of items). Minor modifications are indicated by R-numbers (example: E1R1 facepiece, E1R2 facepiece). Major modifications require new E-number (example: E2 facepiece, E3 facepiece, etc.).

A. Major Components:

A facepiece with a developmental item number may include some standardized components (canisters and carriers have no separate components with model numbers).

B. Minor Components:

An outlet valve, head-harness, hose, or other component of a facepiece is numbered through development in the same manner as a major component.

C. Gas Mask Assembly:

Prior to standardization, a gas mask is identified by its three major components whether they be standard or under development (examples: E1-E2-E3 mask, consisting of E1 facepiece, E2 canister and E3 carrier; also E1-E2-E3R1, E1-M11-M7, E1-M11A1-M7, etc.).

A minor experimental change in the C15R1 carrier of the M9 gas mask would result in the C48R1-M11-E15R2 gas mask.

Standardized Gas Mask:

A. Some developmental models of gas masks eventually became adopted types (whether standard, substitute standard, or limited standard) and an M-number assigned (example: M9 gas mask). Minor modifications are indicated by the addition of A-numbers (example: M17A1 gas mask, M17A2 gas mask).

B. Prior to September 1940, Roman rather than Arabic numerals were used in gas mask model designations, but minor modifications were indicated with Arabic alphanumerics (examples: MI gas mask, MIA1 gas mask, MIA2 gas mask, etc.). After September of 1940, Arabic alphanumerics were used exclusively (examples: M2 gas mask, M2A1 gas mask, M2A2 gas mask, etc.). Designations of masks designed and standardized before September of 1940 retained their original Roman numeral designations even after the September 1940 nomenclature change (the exception is the Training Gas Mask MI, which became known as the Training Gas Mask M2; this occurred due to the fact that the new style fully molded rubber facepieces formed the basis of the entire new line of service gas mask developments which followed from the original MI series masks). The Training Gas Mask MI is usually referred to as the Training Gas Mask MI/M2 (also MIA1/M2A1). This single respirator's hybrid designation has caused some slight confusion owing to its unique place in the U.S. gas mask development hierarchy.

C. Prior to December 1947, standardized gas masks were routinely identified and referred to by three numbers in a manner similar to the system for designating developmental types, although the letter M appeared only before the first number (facepiece) and was not repeated before the second number (which indicated filter), or the third number (which indicated carrier). Examples would be the M8-11-10 gas mask (M8 facepiece, M11 filter canister, and M10 carrier), and the M5-11-7 (M5 facepiece, M11 filter canister, and M7 carrier). All masks designated and in use prior to December of 1947 would continue to bear this designation (this was partly due to the fact that most gas masks of the early decades consisted of three major parts, a faceblank, a filter on a hose, and a carrier).

D. When the M9 gas mask was standardized in December of 1947, a new change in nomenclature was instituted. From that date onwards, the whole respirator assembly (of facepiece, filter and carrier) would be referred to by the model of the facepiece only (examples would be the M9 gas mask, the M17A1 NBC respirator, the M40A1 Field Protective Mask, etc.). After this date, a minor change in a gas mask would be indicated through the use of an A-number after the mask identifier (example: M9A1 mask), and a major change in a gas mask would require an entirely new M-number (example: M14A2 became M25 gas mask).

Standardized Components:

A. Most current components (and all future components) are identified by C-numbers, with minor changes as R-numbers (example: C15 carrier, C15R1 carrier, etc.).

B. Previously standardized major or minor components may be found with M-numbers (example: M11 canister, M8 outlet valve, MIVA1 carrier, MIX filter, M9A1 filter, etc.).

Facepiece Variations (Sizing):

A. In addition to name and number, gas masks are further designated as to facepiece size by a letter or letters on the forehead section of the mask, in combination with the national original designation (U.S.). Examples are S for small, M for Medium, and L for Large sizes. Some models were produced in XS (Extra Small), and early decades featured the so-called Universal facepiece, which is designated by a U character. Manufacturing deviations in the Medium size of masks produced in the 40s led to the markings SU and LU (Small Universal and Large Universal). [As a note of comparative interest, this U.S. sizing letter code may create confusion on occasions when foreign respirators appearing to be marked with an 'S' size code on the faceblank are mistakenly assumed to be *small* sized models. The best examples of this are found on the Serbian M-59 (M1) and M2 masks: in the Serbian alphabet, an 'S' on the facepiece indicates a *medium* size.]

B. Cheek sited filter canister models of older (pre M17 type) masks such as the M9 were made in both left sided filter inlet and right sided inlet faceblank version, with about 7 percent of the total number being produced to accommodate left-handed individuals. The M17 series masks, using internally fitted bilateral filters, required only a standard faceblank for both left and right handed individuals. The latest type NBC respirators feature bilateral filter inlet capability to accommodate both left and right handed individuals, hence only one standard facepiece in three sizes (S, M, L) is required. Respirators which utilize filters attached to hoses pose no problem for left or right hand capability requirements. (Design objectives and standards for current and future mask development projects logically mandate bilateral connector accommodations for filter canisters and accessory communications devices so as to reduce unnecessary cost factors).

APPENDIX III:
U.S. Army Filter Canisters: World War One Through the Present

The earliest U.S. Army filter canisters, used on the American Small Box Respirator or ASBR (which was an ineffectual copy of the BSBR "Box respirator"), were approximately 14cm x 4.7cm x 9.5cm rounded rectangular tin containers filled with about 60% charcoal and 40% soda lime. This ASBR filter was about one fourth again as large as the standard BSBR filter can, due to a fear that American charcoal was inferior to the British type (this was later shown to be an incorrect assumption), and aside from the size clue, is distinguished by its standard black color (frequently found with its top painted red to indicate 'training use only').

The next American Army respirator, the CEM or Corrected English Model, used tin filter box canisters approximately the same size as the BSBR filter (11cm x 4.7cm x 9.5cm) which are distinguished at a glance by their yellow color (the "H" filter). This filter was also used on the KT (Kops-Tissot) and AT (Akron-Tissot) masks, and in January of 1918 had two cotton pads inserted as protection against arsenical type smokes.

When the RFK mask (Richardson, Flory, Kopps) was being produced, the filter canister was about the same size as the yellow CEM filter, but breathing resistance was somewhat lowered due to a reduction of internal contents. These improved canisters are immediately recognized by their green color (the "J" filter).

The final WWI American filter in common use was that found on the Army 1919 Model (later standardized as the Service Gas Mask MI), which incorporated an improved felt smoke filter element, along with soda lime and charcoal, and is recognized by its blue paint. When the 1919 Model became known as the Service Gas Mask MI in 1921, the filter canister adopted initially was designated as the MI Filter. This was the blue tin canister which had been introduced with the 1919 Model. By 1930, no fewer than 4 improved filter canisters had been developed for use with the MI mask, and all measuring approximately 14.7cm x 5.5cm x 9.5cm. These were the entirely blue MI filter (with straight connector outlet), the MII filter (olive drab, with a blue top and straight connector outlet), the MIII filter (completely olive drab and with an angled outlet tube), and the MIV (olive drab, with angled outlet tube).

By 1941, the number of successively improved filter canisters had increased to about 11. They included, in addition to the earliest 4 already referenced, the MIIR (olive drab with two blue stripes and angled connector tube), the MIIIR (olive drab, angled connector tube), the MIV (olive drab, with angled connector tube, slightly smaller size), the MVIII (same color, and tube as preceding, and about the same size as the MIV), the MIX (fractionally shorter in size than the MVIII, same color and angle tube), and the MIXA1 (same color, and angle tube, about 13cm x 6cm x 9cm). Supplementing the boxy "service" filters were the gray cylindrical metal MI Training Filter, and the M1 Optical Filter (olive drab, with inlet holes aligned along its cylindrical length, and outlet tubes at each end).

Whereas the MI, MII and MIII filters featured a top-opening inlet (on the same end as the outlet tube), the MIIR, the MIIIR and the MIV filter featured air inlets (with rubber disc check valves) on the opposing end (bottom) of the filter. The contents of all of these early filters continued to consist of a mixture of soda lime and activated charcoal, and all featured felt smoke filter elements. The M1 Optical filter featured a rubber check valve in each outlet, and the cylindrical MI Training Filter had a rubber check valve in the bottom (opposite end from outlet).

From the MIII Service filter onwards (with the exception of the MI Training Filter, and the M10 and M10A1 cylindrical gray metal filters), all filter canisters were OD in color. The early canisters were constructed from tin and steel, and consequently were quite prone to rust—especially a problem in tropical areas with high humidity levels and excessive rain.

Of all of these, the MIXA1 (M9A1) filter would be used throughout most of the war years as the standard filter found in use with the so-called 'Heavyweight type' gas mask, using the new fully molded M2 type rubber facepiece. As with all of the radial-flow type MI through MIXA1 service-type filters, tin & steel construction was used. In addition to being prone to rusting, they were also quite heavy (about a kilogram in weight when filled with charcoal and soda lime contents). These problems resulted in the requirement for a new lightweight service-type filter, and the M10 type "lightweight" filter resulted, following the construction design of the Training Mask filter (MI).

With the approach of the Second World War, the USCWS's concern with possible chemical threat from the Axis powers resulted not only in the new fully-molded rubber (M2) type facepiece, but more importantly in improved filter capabilities. Filter absorbents were first studied, with an eye to addressing this concern, in fundamental researches conducted at three U.S. universities. Whetlerite, a copper impregnated, activated charcoal was the absorbent utilized in the standard MIXA1 (M9A1) service type filter in service by 1939. Mixed with 20% soda lime, it removed such gases as chloropicrin, phosgene, mustard and lewisite. It furnished only fair protection against hydrogen cyanide, and cyanogen chloride. Studies confirmed the British finding that the addition of silver to charcoal greatly improved canister capabilities against phosgene and hydrogen cyanide, and by 1942 this new composite whetlerite was adopted for use. Further studies conducted later that same year demonstrated that soda lime, a basic component of every filter canister in use since the middle of the First World War (and used to assist adsorption of volatile acid gases and hydrogen cyanide), was no longer needed, hence its use in U.S. Army filter canisters was discontinued.

Continued research at the universities, under Army sponsorship, resulted in the addition of chromium to the silver and copper already used to treat activated charcoal in filters, a measure which considerably improved cyanogen chloride protection capabilities (even under high humidity conditions). This third improved type of impregnated activated charcoal was adopted for use in July of 1943 and was referred to as 'ASC type' absorber. It was incorporated for the first time in the M9A2 filter canister, used with the early lightweight masks. Shortly after this, scientists produced acceptable wood and coal charcoals as substitutes for the pre-war coconut charcoal in wide use prior to the war (WWII).

The result, as determined by USCWS experts, was a filter canister which gave better absorbent protection than that offered by either the contemporaneous German or Japanese filters.

The second phase of wartime (WWII) filter improvement related to aerosol and particulate filter elements used in the canisters. The standard filter element in use in 1940 (MIX type filters) employed a cellulose fiber mat known as "alpha web." A slight improvement of the material had been obtained by impregnating it with fine carbon particles. This assured adequate protection against toxic smokes, but increased breathing resistance and offered only limited liquid particle protection. Furthermore, the development of new mechanical smoke projectors necessitated further work on the filter element of canisters because fine oil particles of the smoke deteriorated the impregnated paper.

New filtering materials were tested, including rock wool, fiberglass, paper substitutes, and finally asbestos (a material used in British, German, Japanese and Russian filters). These tests resulted in three successive types of asbestos-bearing alpha web being produced. After 1942 they were used in place of the carbon-impregnated paper employed in the M9A2 and M10A1 canisters. The harmful properties of respired asbestos fibers ultimately led to the substitution of paper filtering element made from Moroccan esparto grass, which provided less breathing resistance than asbestos and equal filtering capability. The new material was subsequently enhanced by treating it with dimethyl silicone—making the paper highly water resistant. However, many of the M11 type filter canisters produced in the war years contain asbestos, and a substantial proportion of them were issued with the Civil Defense Protective Mask CD V-800. This is confirmed in CD Technical Bulletin TB-11-13, dated 13 June 1959 (No.6 in the CW Warfare Series).

Due to the referenced filtration improvements, the new lightweight filters (M10 type) featured protection just about equal to that offered by the larger, bulkier "heavyweight" filters. However, with the development of the new Army Assault Gas Mask (M5) with its cheek-mounted filter configuration, a new type of aluminum-bodied, lightweight, screw-on filter was designed for use with it. This filter, the M11 'drum' filter, borrowed heavily from the aluminum-bodied German FE-42 filter canister upon which it was modeled, to some degree. Two-thirds lighter than the "lightweight" cylindrical M10 type filter, the M11 featured a very effective, water-repellent mechanical smoke filtering element and a wide, deep bed of ASC type charcoal. Finally, it offered almost as much protection as the older radial-flow type filters. The new M11 canister featured a screw-thread that was identical to and interchangeable with that found on the English Light Type Respirator, which had partly inspired the U.S. M5 respirator design (providing an early, and unusually successful Allied 'interoperability' benefit, something that would only later be achieved in NATO to a widespread degree). Initially produced in 1944, the M11 filter would remain the standard U.S. filter canister in use until the introduction of the M17 series masks of the 60s (the M10A1 filter would remain in use with special types of mask, such as the M24/M25 aircraft and tank respirators, well into the 80s), and since the M9 series were also retained as "special purpose respirators" even after the M17 mask was standardized, the M11 filter has remained in use until the introduction of the latest C-2 type filter (M40 mask). As mentioned in several other parts of the text, the M11 filter design has been adopted in various forms, by most of the foreign nations which produced copies of the American M9 series masks, as well.

One of the more obscure U.S. Army filters of the 1950s, designated the 'Filter, Particulate, 3 CFM, M14' (or 'Canister, Gas Mask, Aerosol, M14') is identified by its red aluminum body. With dimensions similar to the M11 filter, the M14 filter had a standard 2 inch wide male screw on port on one side with a 2 inch wide female screw-on aperture on the other. This enabled it to be used in series for extra protection against aerosols. The filter was not intended to be used with toxic gases and was primarily intended for use by personnel engaged in research and production of biological and radiological agents. The M14 filter was in use mainly during the 1950s and 1960s. A further entry in this category of "obscure" filters is the M12 Dog Gas Mask filter, which resembles the U.S. Navy NC-1 mask's M2 cylindrical filter in both appearance and shape.

With the introduction of the M17 series masks, with their bilateral, internally fitted "pork-chop" filters, a new filtering composite was introduced which featured a semi-triangular, curved sandwich of ASC type charcoal, enclosed within mechanical filtering elements on both sides, and contained with outer wire mesh surfaces that were sealed along the edges with plasticized sealant. These were the M13 (eventually rejected for combat use due to faults), the M13A1 and M13A2 filter unit provided for use with the M17, M17A12 and M17A2 Army respirators. The problem of replacing the filters during a sustained chemical attack has already been discussed, but this inherent filter design concept remains one of the largest criticisms of the M17 mask—despite the fact that the filtering capacity of the units, functionally speaking, was very good. Whereas the M11 type drum filters were packed in hermetically sealed cans for storage until use, the new M13 type filters, presenting an irregular and awkward shape unsuited for containment within cans, were packed in hermetically sealed aluminized *Tyvek*-type packages which conformed to their unusual profiles.

The latest U.S. Army standard filter design is the C-2 series. This STANAG 4155 (40 x 3.63 mm) threaded canister (diam: 106 mm; height: 77 mm; weight 265 gm) was originally developed by the Canadians as part of the initial 70s *joint respirator project*, and is used by both nations (Canada and the USA) today. The original C-2 design was contained in a lightweight aluminum body, but a more recent version in the Racal C-series (C-7) incorporates non-metallic polymeric/glass fiber material in the filter's outer shell .The C-2 filter is manufactured by the Racal Company for Canadian forces and incorporates state-of-the-art impregnated ASC or TEDA, as does the newer plastic-bodied filter, which Canada has temorarily postponed procuring. The U.S. military C-2 filters (both the original C-2 and the current C2A1) are manufactured by MSA, in the U.S. (under license to Racal), and are hermetically sealed in a can for long-term shelf storage capability and protection until use is required. Normally the M40 and MCU-2/AP type US respirators are initially issued with two each of the C-2 filters. The C-2 filter canister is readily identified by its overall subdued black anodized color.

In 1992 the C-2 filter canister was upgraded and redesignated the C-2A1 filter canister. External specifications and dimensions for the C-2A1 filter canister remain unaltered, as do performance parameters. The major difference between the C-2 and the C-2A1 filter is the use of ASZM-T activated charcoal (instead of ASC/TEDA type). The ASZM-T activated charcoal does not contain the element of chromium, which has been identified by the US Army as an environmentally hazardous material. The new C-2A1 filter canister is easily differentiated from the black anodized C-2 by its anodized dark metallic green canister color. There are at present no plans for the U.S. to adopt the C-7, plastic bodied filter canister, despite the fact that most other modern NBC filters now incorporate polymers materials in filter containment bodies. Compatibility and competitive cost factors have been cited as a stumbling block.

One further improvement to the C-2A1 is the use of new polyurethane sealant instead of the mercury-containing sealant used in the original C-2 filter canister; additional toxic waste disposal concerns stemmed from use of the mercury sealed filter canister.

Although Racal Filter Technologies Limited, of Canada, has completed development of a newer NBC filter design, designated the C-7, the United States Army has no immediate plan to procure the NORYL (polyphenyloxide polymer) bodied C-7 canister to either replace or augment the C-2A1 filter standardized for use with the latest U.S. military NBC respirators. Diameter of the C-7 is 115 mm, height is 80 mm, and weight is given as 290 gm; a particular feature of the C-7 is its high efficiency particulate filter media of glass and vinyon fibres, which are co-pleated with polypropylene scrim to provide strong structural support. The new C-7 filter, with a 250 cc charcoal bed, is purported to be highly resistant to mildew and fungal growth, as well. [Racal has successfully acquired the contract for the Swedish M90 military NBC filter and are also producing the AMF-12 filter canister for the Nederlands' use with their new AVON FM-12 masks].

APPENDIX IV: U.S. Army Protective Mask Carriers: Early Types Through the Present

The earliest carrying satchel for U.S. gas masks was modeled directly on the British developed BSBR satchel. All of the early American (WWI) masks, including the ASBR, the CEM, the RFK, the AT, the KT, and the 1919 Model, were contained in this chest style carrier. The carrier, later standardized as the U.S. Army MI carrier (in 1921), measured about 20cm x 18cm x 6cm, and was fabricated from khaki-tan canvas duck material. A top-opening flap, secured by two snaps, allowed access to the interior, which was divided into two compartments by a partition (one side held the box-shaped filter, the other the facepiece). Capable of being worn in two modes (the 'Ready' position, slung over the shoulder and worn on the side, or the 'Alert' position, on the chest, with the single strap slung around the neck), the carrier was well suited for the trench-style warfare of the First World War period. Due to the fact that the filters used with the early American Small Box Respirator were slightly larger than the subsequent (CEM, RFK, KT and AT) types, the earliest carrier is fractionally taller than the succeeding versions.

The chest-worn carrier was obviously unsuited for prone firing positions, and therefore, with the standardization of the Service Gas Mask MI (formerly Army 1919 Model), a new design was introduced which differed considerably from the original British-copied satchel. Designated the Carrier MII, this new style satchel would be subsequently used with all the succeeding MI series and M2 series respirators (in various improved versions). Due to a somewhat irregular shape, the satchel has been referred to as 'kidney-shaped,' although there is nothing about it that suggests the outline of that organ of the body. The MII carrier was designed to be worn on the left side, suspended from an adjustable shoulder strap slung crossways over the neck, and secured below by an adjustable waist strap. This new carrier was much better suited to all combat soldier firing positions, and presented only a moderate protrusion due to its being worn under the arm, and above the hip on the left side. The new carrier required a lengthened hose of 27 inches (contrasted to the 12 inch hose used with the MI carrier) between filter, carried in the satchel, and the facepiece as worn.

As of October of 1941, a total of 5 slightly improved variations of the 'kidney' carrier had been developed, designated MII, MIII, MIIIA, MIV, and MIVA1. Each incorporated small modifications, and were generally quite similar to each other. The carrier satchel identification was stamped in ink under the flap, and the color variations of the un-proofed canvas duck material used for each ranged from khaki-tan to light olive drab. Revisions of the basic respirator filter canisters used with the MI series mask were responsible for a few of the carrier alterations (change in outlet tube shape); other changes were created to increase functional utility (the MIXA1, for example, was identical to the MIV except for the addition of a slightly lengthened waist strap—4 inches longer).

With adoption of the new lightweight type respirator masks in the early 40s (M3, M4) with their M9A1 and M10 cylindrical metal filters, a newer, more compact carrying satchel was provided for use with them. Featuring a three snap top closing flap and carried in the same side position—under the arm on the left-side—the new un-proofed canvas carriers ranged in color from khaki-tan to various shades of olive drab. Two straps inside the carrier secured the M10-type cylindrical filter, while allowing it positional range of motion within the satchel, and a tube containing an anti-dim cloth was provided in a fabric loop inside. Shoulder and waist straps were featured, which were adjustable. The carrier used with both lightweight type respirators was designated the M6.

The new Assault Gas Mask design (later standardized as the Combat Service Gas Mask M5-11-7), with its cheek-mounted canister was issued with a special rubber-proofed carrying satchel that featured a folding flap, secured with snaps, which would make the carrier watertight. This carrier, designated the M7 carrier, could be used as an emergency flotation device by amphibious assault troops—a capability designed with the D-Day invasion in mind, particularly. As such, the M7 carrier is reputed to have served that emergency flotation purpose to save lives during the Normandy assaults and cine footage of U.S. troops forming on the beach after the Normandy invasion show the M7 carrier satchel being worn on the chest, with the strap looped around the neck. The M7 carrier was made of thin fabric, coated on both sides with black butyl rubber. A later version, identical in shape and form, would be used by U.S. Marines with the M9 mask (that carrier was designated the C15R1, and was fabricated of thicker OD colored canvas duck, coated only on the inner side with rubber).

The 1940s model Army optical mask was carried in a special canvas carrier (M5) of its own, whereas the later 'Lightweight Optical Gas Mask' version was carried in a standard M6 canvas carrier, along with the other lightweight (M3, M4) service gas masks.

All of the so-called 'snout-type' masks of the 40s were carried in similar canvas, khaki colored satchels, slung across the neck and worn at the side with a single strap. These were shaped like the inverted frustum of a cone, and in some cases featured a tie-cord for added waist securing. The Training Gas Mask MI/M2 was provided with the MI carrier, and the M8 (late WWII) mask was carried in the M10 satchel.

With the introduction of the M9 series masks, the modified assault style carrier mentioned earlier as being the C15R1 carrier, of one-side-proofed OD canvas, was used. When a new OD colored non-proofed canvas carrier was introduced for use with the M9 mask in the early 50s, the mask was redesignated M9A1 (the M9 and M9A1 facepieces are identical, only the carrier is different). The new M9A1 mask satchel was designated the M11 carrier, and it bore a slight resemblance to the earlier WWII lightweight mask carrier (M6), although it featured a side-opening flap secured by three snaps, and a different arrangement of upper (shoulder) and lower (waist) straps. The M11 carrier was OD in color and, as with virtually all U.S. masks, an anti-dim cloth was supplied.

The M24 aircraft and M25/M25A1 masks were provided with virtually identical carriers made of dark OD canvas duck. Designated the M17 (aviation) and M13A1 (tank) carriers, the only difference between them was that they were worn on opposite sides, and therefore resembled mirrored versions of each other. The two carriers featured circular orifices along the bottom at one end through which the inlet of the M10A1 type filter's inlet adapter/connector could be protruded (for connection to collective protection, blower, or aircraft oxygen breathing systems). The M17 and M13A1 carriers were roughly rectangular in shape, and worn with an adjustable shoulder and adjustable waist strap. The flaps were side-opening, as with the M11 carrier used with the M9A1 Army respirator.

In the early 60s, along with an entirely new respirator design (M17 series), a completely new style carrier was also introduced. This was the M15 carrier, made of OD colored canvas duck (unproofed), which was irregularly shaped, featured a side-opening flap secured with two snaps, and internally sewn-in fiberglass stiffening battens for enhanced protection of carrier contents. The M15 carrier featured a large external pocket on the end opposite the main access flap for the purpose of holding the M13 decontamination set. The carrier was later slightly modified (pocket detail) when the M17A1 mask was introduced, and finally, once again in the mid-80s (M15A1 carrier). The carriers intended for use with each improved M17 mask (M17, M17A1 and M17A2) were originally imprinted with the identifier of the mask each was specifically intended to hold; in the mid-80s, this procedure was abandoned with the production of one replacement carrier imprinted "Carrier, M17 Field Protective Mask Series." The carrier was virtually identical to the two earlier versions, but very slightly more capacious. Two other smaller external pockets were provided on the M15 type carriers, as well as an internal pocket in which lens outserts, MI waterproofing bag, etc., could be placed. The carriers were worn in the conventional, standard manner (left side, suspended with a shoulder and waist strap), or could be worn around the waist and leg, through the use of the adjustable attachments. These carriers would accommodate an M17 type mask with the M6A1 chemical hood installed and folded into it, providing quick donning access. When placed in the carrier thusly, the front of the mask faced forward. The last carriers of this type were fabricated entirely of OD nylon duck material.

The M28 Riot Control Agent mask was provided with a plastic-lined (vinyl) OD nylon carrier pouch, which lacked straps but rather was worn on the utility belt with Alice-style clips. The pouch featured Velcro for closure, after the mask was folded in upon itself and placed within the pouch.

A carrier shaped in a 'semi-crescent' form was provided for the MCU-2/P and MCU-2A/P type modern NBC respirators in use at the present time. This carrier, constructed of rugged nylon duck material (unproofed), and worn in the standard side position via upper and lower straps, featured a front opening flap secured solely with Velcro. A pull tab facilitated access to the interior, helping to release the Velcro hook and loop secured flap, and an exterior pocket was provided for use with the M258A1 or late model M291 decontamination sets. Additionally, a clear window on the carrier is provided for removable personal identification, and a lengthwise internal Velcro secured pocket is also provided.

The latest carrier, provided with both the M40 and M42 (standard and tank) masks, is similar in design to the carrier provided for the MCU-2A/P mask, although it is somewhat more rectangular than the former. In the current manner, fiberglass internal side inserts are provided in the carrier walls to help protect the mask contained within, and a large exterior pocket is sewn in to hold the M291 (or M258A1) decon sets. A special, Velcro-closed circular filter inlet orifice is featured on this carrier, which allows it to be used with the M42's filter adapter connection (for collective protection system hookup), hence the carrier is issued unchanged for use with both M40 and M42 masks. A transparent plastic panel allows for insertion of personal identification data.

The M40/M42 type carrying satchel is identified by the stenciled designation "Carrier, M40/M42 Mask" on its exterior, and is intended for use with all M40/M40A1 and M42/M42A1 respirators.

APPENDIX V: Notes on U.S. Chemical and Biological Respirators as Collectible Militaria

Whether stemming from military history, academic or purely a vocation or hobby interests, the pursuit of respirator *collecting* as a special area within the field of general militaria is a relatively rare one. Chemical and biological warfare artifacts such as 'gasmasks' lack the attractive *elàn* of aeronautical and aviation memorabilia and instead seem to evoke an association with unspeakable horrors and near criminal acts of barbarity. There is, however, a simultaneous fascination with these items of personal protection that prompts deeper interest in the circumstances which necessitated their development. As an expression of exotic technology, the NBC respirator is singular; as artifacts of one of the more arcane areas of modern warfare they are unique.

There are very few collections of NBC respirators in existence in the United States. Although there are a few such items in all the major museums, there is, to the best of my knowledge, no significant museum dedicated solely to military respirators and individual CBW warfare protection technology other than the U.S. Army Chemical Corps Museum at Ft. McClellan, Alabama. Modest sized private collections of such items undoubtedly exist, but again the number of collectors of such things is in all likelihood very small.

Unfortunately, due to their being constructed of relatively fragile materials (rubber, fabric, leather, etc.) that are susceptible to deterioration from exposure to ultraviolet light, ozone, heat and other environmental elements (petroleum products, among many), many respirators which are products of earlier decades are now in very poor condition. This is especially true of World War One vintage masks, but also particularly of masks produced in the 30s, 40s and 50s. Only occasionally does one locate examples of earlier respirators which are in unissued condition, or still in their original storage packaging. Early U.S. Army chemical respirators such as the Corrected English Mask, KTM and RFK masks vary in their state of preservation but are almost uniformly in very poor condition. With regard to the WWI masks, the usual deterioration found include eye lens laminations which have become clouded, face-pieces in which the interior rubber coating has become desiccated, stiff, or entirely flaked off the fabric, head-harness bands dried out and no longer elastic, and stockinet-covered hoses deformed and stiffened.

Similar problems are found with the next generation masks (MI/Model 1919, MIA1 and MIA2, etc.), although occasional examples are turning up, now and again, still sealed in their original metal (MI or MII) storage cases (unissued); the condition of the masks within such cases is open to speculation, although there is a distinct possibility that external ambient temperature changes and 'sweating effects' of the metal cases have not significantly harmed the contents.

M2 (Heavyweight), M3 and M4 (Lightweight) series masks are generally found in fair condition, although examples of brand-new, unissued M4 masks in SS sizes are occasionally discovered today. Examples of the synthetic (Neoprene) rubber M3 and M5 (Assault Gas Mask) are generally severely afflicted with "cold set" deformation when found, although occasional good examples are surprisingly still in circulation. In connection with the M3 Lightweight Gas Mask, it is worthy to note that these masks were assembled with a variety of components, some new and some refurbished, due to the expediencies of wartime production. All natural rubber M3 masks have been found, as well as M3 masks with Neoprene face blanks and natural rubber hoses, and M3 masks manufactured with both Neoprene facepieces and hoses. Naturally, an all-Neoprene mask assembly is more of a rarity, due to the unsuitable nature of the material and the fact that they were invariably withdrawn from service. Far more good examples of the later M3 and M4 series masks are to be found today than the earlier M2 type (this includes the "Training Gas Mask" and the Heavyweight Army Service Gas Mask models), as might be expected from numbers produced and aging effects.

Examples of the M8 'snout-type' mask are rare and usually found in fair condition, if that, while the M9 series masks of the late 40s, 50s and early 60s are plentiful and range in condition from very poor to brand new. It is worth noting that only 300,000 of the M8-11-10 Snout-type masks were produced before V-J Day halted their production (most M8 masks used a reconditioned rubber faceblank in the same manner as had the M4-10A1-6 lightweight service gas mask—these were frequently refurbished M2A2 facepieces)

Examples of the M17 type masks of the 60s and 70s are again plentiful and range from very poor to excellent or unissued (mint). The M28 Riot Agent Mask (the so-called "Grasshopper Mask") is a bit rarer, but examples are to be found in unissued (new), storage-packed condition. M14, M24 and M25 type respirators (aircraft/tank) are not hard to find in average to good condition, while stocks of old Civil Defense (CDV-800) and earlier MIA1 type Noncombatant (40s) masks are occasionally found in new or excellent condition at militaria shows, surplus stores and flea markets. The unusual CD V-805 mask is one of the rarer finds today, however.

Undoubtedly one of the rarest of all U.S. chemical warfare respirators, from a collecting standpoint, is the World War Two vintage M5 Assault Gas Mask (less than 550,000 were made). Due to the problem-plagued nature of the Neoprene synthetic rubber used in these masks, and the fact that very few survived their recall and consequent destruction, their value as collectibles has risen considerably. Examples of the early World War One masks in excellent condition are also extremely rare, a fact reflected in their value today. Another interesting and somewhat scarce respirator is the Dog Gas Mask, M6, in use at least as late as the early 1950s; they are somewhat hard to locate, as might be imagined.

Least valuable in terms of collectibility are the M9 and M17 series masks, although the latter, while plentiful, are still bringing a good price (from the public—survivalists, paramilitary groups, etc.) due to their serviceable nature and overall basically good design. Although the M17 design's military value today is somewhat lessened by its internally fitted filters (requiring a gas-safe filter changing area in the event of a prolonged attack with CBW agents), both it and the Czech M10M mask (which is an M17 copy) are very effective masks for civilian defense or limited use CBW defense purposes.

As regards the current MCU-2/P and M40/M42 type masks, they are currently available on the black market, demanding prices from about $75 for examples of the former in excellent condition, to about $150 for examples of the M40/M42 in a similar state of repair. The value of these latest, current-issue masks lies in the fact that they are considered very desirable items by survivalists, law enforcement types, and others who wish to acquire these units owing to a perception that they represent the finest state of CBW protection available in the United States. The legality of business in current issue MCU-2/P and M40/M42 type masks is subject to serious reflection as many of the masks have been 'borrowed' from the U.S. Government by military personnel interested in making a few dollars through their sale to surplus outlets and militaria businesses (where they end up being resold to the public).

Of the wartime (considered here to be from 1940 through V-J Day) respirator types (this includes the MIA2, M2 service and training masks, the M3, M4, M5, M8 and noncombatant models) it has been stated that there were in excess of 30 million private industry produced gas masks manufactured, in addition to those produced by the U.S. Army production facilities at the Edgewood Arsenal.

Of special interest, as much to collectors of militaria as to historians, are the various methods employed over the past decades to package, preserve, protect and ship American respirators (prior to issue or actual use). The earliest method used to protect respirators consisted of packaging the masks in hermetically sealed metal cans—very much in the manner food is preserved in tins. The first such metal container was designated the Unit Container MI. It consisted of a flat, tin-plate (approximately 13" by 15" by 4") case made in two halves. After the mask, carrier and accessories were placed within the case halves, the unit was sealed by a soldered tear-strip around the periphery. Next the air was withdrawn from the case and replaced with nitrogen gas through a small orifice which was subsequently also sealed. Owing to the fact that these cases were prone to leakage, a second container was standardized designated the Unit Container MII. This container, roughly 4" by 15" by 13", was fabricated in the shape of what is described by Army TM 3-205 (9 Oct 41) as a 'flattened cylinder' shape. The sides of the container were corrugated for strength and the top and bottom plates were double seamed to the body of the case. The body and bottom plate were joined first, the mask in its carrier placed within, and the top plate was then joined and sealed. As with the Unit Container MI, a small hole in the top plate allowed withdrawal of air and replacement with nitrogen gas, with subsequent closure and sealing. The MII containers were opened with a machine functioning very much like a large, complex can opener. Early U.S. Army gas masks, such as the MI Service Gas Mask (standardized 1919 Model) may still be found sealed in the Unit Container MI type cans. Unfortunately, they are more than likely to have lost their original airtight integrity, although their contents may still be in excellent condition (depending on storage and handling over the years). U.S. Army Service Gas Mask MIA1 and M1A2 models are also to be found in their original Unit Container MII cases on occasion, although again the hermetic seals may no longer be functional.

Later model WWII gas masks such as the M2, M3, M4, and subsequent types, were usually packaged in *pliofilm* (an early form of transparent plastic) or in cellophane sacks, which were then placed in cardboard boxes. After the war, tinned metal cases were again used to pack and protect the M9 mask and its contemporaries. These were usually OD colored and rectangular in shape. Occasionally, one will find these intact and complete—certainly to a far greater extent than the earlier types. Respirators from the M17 through the latest types (M40/MCU-2A/P series) are packaged in aluminized plastic sacks, hermetically sealed and placed in cardboard boxes. Shelf life for materials protected in this last manner is estimated to be from 10 to 20 years, on average.

Early American gas mask filters (such as the M10 and early M10A1 service mask types) were packaged in waxed cardboard cylinders with metal ends. From the M11 filter onwards, sealed cylindrical metal cans have been used; this technique is still in use today with the latest C-2A1 filters.

While it is doubtful that the collecting of chemical and biological respirators shall ever become a major phenomenon within the field of militaria or historical military memorabilia collecting, interest in these unique defense artifacts produces many valuable, interesting insights into the technological process of warfare materiel development and richly enhances understanding of the history of modern warfare in ways that make it a very worthwhile undertaking.

APPENDIX VI: CBW Respirators Not Covered by this Reference

A number of special masks which were either developed and/or used in special applications throughout the last 80 years include those designed and produced for animals (dogs and horses employed during the Second World War) and modern aircraft NBC protection systems of the present decade for high-performance fixed wing aircraft.

The U.S. Army WWI horse gas mask has not been described in this text, nor have the U.S. Army WWII animal respirators (Horse Gas Mask models M4 and M5, and the Dog Gas Mask model M6-12-8). Two other protective masks which have not been examined or referenced are the U.S. Army M-21 Rocket Propellant Gas Mask, and the WWII U.S. Navy Submarine Gas Mask (model NS-1).

One further respirator which has not been described or illustrated is the "Mask, Chemical and Biological Oxygen", a pressure-demand oxygen mask intended for use in aircraft, and integrated to a special, purpose-modified (visorless) SPH-5 type helicopter helmet, fitted with standard USAF oxygen mask bayonet receivers. This mask, incorporating a single large panoramic visor and made of OD silicone rubber, came into use in the mid 80s, presaging subsequent and far more sophisticated systems which are now either being developed or already in use in aircraft. It bears a striking resemblance to the commercial *Demand Flow Airline Respirator*, manufactured for airline crew use in the 1970s and 1980s utilizing the MSA Clearview Facepiece.

Undoubtedly, in the preparation of this text, there will have been more than a few oversights. The writer of this reference acknowledges responsibility for any errors appearing herein, and hopes that anyone having information concerning possible errors of omission or misidentification of U.S. designed and developed NBC respirators will kindly communicate them so that corrections may be made in any future revisions of this book that might be forthcoming.

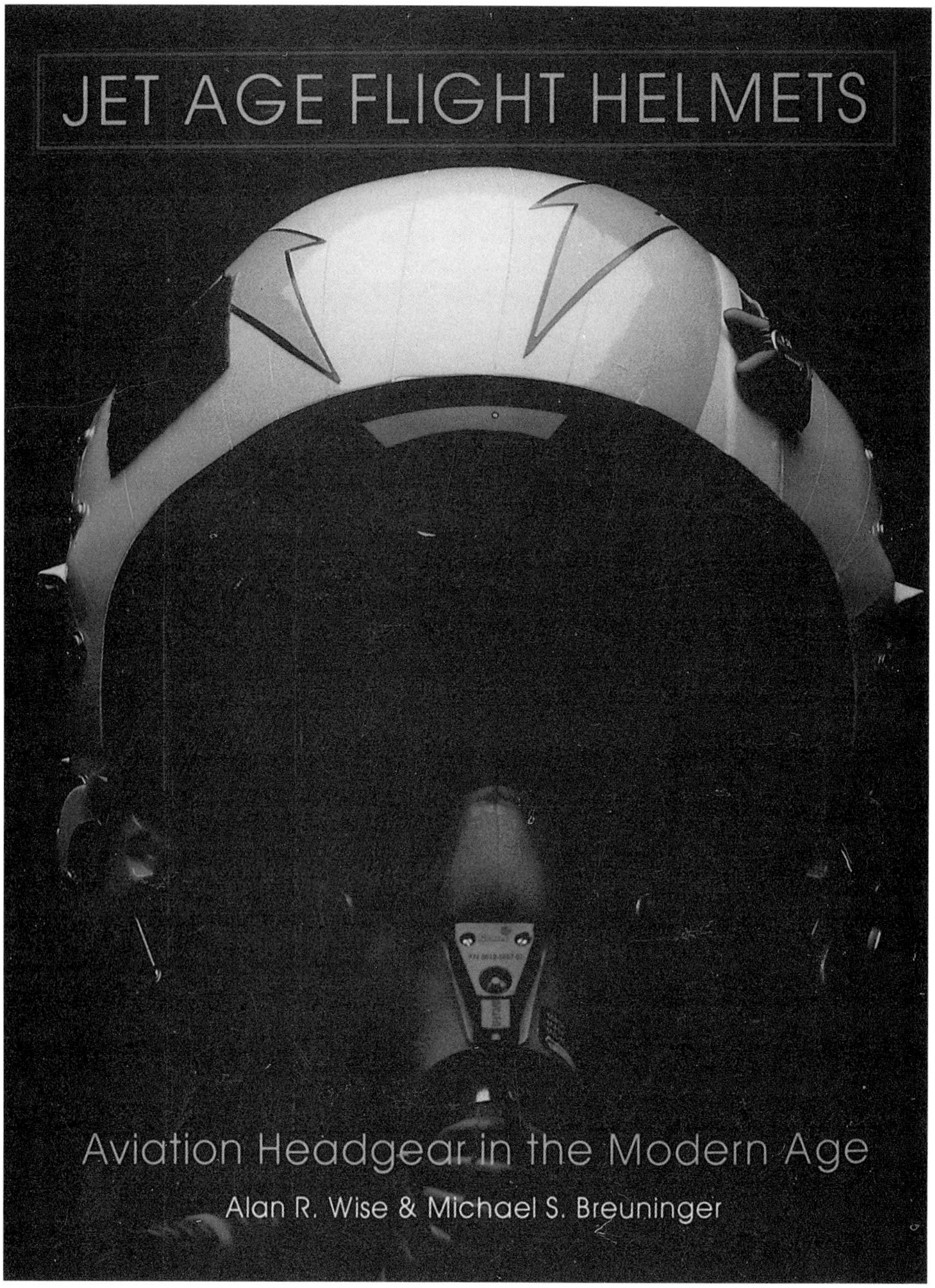

JET AGE FLIGHT HELMETS:

Aviation Headgear in the Modern Age

Alan R. Wise & Michael S. Breuninger

This new photo documentation is the first book ever to cover in detail the history and development of military flight helmets from the post-World War II era to the present, and includes over 120 different helmets and their associated equipment such as oxygen masks, boom microphones, inner helmets, etc. Extensively researched this book contains over 1000 images, most in color, and includes multiple-view photographs as well as detail views. Specific details of each helmet include manufacturer, proper designation, unique features, accessories, periods of use, branch of service(s), and aircraft in which it was used.

Size: 9" x 12" over 1000 color and b/w photographs

248 pages, hard cover

ISBN: 0-7643-0070-9 $75.00